SpringerWienNewYork

Acta Neurochirurgica
Supplements

Editor: H.-J. Steiger

Hydrocephalus

Selected Papers from the International Workshop in Crete, 2010

Edited by
G.A. Aygok, H.L. Rekate

Acta Neurochirurgica
Supplement 113

SpringerWienNewYork

Gunes A. Aygok
VCU Medical Center, Department of Neurosurgery, East Marshall Street 1250, 23294 Richmond Virginia, USA
gaaygok@vcu.edu

Harold L. Rekate
The Chiari Institute, Hofstra, Northshore LIJ College of Medicine, 865 Northern Boulevard, 11021 Great Neck NY, USA
haroldrekate@gmail.com

This work is subject to copyright.
All rights are reserved, whether the whole or part of the material is concerned, specifically those of translation, reprinting, re-use of illustrations, broadcasting, reproduction by photocopying machines or similarmeans, and storage in data banks.

Product Liability: The publisher can give no guarantee for all the information contained in this book. This does also refer to information about drug dosage and application thereof. In every individual case the respective user must check its accuracy by consulting other pharmaceutical literature. The use of registered names, trademarks, etc. in this publication does not imply, even in the absence of a specific statement, that such names are exempt from the relevant protective laws and regulations and therefore free for general use.

©2012 Springer-Verlag/Wien
Printed in Germany
SpringerWienNewYork is part of Springer Science+Business Media
springer.at

Typesetting: SPI, Pondichery, India

Printed on acid-free and chlorine-free bleached paper
SPIN: 80022360

Library of Congress Control Number: 2011940862

With 117 (partly coloured) Figures

ISSN 0065-1419
ISBN 978-3-7091-0922-9   e-ISBN 978-3-7091-0923-6
DOI 10.1007/978-3-7091-0923-6
SpringerWienNewYork

Preface

The 5th International Hydrocephalus Workshop was held May 20-23, 2010, in the Aegean island of Crete, Greece. The workshop was preceded by the 24th Annual Hellenic Congress of Neurosurgery and the 4th Annual Neurosurgery Nurses Meeting as well. This volume includes papers presented at the 5th Hydrocephalus Workshop which recent updates and new concepts in hydrocephalus were introduced.

Under the leadership of Dr. Anthony Marmarou there have been two previous Hydrocephalus Workshops on beautiful Greek islands, the 3rd International Hydrocephalus Workshop on the Island of Kos in 2001 and the 4th on the Island of Rhodes in 2007. The planning for the 5th International Workshop was well along when unexpectedly Professor Marmarou died. His last wish was that his work and especially the tradition of International Hydrocephalus Workshops "continue." With that in mind and with the help and support of the Hellenic Neurosurgical Society, the hydrocephalus study group at the Medical College of Virginia, the International Society for Hydrocephalus and Cerebrospinal Fluid Disorders and the very professional congress organization of Artion, we were able to continue with Professor Marmarou's vision of getting together the leaders in clinical and basic science research in the field of hydrocephalus.

We believe that this workshop was a major turning point, and made a significant contribution to the effort to ensure further understanding of timely diagnosis and treatment of hydrocephalus. The wide number of topics covered, including advances in management of both pediatric and adult hydrocephalus, identifying shunt responders, clinical experiences in endoscopic third ventriculostomy, clinical trials, pathophysiology, experimental studies, introducing the new classification for hydrocephalus and the option of all workshop participants to become actively involved in its proceedings, guaranteed that this objective was achieved.

As Professor Kouzelis stated in his opening remarks, during this meeting, our participants were able to follow Ariadne's lost thread through the ruins of the ancient Minoan labyrinth on the mythical island of Crete, and find the much sought-after solution to the ancient Hippocratic riddle of hydrocephalus.

November 2011   Gunes A. Aygok and Harold L. Rekate

Acknowledgments

The meeting would not have been possible without the hard work of Despina Amarantidou as workshop coordinator, Matina Katsarou and Niki Chatziilia as organizing secretariat, Marianna Georgitseli, Maria Kantziari, Ioanna Kazantzidou as sponsorship and publications & website coordinators.

We would like to express our sincere thanks to the Hellenic Neurosurgical Society for their enormous support during the international hydrocephalus workshops and for their enthusiasm to continue Professor Marmarou's tradition of hosting the international hydrocephalus workshops.

We would also like to thank Codman & Shurtleff and Dr. Sean Lilienfeld who serves as the vice president for clinical research & medical affairs of Codman & Shurtleff, for providing educational grant in support of the meeting.

The publication of this volume became possible with the commitment of Professor Hans-Jakob Steiger and the staff of Springer – Verlag.

Contents

Importance of the Work of Professor Marmarou

Fifth International Hydrocephalus Workshop, Crete, Greece, May 20–23, 2010: Themes and Highlights.. 1
Harold L. Rekate, Gunes A. Aygok, Kostantinos Kouzelis, Petra M. Klinge, and Michael Pollay

Modeling of CSF Dynamics: Legacy of Professor Anthony Marmarou.......... 9
Marek Czosnyka, Zofia Czosnyka, Kiran J. Agarwal-Harding, and John D. Pickard

Importance of Data, Especially from Randomized Controlled Trials

Ethical Considerations in Hydrocephalus Research That Involves Children and Adults... 15
Michael A. Williams

Conservative Versus Surgical Management of Idiopathic Normal Pressure Hydrocephalus: A Prospective Double-Blind Randomized Controlled Trial: Study Protocol... 21
Ahmed K. Toma, Marios C. Papadopoulos, Simon Stapleton, Neil D. Kitchen, and Laurence D. Watkins

Ten Years of Clinical Experience in the Use of Fixed-Pressure Versus Programmable Valves: A Retrospective Study of 159 Patients.................. 25
Maria Mpakopoulou, Alexandros G. Brotis, Haralampos Gatos, Konstantinos Paterakis, and Kostas N. Fountas

Magnetic Resonance Imaging as a Powerful Tool

Changes of Fractional Anisotropy and Apparent Diffusion Coefficient in Patients with Idiopathic Normal Pressure Hydrocephalus.................. 29
Koichiro Demura, Mitsuhito Mase, Tosiaki Miyati, Tomoshi Osawa, Manabu Hattori, Harumasa Kasai, Masaki Hara, Yuta Shibamoto, and Kazuo Yamada

Virchow-Robin Spaces in Idiopathic Normal Pressure Hydrocephalus: A Surrogate Imaging Marker for Coexisting Microvascular Disease?........... 33
Andrew Tarnaris, J. Tamangani, O. Fayeye, D. Kombogiorgas, H. Murphy, Y.C. Gan, and G. Flint

Quantification of Normal CSF Flow Through the Aqueduct Using PC-Cine MRI at 3T 39
Eftychia Kapsalaki, Patricia Svolos, Ioannis Tsougos, Kyriaki Theodorou, Ioannis Fezoulidis, and Kostas N. Fountas

Correlation Between Tap Test and CSF Aqueductal Stroke Volume in Idiopathic Normal Pressure Hydrocephalus 43
Souraya El Sankari, A. Fichten, C. Gondry-Jouet, M. Czosnyka, D. Legars, H. Deramond, and Olivier Balédent

Basic Science: The Aquaporin Story

Overview of the CSF Dual Outflow System 47
Michael Pollay

Hydrocephalus and Aquaporins: The Role of Aquaporin-1 51
M.Y.S. Kalani, A.S. Filippidis, and H.L. Rekate

Hydrocephalus and Aquaporins: The Role of Aquaporin-4 55
A.S. Filippidis, M.Y.S. Kalani, and H.L. Rekate

Effect of Acetazolamide on Aquaporin-1 and Fluid Flow in Cultured Choroid Plexus 59
Pouya A. Ameli, Meenu Madan, Srinivasulu Chigurupati, Amin Yu, Sic L. Chan, and Jogi V. Pattisapu

Experimental Studies: Hydrocephalus

Physical Phantom of Craniospinal Hydrodynamics 65
R. Bouzerar, M. Czosnyka, Z. Czosnyka, and Olivier Balédent

Programmable Shunt Assistant Tested in Cambridge Shunt Evaluation Laboratory 71
Marek Czosnyka, Zofia Czosnyka, and John D. Pickard

Simulation of Existing and Future Electromechanical Shunt Valves in Combination with a Model for Brain Fluid Dynamics 77
Inga Margrit Elixmann, M. Walter, M. Kiefer, and S. Leonhardt

Examination of Deposits in Cerebrospinal Fluid Shunt Valves Using Scanning Electron Microscopy 83
Constantinos Charalambides and Spyros Sgouros

Microstructural Alterations of Silicone Catheters in an Animal Experiment: Histopathology and SEM Findings 87
Regina Eymann, Yoo-Jin Kim, Rainer Maria Bohle, Sebastian Antes, Melanie Schmitt, Michael Dieter Menger, and Michael Kiefer

Expression Analysis of High Mobility Group Box-1 Protein (HMGB-1) in the Cerebral Cortex, Hippocampus, and Cerebellum of the Congenital Hydrocephalus (H-Tx) Rat 91
Mitsuya Watanabe, Masakazu Miyajima, Madoka Nakajima, Hajime Arai, Ikuko Ogino, Sinji Nakamura, and Miyuki Kunichika

Brain Localization of Leucine-Rich α2-Glycoprotein and Its Role 97
Madoka Nakajima, M. Miyajima, I. Ogino, M. Watanabe, Y. Hagiwara, T. Segawa, K. Kobayashi, and H. Arai

Role of Artificial Cerebrospinal Fluid as Perfusate in Neuroendoscopic Surgery: A Basic Investigation 103
Masakazu Miyajima, Kazuaki Shimoji, Misuya Watanabe, Madoka Nakajima, Ikuko Ogino, and Hajime Arai

Subdural or Intraparenchymal Placement of Long-Term Telemetric Intracranial Pressure Measurement Devices? 109
Melanie Schmitt, Regina Eymann, Sebastian Antes, and Michael Kiefer

Clinical Studies: Hydrocephalus

Twelve-Year Hospital Outcomes in Patients with Idiopathic Hydrocephalus 115
George Stranjalis, T. Kalamatianos, C. Koutsarnakis, M. Loufardaki, L. Stavrinou, and D.E. Sakas

What Is the Appropriate Shunt System for Normal Pressure Hydrocephalus? 119
Christos Chrissicopoulos, S. Mourgela, K. Kirgiannis, A. Sakellaropoulos, N. Ampertos, K. Petritsis, and A. Spanos

Indications for Endoscopic Third Ventriculostomy in Normal Pressure Hydrocephalus 123
Nikolaos Paidakakos, S. Borgarello, and M. Naddeo

Role of Endoscopic Third Ventriculostomy in Treatment of Selected Patients with Normal Pressure Hydrocephalus 129
Kostas N. Fountas, Eftychia Z. Kapsalaki, Konstantinos N. Paterakis, Gregory P. Lee, and Georgios M. Hadjigeorgiou

Endoscopic Third Ventriculostomy in Obstructive Hydrocephalus: Surgical Technique and Pitfalls 135
D. Bouramas, Nikolaos Paidakakos, F. Sotiriou, K. Kouzounias, M. Sklavounou, and N. Gekas

Benign Cerebral Aqueductal Stenosis in an Adult 141
Christos Chrissicopoulos, S. Mourgela, N. Ampertos, A. Sakellaropoulos, K. Kirgiannis, K. Petritsis, and A. Spanos

Efficacy and Versatility of the 2-Micron Continuous Wave Laser in Neuroendoscopic Procedures........ 143
Florian H. Ebner, Christoph Nagel, Marcos Tatagiba, and Martin U. Schuhmann

Complications of Endoscopic Third Ventriculostomy: A Systematic Review....... 149
Triantafyllos Bouras and Spyros Sgouros

Syndrome of Inappropriately Low-Pressure Acute Hydrocephalus (SILPAH).... 155
Mark G. Hamilton and Angel V. Price

Lhermitte–Duclos Disease Presenting with Hydrocephalus................... 161
Mun Sul Yang, Choong Hyun Kim, Jin Hwan Cheong, and Jae Min Kim

Atypical Meningioma in the Posterior Fossa Associated with Colpocephaly and Agenesis of the Corpus Callosum........................ 167
Jin Hwan Cheong, Choong Hyun Kim, Mun Sul Yang, and Jae Min Kim

Management of Intraventricular Hemorrhage in Preterm Infants with Low Birth Weight........................ 173
Takayuki Inagaki, Takuya Kawaguchi, Takahiro Yamahara, Naoyuki Kitamura, Takashi Ryu, Yo Kinoshita, Yasuo Yamanouchi, Kazunari Kaneko, and Keiji Kawamoto

Pathophysiology of Brainstem Lesions Due to Overdrainage......... 177
Sebastian Antes, Regina Eymann, Melanie Schmitt, and Michael Kiefer

Dynamics of Cerebrospinal Fluid Flow in Slit Ventricle Syndrome............. 181
Regina Eymann, Melanie Schmitt, Sebastian Antes, Mohammed Ghiat Shamdeen, and Michael Kiefer

Quality and Safety of Home ICP Monitoring Compared with In-Hospital Monitoring........................ 187
Morten Andresen, Marianne Juhler, and Tina Nørgaard Munch

Author Index........................ 193

Subject Index........................ 195

Fifth International Hydrocephalus Workshop, Crete, Greece, May 20–23, 2010: Themes and Highlights

Harold L. Rekate, Gunes A. Aygok, Kostantinos Kouzelis, Petra M. Klinge, and Michael Pollay

Abstract The purpose of the Fifth International Hydrocephalus Workshop was to allow clinicians and basic science researchers to educate each other in the advances that have been and are being made in the understanding and treatment of hydrocephalus and related disorders. This vision of the meeting was the work of Dr. Anthony Marmarou, who died a few months before the meeting was held. The presentations on all aspects of the study of hydrocephalus can be roughly grouped into seven basic themes. These themes are a summary of the important lifelong work of Professor Marmarou himself, including mathematical modeling, clinical selection of patients for the treatment of normal pressure hydrocephalus, and the development of international guidelines for the management of this condition. Other themes included the gathering of data, and in particular, randomized controlled trials; the use of magnetic resonance imaging for basic research in hydrocephalus, basic science and in particular the role of aquaporins; reports on clinical studies; and the late outcomes for patients treated in infancy. Finally, a report on the development of a consensus on the definition and classification of hydrocephalus based on the point of obstruction to flow of cerebrospinal fluid was presented.

Keywords Hydrocephalus • Classification • Normal pressure hydrocephalus • Third ventriculostomy • MRI • Aquaporins

H.L. Rekate (✉)
The Chiari Institute,
Hofstra, Northshore LIJ College of Medicine,
865 Northern Boulevard, 11021 Great Neck NY, USA
e-mail: haroldrekate@gmail.com

G.A. Aygok
Department of Neurosurgery,
Medical College of Virginia Commonwealth University, Richmond, VA, USA

K. Kouzelis
Department of Neurosurgery, Thriasio General Hospital, Athens, Greece

P.M. Klinge
Department of Neurosurgery, Warren Alpert Medical School of Brown University, Rhode Island Hospital, Providence, RI, USA

M. Pollay
University of Oklahoma School of Medicine (Ret), Pediatric Neurosurgery, Sun City West, AZ, USA

Introduction

Under the leadership of Professor Anthony Marmarou, there have been two previous Hydrocephalus Workshops on two beautiful Greek islands: the third International Hydrocephalus Workshop on the island of Kos in 2001 and the fourth on the island of Rhodes. The planning for the fifth International Workshop was well along when, tragically, Professor Marmarou died. His last wish was that his work, and especially this meeting, should "continue." With that in mind, and with the help and support of the Hellenic Neurosurgical Society and its president, Professor Konstantinos Kouzelis; the hydrocephalus group at the Medical College of Virginia with Professor Marmarou's colleagues Drs. Gunes Aygok and Harold Young; and the professional organization, the Artion Company, we were able to continue with Professor Marmarou's vision of bringing together the leaders in clinical and basic science research in the field of hydrocephalus. The Workshop was attended by almost 400 participants and by all measures was extremely successful. This success is a tribute to the vision of this leader in hydrocephalus. What follows is a brief summary of the themes that wound themselves throughout the meeting like the legendary thread of Ariadne in Cretan mythology. We will also attempt to explain what was accomplished during the 3 days of the Workshop. A comprehensive discussion of the entire program is beyond the scope of this summary, but we will attempt to emphasize the most important aspects.

Importance of the Work of Professor Marmarou

Professor Marmarou will be remembered for his continuing commitment to the study of intracranial pressure dynamics, and especially apropos of this meeting, hydrocephalus, over a 40-year career. The importance of his work was celebrated at this meeting relative to three areas of leadership. By his work on a novel mathematical model of intracranial pressure dynamics that formed the basis of his Ph.D. thesis,

Professor Marmarou was responsible for providing students of intracranial pressure with a tool to understand the complex interaction of elements within the central nervous system. That tool was the pressure volume index (PVI). This measurement represents the amount of volume that must be added to the intracranial compartment to raise intracranial pressure by a factor of 10 [9, 14, 15]. The ability of the PVI measurement to define cerebral compliance and to determine the effect of abnormal cerebrospinal fluid (CSF) dynamics on an individual was discussed by Dr. Marek Czosnyka and his colleagues from the University of Cambridge. The concept of PVI led to an improved understanding of the various forms of hydrocephalus, allowed improved prediction of outcome, and provided guidelines for management of increased intracranial pressure in traumatic brain injury.

Professor Marmarou directed a 3-year effort to develop guidelines for the diagnosis and management of normal pressure hydrocephalus (NPH). He led a continuing cooperative study on the level of evidence regarding all aspects of NPH among a large number of recognized experts in a number of fields. The outcome of this work was the publication of the Guidelines for the Diagnosis and Management of Normal Pressure Hydrocephalus, which was published as a special supplement to Neurosurgery [7, 8, 10]. The process and Professor Marmarou's critical role in it were described by Dr. Petra Klinge of Brown University in the United States. These guidelines were published in 2005 and revolutionized the management of patients with NPH.

Dr. Gunes Aygok, who became Dr. Marmarou's associate after training under his mentorship at the Medical College of Virginia (MCV) in Richmond, Virginia, described the working of the NPH assessment at the treatment program at MCV. Since 1992, under the leadership of Drs. Harold Young and Anthony Marmarou, this clinic has provided critical documentation of their approach to the diagnosis and management of NPH and the value of their testing methods, including the 3-day lumbar drainage assessment and the high-volume tap test [1]. External lumbar drainage and the high-volume tap test has become a highly prognostic and safe procedure, with a sensitivity of 92% and a specificity of 80%, for identifying patients with NPH most likely to benefit from shunt surgery. CSF resistance testing provides a predictive accuracy of 72% and remains useful as an outpatient supplementary test. The experience at MCV was presented at the third and fourth International Hydrocephalus Workshops by Dr. Marmarou. The most recent updates concluded that despite the prevalence of confounding comorbidities in the elderly population, appropriate diagnosis coupled with supplementary testing allows clinicians to accurately identify shunt responders, leading to sustained long-term improvement.

Importance of Data, Especially from Randomized Controlled Trials

Two of the initial invited talks dealt with the importance of randomized controlled trials (RCTs). Dr. John Kestle has been involved in the design of very important RCTs related to both hydrocephalus and pediatric neurosurgical issues. He was one of the authors of the Shunt Design Trial comparing the results of three different shunt designs related to the outcome of treatment for children treated with a first shunt. Dr. Kestle reported that several large children's hospitals with dedicated and active pediatric neurosurgical faculties have created a consortium to work together to perform clinical trials on the treatment of hydrocephalus [6]. The first step, as defined by Dr. Kestle, would be to standardize treatment across institutions and the entire faculty to obtain baseline information. Such baseline information is essential in the planning of RCTs and in the assessment of their feasibility, by providing information about the design of the trial, including the number of participants that would be needed. Next, a proposed change to the protocol would be studied in an RCT. Proposals for study include the treatment of shunt infections, the use of antibiotic-impregnated catheters, and the management of posthemorrhagic hydrocephalus of the premature newborn. Dr. Kestle not only emphasized the importance of committing ourselves to these RCTs but was also realistic about the difficulties involved given the chronic nature of hydrocephalus and the relatively small numbers of cases from single institutions.

The second presentation was by Professor Shlomi Constantini from Israel who reported on the challenges and successes related to the planning and execution of RCTs related to neuroendoscopy. With the encouragement of the International Federation of Neuroendoscopy, a prospective multicenter trial was completed related to the efficacy of endoscopic third ventriculostomy (ETV) in the treatment of hydrocephalus related to subarachnoid hemorrhage and infection [16]. This important study showed that patients with either posthemorrhagic hydrocephalus or hydrocephalus after meningitis can be managed with ETV with a high-likelihood of success, but if both hemorrhage and infection are present, such treatment is likely to be futile. The same group of active centers has embarked on an RCT to study outcomes for pediatric hydrocephalus, comparing a shunt group with an ETV group. We anxiously await the outcome of that study.

During the course of the Workshop, two well-structured RCTs were reported by oral presentation. In the first presentation, Mr. Richard Edwards and colleagues from Bristol in the United Kingdom reported a prospective trial of the use of ETV in the treatment of idiopathic NPH. This well-designed study, in which the analysts of the outcome measures were blinded to the treatment method of ETV or shunting with a programmable valve, was stopped early due to a lack of efficacy of ETV.

While there were some early successes, all patients in the ETV group crossed over into the shunt group within the first year. The discussion after the presentation emphasized the need to develop specific inclusion criteria if there are to be future studies on the use of ETV to treat idiopathic NPH.

A device-based efficacy trial for the treatment of Alzheimer's disease (AD) utilizing a specially designed shunt system to clear specific neurotoxins from patients was presented by Professor Silverberg from Brown University. The presentation was a post hoc analysis of the outcomes of the study, which is now closed due to the failure to show a benefit from the shunt-clearance technique. Subsequent analysis showed that several problems with the study might have led to the negative outcome. Early AD patients received a positive benefit from the shunting, but there were no improvements in patients with moderate and severe AD. The results suggest that if future studies are planned, only mild early AD patients should be studied. Furthermore, the shunt used in the study did not conform to the parameters chosen for rates of flow. Finally, the primary end points were insensitive to the changes seen in the short period of the study. For large and expensive studies such as this one, it is essential to have clear expectations of the data related to the outcome measures that are to be used.

Finally, presentations on almost all of the other clinical studies concluded with the statement that an RCT is necessary to assess these outcomes. There is a very small reservoir of energy and funding for a large number of RCTs in the context of hydrocephalus. It is unlikely that there will be RCTs to study most of the questions that need answering in this field. Unless the leaders in the field commit to these studies in a cooperative way, we will not likely find answers to these problems and progress in the near future.

Magnetic Resonance Imaging as a Powerful Tool for Investigating Basic Mechanisms of Hydrocephalus

In his invited presentation, Dr. Norman Relkin from Cornell in New York discussed exciting developments related to the use of magnetic resonance imaging (MRI) as a research tool, not only in the diagnosis of hydrocephalus, but also in understanding the actual effects of the distortion caused by hydrocephalus and by the presumed changes in the chemical milieu of the brain in patients with hydrocephalus.

There were four other presentations on this exquisite potential tool for the study of what actually happens in hydrocephalus of various types. Professor Mitsuhito Mase and colleagues from Nagoya, Japan, presented their study on changes in fractional anisotropy (FA) in idiopathic NPH.

After a tap test, there were significant changes in FA in the idiopathic NPH patients. These results suggest that a packing effect may lead to decreased random water movement that can be reversed by draining CSF.

Subsequently Professor Sprung from Berlin, Germany, measured MR elastography and its importance in defining basic mechanisms in idiopathic NPH. This measurement relates to the viscoelastic properties of the living brain. He found changes in the viscoelastic properties of idiopathic NPH patients. While the changes did not relate to the severity of the disease, they did differ from age-matched controls and tended to improve after treatment with a shunt.

Dr. Niklas Lenfeldt and colleagues from Umea in Sweden presented measured diffusion tensor imaging (DTI) in patients with idiopathic NPH before and after extended lumbar drainage. Again, in idiopathic NPH, FA was decreased, as shown by Prof. Mase. However, this finding was limited to specific white matter areas that may correspond to regions that relate specifically to clinically relevant findings in such patients. These observations are clearly very important, but the mechanisms involved and what actually happens related to the movement of water molecules still require explanation.

Finally, higher field magnets are likely to lead to more elegant information related to the study of what is happening in the brain affected by hydrocephalus. Dr. Eftychia Kapsalaki and her colleagues at the University of Thessaly School of Medicine, in Larissa, Greece, used a 3-T magnet to study the complex geometry of the CSF circulation with great precision. The anatomy of the ventricle and subarachnoid space as well as the pulsatile action of the CSF can be defined precisely, giving insight into normal and abnormal flow dynamics, points of obstruction, and water distribution.

These new techniques involving MRI are extremely exciting in terms of defining what actually occurs in brains affected by hydrocephalus, with resolution approaching the cellular level. The discussions, however, pointed out a great challenge. Very few physicists or neuroradiologists participated in the Workshop. The language used in these studies is not comfortable for clinicians and neurobiologists who are not involved in MRI programming. Understanding the techniques, their potentials, and their limitations requires hours of study, if indeed a dictionary of the terminology and discussion of the techniques used can be found. There are a limited number of scientists in this rapidly progressing field and fewer still who have collaborators who understand the issues that require these tools for study. Perhaps the most compelling achievement of the Workshop relates to creating an active dialogue among these individuals and scientists in other areas studying hydrocephalus. We strongly suggest that the small number of these physicist/neuroradiology leaders be identified and recruited to participate actively with established investigators so that these tools can be made available and appropriate studies can be designed to test the strength of the techniques and to develop testable hypotheses that can use these techniques.

Basic Science: The Aquaporin Story

The role of aquaporins (AQPs) in fluid management has been recently defined in a number of articles (both the physical configuration of AQPs and their biochemical and physiological characteristics) [4]. At this meeting, there was a series of papers describing the role of the AQP water channels in water transport at the brain-barrier systems.

The first two papers presented by Dr. M. Kalani and colleagues provided excellent reviews of the literature and demonstrated the importance of AQP-1 and AQP-4 on water transport at the blood–brain and blood–CSF (choroid plexus) barriers, with emphasis on their potential role in ameliorating the effects associated with hydrocephalus. AQP-1, which is associated with water transport at the choroid plexus under normal physiological conditions, is down-regulated in hydrocephalus and up-regulated in cases of human choroid plexus tumors. These observations suggest a compensatory role for AQP-1 in hydrocephalus and the basis for excess CSF production in choroid plexus papillomas. The second paper from this group reviewed the literature concerned with AQP-4 and its role in hydrocephalus. Based on their review, AQP-4 expression is up-regulated at the blood–brain and blood–CSF barriers. They concluded that AQP-4 has an adaptive and protective role in hydrocephalus.

Skjolding and colleagues studied the changes in AQP-4 expression on induced hydrocephalus in rats. Under normal conditions, AQP-4 is expressed in astrocytes and ependymal cells. In hydrocephalic animals, the periventricular AQP-4 is initially reduced and then elevated. This increase could represent a compensatory response. The differential roles of AQP-4 in hydrocephalus suggested to these authors that this protein may be a possible target for pharmacological agents.

Dr. Pouya Ameli and colleagues from Orlando, Florida, studied the effect of acetazolamide (AZA) on AQP-1 located in the apical membrane of the choroid plexus. They noted that AZA decreases CSF production, which could be due to an effect on AQP-1 expression in choroid plexus tissue. A monolayer of choroidal cells was produced for this study, and tissue viability and extent and direction of fluid flow across the monolayer were documented. Treatment of the monolayer with 10 µm of AZA resulted in a reduction of the AQP-1 protein, which returned to baseline in 12 h. These results indicate the possible clinical utility of modulating AQP-1 protein expression in the choroid plexus by pharmacological agents in the treatment of hydrocephalus.

The general conclusion from all of these interesting presentations is that an understanding of CSF movement across the brain-barrier systems due to AQP-1 and AQP-4 may be important to our understanding of the pathophysiology of hydrocephalus and possible treatments by modulating the expression of these proteins.

Clinical Studies

One of the important subjects evaluated at this Workshop related to neuroendoscopy, particularly ETV. As mentioned earlier, an RCT is underway under Professor Constantini's direction related to the efficacy of ETV compared to ventricular shunting in children. When completed, this RCT will add immeasurably to our understanding of the role of neuroendoscopy. In general, the work related to endoscopic management of hydrocephalus has been under the purview of the pediatric neurosurgeon. At this Workshop the emphasis was on the use of ETV to treat NPH. As discussed, in a well-controlled study, Edwards and his colleagues were unable to demonstrate prolonged improvement in patients with idiopathic NPH. Their intention-to-treat study selected patients based on the generally accepted criteria for idiopathic NPH and excluded patients with aqueductal stenosis and with clear-cut secondary NPH.

Dr. Nikolaos Paidakakos and his colleagues from Turin, Italy, performed both intraventricular and lumbar infusion tests and shunted patients, with no difference in the measurement of resistance to CSF outflow from the ventricle and lumbar theca. Their study was neither randomized nor blinded, but their results did show a significant improvement in the patient group undergoing ETV selected on the basis of a high ventricular resistance to CSF outflow but a normal lumbar resistance to outflow. The complication rate of ETV in these patients was significantly lower than that of the shunted group. They had a large number of exclusion criteria, but their most important inclusion criterion was a hyperdynamic pulse flow through the aqueduct as measured on a 3-T MRI. Improvement in urinary continence and gait was substantial, but any improvement in cognitive difficulties was less convincing.

A few pieces of information can be gleaned from these three presentations. If all patients with presumed NPH are treated with ETV, the results will be disappointing. The results of the second and third presentation support the probability that there is a subset of idiopathic NPH patients with a definable obstructive component to their hydrocephalus that may be treated effectively with ETV. The Paidakakos study shows that if high-grade stenosis is present at the aqueduct of Sylvius and differences between the outflow resistances measured above and below the aqueduct are shown, the patients can benefit from ETV. In a study by Dr. Kostas Fountas and colleagues, the authors laid emphasis on the rate of pulsatile flow through the aqueduct of Sylvius. This particular measurement remains controversial. The cause of this hyperdynamic flow is also somewhat controversial. Further studies are needed to define the role of ETV in idiopathic NPH and to understand why it works, if, indeed, it does.

In a study of autopsy material from patients who improved after shunting and who died from unrelated causes, Di Rocco and colleagues found a dense thickening of the arachnoid around the base of the brain and encompassing the cerebellar tonsils [3]. Before MRI was available, radionucleotide cisternography was considered an effective tool in selecting patients for shunting. In this test if the protein-bound tracer entered the ventricles quickly but flow became restricted over the convexities and required several days to clear, the patient would be very likely to improve with a shunt [5, 11, 13]. Together, these two observations suggest that there is a resistance element between the spinal and cortical subarachnoid space. In such a case the blockage would be proximal to the interpeduncular cistern, making this study potentially useful in choosing patients with idiopathic NPH who could be offered ETV.

Clinical studies for idiopathic NPH were also discussed. There has been tremendous effort since the Kos meeting, and the first guidelines for the diagnosis and management of idiopathic NPH were introduced at the Workshop. Multiple lines of evidence presented by Dr. Graff-Radford indicated that hypertension and cerebrovascular disease are associated with NPH. Furthermore, coexisting comorbidities such as Alzheimer's, Binswanger's, or Parkinson's disease have been identified as independent covariables associated with idiopathic NPH. These findings led to the classification, imaging, and supplementary tests recommended in the guidelines for patients suspected of having idiopathic NPH. As described by Dr. Michael Williams, in clinical studies of hydrocephalus ethical considerations have to be addressed, and treatment has to be offered to patients who fulfill the diagnostic criteria. All of these efforts will help increase the success rate of treatment in using the right shunt option.

Carsten Wikkelsø and colleagues presented preliminary data from an ongoing two-center (Oslo and Gothenburg), prospective, double-blind, randomized study of patients with idiopathic NPH comparing "fixed" and adjustable shunts. The purpose of this trial was to answer the question of what we would like adjustable valves to do. They concluded that treatment of the idiopathic NPH patients at the optimal pressure setting via an adjustable valve offered the best possible effect of shunting. This strategy also reduced the frequency of complications that often occur in patients treated with fixed shunts and enabled the noninvasive treatment of those complications. When revision was the concern, adjustable valves were associated with a lower risk for shunt revision.

Late Outcomes for Patients Treated in Infancy

The issue of what happens to patients with hydrocephalus who are treated in infancy is troubling. Many, if not most, of these patients will need to change their care center when they become too old to receive care in their original children's hospital. Three very important presentations at this Workshop dealt with this issue.

Persson and colleagues from Gothenburg, Sweden, presented the late follow-up of patients treated between 1967 and 1978 and followed until now. All patients in the study were seen and underwent thorough assessments in the 1980s. To be included in the study, the patient had to have an IQ >73 measured at the time of entry. Of the 43 patients, 28 agreed to be part of this long-term outcome study. All had experienced shunt complications that required surgical intervention, and 41% also had cerebral palsy. Almost two-thirds of the patients had finished secondary school and were working and living with a partner. The authors concluded that normally bright children who are shunted for hydrocephalus can grow up in Sweden to be productive citizens with relatively normal lives. The authors are planning to repeat these studies in more severely involved individuals, particularly those with spina bifida.

Schuhmann and colleagues from Tubingen, Germany, sounded a somewhat cautious note regarding the long-term follow-up of shunted individuals. They identified 15 children with long-term shunts and no evidence of overtly increased intracranial pressure or outward signs of shunt failure. The patients had enlarged ventricles and developmental delays. Investigation of intracranial pressure and CSF dynamics revealed significantly abnormal parameters in 10 of the 15 children. These ten children, who were offered and accepted treatment either with a shunt or ETV, showed cognitive improvement after treatment despite having been considered asymptomatic.

Juhler and colleagues in Copenhagen, Denmark, studied a group of patients who had undergone one or several shunt surgeries for presumed shunt malfunction where the symptoms related specifically to headache. At surgery it could not be determined with certainty that the shunts had actually failed. Based on the International Classification of Headache Disorders-11 criteria, medication overuse headaches were diagnosed. The patients were referred to specialized headache management clinics where the first step is withdrawal of all pain medications. This procedure markedly improved their quality of life, significantly decreased the severity and duration of their headaches, and markedly decreased their need for surgical intervention and utilization of medical resources. Medication overuse headaches are common in the young adult population of shunted individuals, and analgesics, especially narcotic analgesics, should be avoided at all costs in these individuals.

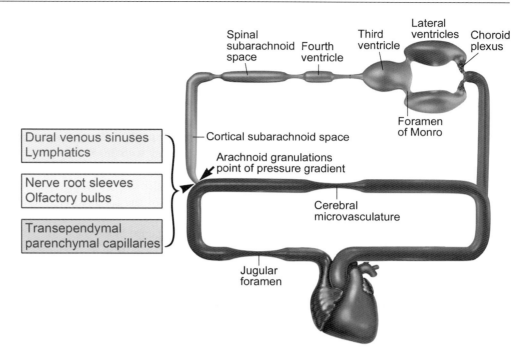

Fig. 1 The cerebrospinal fluid (CSF) system as a circuit diagram of flow from point of production in the cerebral ventricles to its point of absorption into the systemic circulation. Potential sites of that absorption are noted in the diagram. (Used with permission from Barrow Neurological Institute)

Definition and Classification of Hydrocephalus

At the first meeting of the International Society for Hydrocephalus and Cerebrospinal Fluid Disorders (ISHCSF) in Hannover, Germany, the president of this international workshop, Dr. Harold Rekate, presented a proposal to develop a consensus statement on a contemporary definition and classification of hydrocephalus. In preparation for that meeting, he published his concepts in *Cerebrospinal Fluid Research (CSFR)*, the online open-access journal devoted to research in hydrocephalus [12]. This proposal, by definition, was designed to serve as a "straw man" that would lead to a broad consensus on this important subject.

In the intervening 2 years, researchers and clinicians have met in Los Angeles at the International Society of Pediatric Neurosurgery meeting and in Phoenix, Arizona. As a result of these meetings, a consensus on the definition and classification of hydrocephalus has been reached. It was impossible to obtain a consensus on a single definition of hydrocephalus. Therefore, as in most dictionaries, more than one definition was needed. The two definitions are as follows:

1. Hydrocephalus is a condition characterized by a dynamic imbalance between the formation (production) *and absorption* of spinal fluid resulting in an increase in the size of the fluid cavities (ventricles) within the brain. Note: This definition would serve for general use of all readers.
2. Hydrocephalus is a condition characterized by a dynamic imbalance between the formation (production) *and absorption* of spinal fluid that results in an increase in the size of the fluid cavities within the brain and, in some situations, in an expansion of the spaces outside the brain, with or without an increase in the size of the ventricles. Note: This definition is most heuristic for those treating or studying this condition.

The currently accepted classification of hydrocephalus was initially proposed by Dandy 97 years ago and has not been modified since then [2]. The classification originally presented in the *CSFR* was accepted by consensus with the following exception. Multiple sites of absorption of CSF after it flows into the cortical subarachnoid spaces were identified and would require individual study, including the lymphatic system, nerve root sleeves, paranasal sinuses, and the brain itself.

The consensus is described briefly in Fig. 1. Dr. Michael Pollay's invited presentation thoroughly evaluated the evidence for pathways other than the dural venous sinuses, and these proven and potential sites are included in the figure. The utility of this classification system to drive clinical decision-making, as well as its use to plan and analyze basic science studies on animal models, was discussed thoroughly.

Conclusion

Professor Marmarou's instructions to "continue" led to this very successful meeting. Much was accomplished and much is left to be done. Areas of both basic science and clinical research have been defined, and work in these areas continues.

Plans are well underway for the next hydrocephalus meeting under the auspices of the International Society for Hydrocephalus and Cerebrospinal Fluid Disorders (ISHCSF) to be held in Copenhagen from September 4–7th of this year. Thank you, Tony.

The following members of the Hydrocephalus Classification Study Group worked diligently to come up with this consensus statement:

Harold L. Rekate, M.D. (Chairman)	Phoenix, AZ, USA
Petra Klinge, M.D.	Providence, RI, USA
J. Patrick (Pat) McAllister, Ph.D.	Salt Lake City, UT, USA
Concezio Di Rocco, M.D.	Rome, Italy
Charles Teo, M.D.	Sydney, Australia
Shizuo Oi, M.D., Ph.D.	Juntendo University, Japan
Osamu Sato, M.D.	Tokyo, Japan
Marion (Jack) Walker, M.D.	Salt Lake City, Utah, USA
Michael Pollay, M.D.	Phoenix, AZ, USA
Spyros Sgouros, M.D.	Athens, Greece
Conrad Johansson, Ph.D.	Providence, RI, USA
Martina Messing-Jünger, M.D.	Dusseldorf, Germany
John Picard, M.D.	Cambridge, UK
Gordon McComb, M.D.	Los Angeles, CA, USA

Conflicts of interest statement We declare that we have no conflict of interest.

References

1. Aygok G, Marmarou A, Young HF (2005) Three-year outcome of shunted idiopathic NPH patients. Acta Neurochir Suppl 95: 241–245
2. Dandy WE, Blackfan KD (1914) Internal hydrocephalus, an experimental, pathological and clinical study. Am J Dis Child 8:406–482
3. Di Rocco C, Di Trapani G, Maira G, Bentivoglio M, Macchi G, Rossi GF (1977) Anatomo-clinical correlations in normotensive hydrocephalus. Reports on three cases. J Neurol Sci 33:437–452
4. Filippidis AS, Kalani MY, Rekate HL (2011) Hydrocephalus and aquaporins: lessons learned from the bench. Childs Nerv Syst 27:27–33
5. James AE Jr, DeLand FH, Hodges FJ III, Wagner HN Jr (1970) Normal-pressure hydrocephalus. Role of cisternography in diagnosis. JAMA 213:1615–1622
6. Kestle J, Drake J, Milner R, Sainte-Rose C, Cinalli G, Boop F, Piatt J, Haines S, Schiff S, Cochrane D, Steinbok P, MacNeil N (2000) Long-term follow-up data from the Shunt Design Trial. Pediatr Neurosurg 33:230–236
7. Marmarou A, Bergsneider M, Relkin N, Klinge P, Black PM (2005) Development of guidelines for idiopathic normal-pressure hydrocephalus: introduction. Neurosurgery 57:S1–S3
8. Marmarou A, Black P, Bergsneider M, Klinge P, Relkin N (2005) Guidelines for management of idiopathic normal pressure hydrocephalus: progress to date. Acta Neurochir Suppl 95:237–240
9. Marmarou A, Shulman K, LaMorgese J (1975) Compartmental analysis of compliance and outflow resistance of the cerebrospinal fluid system. J Neurosurg 43:523–534
10. Marmarou A, Young HF, Aygok GA, Sawauchi S, Tsuji O, Yamamoto T, Dunbar J (2005) Diagnosis and management of idiopathic normal-pressure hydrocephalus: a prospective study in 151 patients. J Neurosurg 102:987–997
11. Patten DH, Benson DF (1968) Diagnosis of normal-pressure hydrocephalus by RISA cisternography. J Nucl Med 9:457–461
12. Rekate HL (2008) The definition and classification of hydrocephalus: a personal recommendation to stimulate debate. Cerebrospinal Fluid Res 5:2
13. Rossi GF, Galli G, Di RC, Maira G, Meglio M, Troncone L (1974) Normotensive hydrocephalus. The relations of pneumoencephalography and isotope cisternography to the results of surgical treatment. Acta Neurochir (Wien) 30:69–83
14. Shapiro K, Marmarou A (1982) Clinical applications of the pressure-volume index in treatment of pediatric head injuries. J Neurosurg 56:819–825
15. Shapiro K, Marmarou A, Shulman K (1980) Characterization of clinical CSF dynamics and neural axis compliance using the pressure-volume index: I. The normal pressure-volume index. Ann Neurol 7:508–514
16. Siomin V, Cinalli G, Grotenhuis A, Golash A, Oi S, Kothbauer K, Weiner H, Roth J, Beni-Adani L, Pierre-Kahn A, Takahashi Y, Mallucci C, Abbott R, Wisoff J, Constantini S (2002) Endoscopic third ventriculostomy in patients with cerebrospinal fluid infection and/or hemorrhage. J Neurosurg 97:519–524

Modeling of CSF Dynamics: Legacy of Professor Anthony Marmarou

Marek Czosnyka, Zofia Czosnyka, Kiran J. Agarwal-Harding, and John D. Pickard

Abstract The mathematical model of cerebrospinal fluid (CSF) pressure volume compensation, introduced by Anthony Marmarou in 1973 and modified in later studies, provides a theoretical basis for differential diagnosis in hydrocephalus. The Servo-Controlled Constant Pressure Test (Umea, Sweden) and Computerised Infusion Test (Cambridge, UK) are based on this model and are designed to compensate for inadequate accuracy of estimation of both the resistance to CSF outflow and elasticity of CSF pressure volume compensation.

Dr. Marmarou's further works introduced the pressure volume index (PVI), a parameter used to describe CSF compensation in hydrocephalic children and adults. A similar technique has been also utilized in traumatic brain injury (TBI).

The presence of a vascular component of intracranial pressure (ICP) was a concept proposed in the 1980s. Marmarou demonstrated that only around 30% of cases of elevated ICP in patients with TBI could be explained by changes in CSF circulation. The remaining 70% of cases should be attributable to vascular components, which have been proposed as equivalent to raised brain venous pressure.

Professor Marmarou's work has had a direct impact in the field of contemporary clinical neurosciences, and many of his ideas are still being investigated actively today.

Keywords Cerebrospinal fluid • Intracranial pressure • Hydrocephalus • Mathematical modeling

M. Czosnyka (✉)
Department of Clinical Neuroscience, Neurosurgical Unit, University of Cambridge, Cambridge, UK and
Academic Neurosurgery, Addenbrooke's Hospital, Cambridge, UK
e-mail: mc141@medschl.cam.ac.uk

Z. Czosnyka and J.D. Pickard
Department of Clinical Neuroscience, Neurosurgical Unit, University of Cambridge, Cambridge, UK

K.J. Agarwal-Harding
Harvard Medical School,
Harvard University, Cambridge, MA, USA

Introduction

Models of cerebrospinal fluid (CSF) circulation usually differ from models simulating brain tissue displacement. Anatomical structure and distribution of stress-strain in the tissue are not of interest here compared with the hydrodynamics of CSF flow. Dynamics of intracranial pressure (ICP) may be monitored invasively in clinical practice with a pressure transducer, and dynamics of CSF flow can be measured noninvasively with phase-coded magnetic resonance imaging (MRI). Therefore, models of CSF dynamics have an established clinical application in diagnosis and management of several diseases such as hydrocephalus, idiopathic intracranial hypertension, and syringomyelia.

Many theoretical/modeling studies on CSF dynamics were published before the 1970s [3, 6, 8, 10]. However, Professor Anthony Marmarou was one of the first [11, 13] who integrated all components – CSF production, circulation, absorption, and storage – in one elegant theoretical structure expressed as an electrical circuit (see Fig. 1). He analyzed theoretically three basic maneuvers: bolus CSF withdrawal, addition, and constant rate infusion. This model has withstood the test of time and, with only a very few 'cosmetic' modifications, it is still used today. Consequently, hydrocephalus and other disorders of CSF circulation are now characterized using parameters from this model such as resistance to CSF outflow, elasticity, and pressure volume index (PVI). These parameters were introduced into clinical practice by Marmarou et al. in 1975 [12]. He also proposed a mathematical explanation of the linear relationship between pulse amplitude and mean ICP [12], which was later elaborated by Avezaat and Eijndhoven [2]. In 1987, he described the "vascular component" of ICP [14]. In patients with traumatic brain injury (TBI), only 30% of cases of elevated ICP can be explained by changes in CSF circulation. Therefore, Marmarou concluded that the remaining 70% of cases of elevated ICP are derived from changes in the intracranial vascular component.

All three of these milestone achievements in the area of CSF dynamics are used today. The mathematical model of CSF dynamics will be presented briefly in the next section followed by a synopsis of the legacy of Marmarou's works in contemporary clinical neuroscience.

Fig. 1 Electrical model of cerebrospinal fluid (CSF) dynamics according to (**a**) Marmarou. *Upper panel*: Current source represents formation of CSF, resistor, and diode – unilateral absorption to sagittal sinus (voltage source p_{ss} represents sagittal sinus pressure). Capacitor – nonlinear compliance of CSF space. *Lower panel*: Extended model showing hydrodynamic consequence of shunting

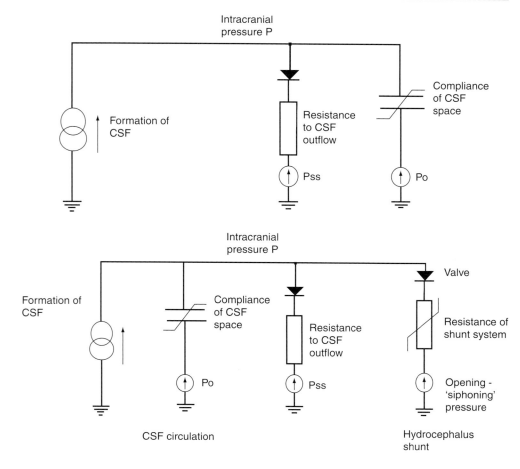

Marmarou's Model of CSF Dynamics

The mathematical model of CSF pressure volume compensation, introduced by Marmarou [11, 13] and modified in later studies [2, 16], provides a theoretical basis for differential diagnosis in hydrocephalus.

Under normal conditions, without long-term fluctuations of the cerebral blood volume, production of CSF is balanced by its storage and reabsorption in the sagittal sinus:

$$\text{Production of CSF} = \text{Storage of CSF} + \text{Reabsorption of CSF} \quad (1)$$

Production of CSF is assumed to be constant, although it may not always be the case. Reabsorption is proportional to the gradient between CSF pressure (p) and pressure in the sagittal sinuses (p_{ss}):

$$\text{Reabsorption} = \frac{p - p_{ss}}{R} \quad (2)$$

p_{ss} is considered to be a constant parameter determined by central venous pressure. However, it is not certain whether an interaction between changes in CSF pressure and p_{ss} exists in all circumstances: in patients with benign intracranial hypertension p_{ss} is frequently elevated due to fixed or variable stenosis of transverse sinuses, and a similar situation can be seen in venous sinus thrombosis.

The coefficient R (symbol R_{CSF} is also used) refers to the resistance to CSF reabsorption or outflow (units: mmHg/(mL/min)).

Storage of CSF is proportional to the cerebrospinal compliance C (units: mL/mmHg) and the rate of change of CSF pressure dp/dt:

$$\text{Storage} = C \cdot \frac{dp}{dt} \quad (3)$$

The compliance of the cerebrospinal space is inversely proportional to the gradient of CSF pressure p and the reference pressure p_0 (4):

$$C = \frac{1}{E \cdot (p - p_0)} \quad (4)$$

Some authors suggest that relationship (4) is valid only above a certain pressure level called the "optimal pressure" [16]. The coefficient E is termed the cerebral elasticity (or elastance coefficient) (unit: mL^{-1}). Elevated elasticity (>0.18 mL^{-1}) signifies a poor pressure volume compensatory

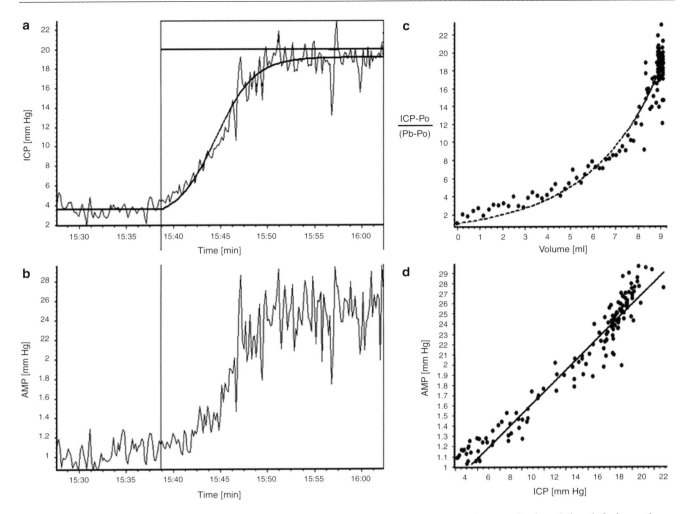

Fig. 2 Methods of identification of the model of cerebrospinal fluid (CSF) circulation during constant rate infusion study. (**a**) Recording of CSF pressure (*ICP*) versus time increasing during infusion with interpolated modeling curve (7) Infusion of constant rate of 1.5 mL/min starts from vertical line. (**b**) Recording of pulse amplitude (*AMP*) during infusion. Rise in AMP is usually well correlated with rise in ICP. (**c**) Pressure volume curve. On the x-axis, effective volume increase is plotted (i.e., infusion and production minus reabsorption of CSF). On y-axis, the increase in pressure is measured as a gradient of current pressure minus reference pressure p_0, relative to baseline pressure p_b. (**d**) Linear relationship between pulse amplitude and mean ICP. Intercept of the line with x-axis (ICP) theoretically indicates the reference pressure p_0

reserve [2]. This coefficient has recently been confirmed to be useful in predicting a patient's response to third ventriculostomy [17]. Relationship (4) expresses the most important law of the cerebrospinal dynamic compensation: When the CSF pressure increases, the compliance of the brain decreases.

A combination of (1) with (2) and (4) gives a final equation (5):

$$\frac{1}{E \cdot (p - p_0)} \cdot \frac{dp}{dt} + \frac{p - p_b}{R} = I(t) \quad (5)$$

where $I(t)$ is the rate of external volume addition and p_b is a baseline CSF pressure.

The model described by this equation may be presented in the form of its electric circuit equivalent [11] (Fig. 1).

Equation (5) can be solved for various types of external volume additions $I(t)$. The most common in clinical practice is (a) A constant infusion of CSF ($I(t)=0$ for $t<0$ and $I(t)=I_{inf}$ for $t>0$) – see Fig. 2:

$$P(t) = \frac{\left[I_{inf} + \frac{p_b - p_0}{R} \right] \cdot \left[p_b - p_0 \right]}{\frac{p_b - p_0}{R} + I_{inf} \cdot \left[e^{-E\left[\frac{p_b - p_0}{R} + I_{inf} \right] \cdot t} \right]} + p_0 \quad (6)$$

The analytical curve (6) can be matched to the real recording of the pressure during the test, which results in an estimation of the unknown parameters: R, E, and p_0 (see Fig. 2a).

(b) A bolus injection of CSF (volume ΔV):

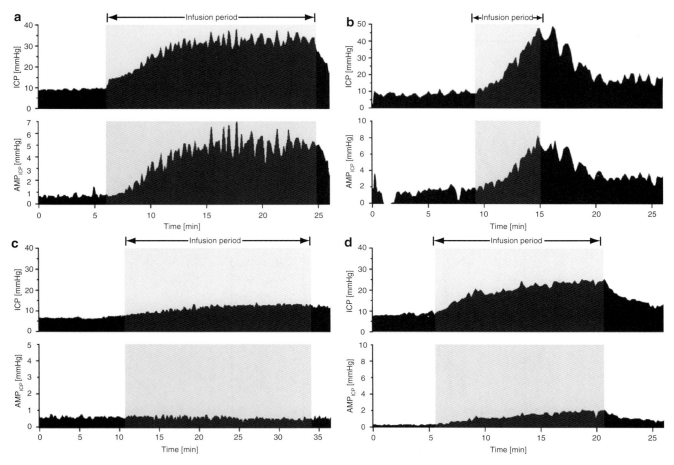

Fig. 3 Examples of a constant rate infusion test. *ICP* mean ICP (10-s average), *AMP* pulse amplitude of ICP. The blue section is the duration of infusion. (**a**) Normal pressure hydrocephalus (NPH): Although the base line pressure is normal, the resistance to cerebrospinal fluid (CSF) outflow increased, there are lots of strong vasogenic waves, and changes in pulse amplitude are fairly well correlated with changes in mean ICP. (**b**) Acute hydrocephalus post-subarachnoid hemorrhage (SAH): The normal baseline pressure was measured, but the resistance to CSF outflow is high. Good response of shunt surgery was expected. (**c**) Cerebral brain atrophy: the base line pressure is low, but the resistance to CSF outflow is low. No vasogenic waves were recorded, and pulse amplitude does not respond. (**d**) Normal: the base line pressure, the resistance to CSF outflow, and other parameters are normal, and thus the result demonstrates normal CSF circulation

$$p(t) = \frac{(p_b - p_0) \cdot e^{E\left[\Delta V + \frac{p_b - p_0}{R} \cdot t\right]}}{1 + e^{E\Delta V} \cdot \left[e^{E \cdot \frac{p_b - p_0}{t} \cdot t} - 1\right]} + p_0 \quad (7)$$

The bolus injection can be used for calculation of the PVI, defined as the volume added externally to produce a tenfold increase in the pressure [12]:

$$\text{PVI} \stackrel{\text{def}}{=} \frac{\Delta V}{\log_{10}\left(\frac{p_p - p_0}{p_b - p_0}\right)}; \quad \text{PVI} \cong \frac{1}{0.434 \cdot E} \quad (8a,b)$$

p_p in the formula (8a) is peak pressure recorded just after addition of the volume ΔV. The PVI is theoretically proportional to the inverse of the brain elastance coefficient E. The pressure volume compensatory reserve is insufficient when PVI <13 mL, and a PVI value above 26 mL signifies an "over-compliant" brain. These norms are valid for the PVI calculated as an inverse of E (according to 8b) using slow infusion. If the bolus test is used, norms for PVI are higher (the threshold equivalent to 13 mL is around 25 mL [15]).

The formula (7) for time $t=0$ describes the shape of the relationship between the effective volume increase ΔV and the CSF pressure, called the pressure volume curve (Fig. 2c):

$$p = (p_b - p_0) \cdot e^{E\Delta V} + p_0 \quad (9)$$

Finally, Eq. (7) can be helpful in the theoretical evaluation of the relationship between the pulse wave amplitude of ICP and the mean CSF pressure. If we presume that the rise in blood volume after a heart contraction is equivalent to a rapid bolus addition of CSF fluid at the baseline pressure p_b, the pulse amplitude (AMP) can be expressed as:

$$\text{AMP} + p_p - p_b = (p_b - p_0) \cdot (e^{E\Delta V} - 1) \qquad (10)$$

In almost all cases, when CSF pressure is being increased by the addition of an external volume, the pulse amplitude rises [2, 12] – see Fig. 2b, d. The gradient of the regression line between AMP and p is proportional to the elasticity. The intercept, theoretically, marks the reference pressure p_0.

Synopsis of Clinical Applications of the Model

- The Servo-Controlled Constant Pressure Infusion Test [7] is used for assessment of CSF disorders. Its aim is to evaluate the resistance to CSF outflow in a repetitive and reliable way.
- Full identification of the model, including elasticity, can be made using a computerized constant rate infusion test [4] supported by the dedicated software ICM+ (http://www.neurosurg.cam.ac.uk/icmplus/).
- Use of the constant rate infusion test in many centers contributed to a definition of profiles of ICP and its pulse amplitude in different possible clinical scenarios, including normal pressure hydrocephalus, brain atrophy, acute hydrocephalus, and in nondisturbed CSF circulation (see Fig. 3).
- Analysis of the constant rate infusion test in shunted patients can be helpful in shunt assessment in vivo. The electrical circuit model proposed by Professor Marmarou, supplemented by a branch-defining nonlinear pressure flow performance curve, is presented in Fig. 1. Direct knowledge of the curve, as assessed in shunt evaluation laboratories [1, 5] allows in vivo identification of the model and sensitive prediction whether the shunt is working properly, underdraining, or overdraining.
- The proportional increase of the pulse waveform of ICP with mean ICP, has been explained by Marmarou [12] as a consequence of the exponential pressure volume curve. Although further works demonstrated that in a system with a good pressure volume compensatory reserve, the pressure volume curve is linear [2, 16], at higher pressures, the curve becomes exponential [2] This led to analysis of a moving correlation coefficient (20-s to 2-min period) between mean ICP and AMP. The resulting RAP coefficient indicates the state of compensatory reserve. RAP = 0 suggests good compensatory reserve; RAP = 1, poor compensatory reserve [9].
- The idea of a vasogenic component of ICP led to modification of Davson's equation: $\text{ICP} = R_{CSF} * \text{CSF}_{formation} + p_{ss} +$ 'Arterial vasogenic component'
- The "arterial vasogenic component" is a component of ICP which is derived by detection of pulsatile blood flow in nonlinear components of cerebrospinal space (intracranial and arterial bed compliance, resistance of collapsible bridging veins, and autoregulation-controlled main cerebrovascular resistance).

Conclusion

When Professor Marmarou was terminally ill and was asked by his coworkers what they should do in future years, he simply said "Continue" (Dr. G. Aygok, personal communication). There are certainly a lot of directions to continue in and many questions initiated by Anthony Marmarou in the field of clinical neurosciences that remain unanswered.

Acknowledgements This work was supported by the National Institute of Health Research, Biomedical Research Centre, Cambridge University Hospital Foundation Trust – Neurosciences Theme, and a Senior Investigator Award (to J. D. P.).

Disclosure ICM+ is a software for brain monitoring in clinical/experimental neurosciences (http//www.neurosurg.cam.ac.uk/icmplus/). It is licensed by the University of Cambridge (Cambridge Enterprise Ltd). M.C. has a share in a fraction of the licensing fee.

Conflicts of interest statement what is in Disclosure may be in Conflict of interest.

References

1. Aschoff A, Kremer P (1998) Determining the best cerebrospinal fluid shunt valve design: the pediatric valve design trial. Neurosurgery 42(4):949–951
2. Avezaat CJJ, Eijndhoven JHM (1984) Cerebrospinal fluid pulse pressure and craniospinal dynamics. Ph.D. thesis, The Jongbloed an Zoon Publishers, The Hague
3. Benabid AL (1970) Contribution a l'etude de l'hypertension intracranienne modele mathematique. M.D. thesis, Grenoble University
4. Czosnyka M, Whitehouse H, Smielewski P et al (1996)Testing of cerebrospinal compensatory reserve in shunted and non-shunted patients: a guide to interpretation based on an observational study. J Neurol Neurosurg Psychiatry 60:549–558
5. Czosnyka Z, Czosnyka M, Richards HK et al (1998) Posture-related overdrainage: comparison of the performance of 10 hydrocephalus shunts in vitro. Neurosurgery 42(2):327–333
6. Davson H, Hollingsworth JR, Segal MD (1970) The mechanism of drainage of the cerebrospinal fluid. Brain 93:665–678
7. Eklund A, Lundkvist B, Koskinen LO, Malm J (2004) Infusion technique can be used to distinguish between dysfunction of a hydrocephalus shunt system and a progressive dementia. Med Biol Eng Comput 42(5):644–649

8. Guinane JE (1972) An equivalent circuit analysis of cerebrospinal fluid hydrodynamics. Am J Physiol 223:425–430
9. Kim DJ, Czosnyka Z, Keong N et al (2009) Index of cerebrospinal compensatory reserve in hydrocephalus. Neurosurgery 64(3):494–501
10. Lofgren J, Zwetnow NN (1973) The pressure-volume curve of the cerebrospinal fluid space in dogs. Acta Neurol Scand 49:557–574
11. Marmarou A (1973) A theoretical and experimental of cerebrospinal fluid system. Ph.D. thesis, Drexel University
12. Marmarou A, Schulman K, LaMorgese J (1975) Compartmental analysis of compliance and outflow resistance of cerebrospinal fluid system. J Neurosurg 43:523–534
13. Marmarou A, Shulman K, Rosende RM (1978) A non-linear analysis of CSF system and intracranial pressure dynamics. J Neurosurg 48:332–344
14. Marmarou A, Maset AL, Ward JD, Choi S, Brooks D, Lutz HA, Moulton RJ, Muizelaar JP, DeSalles A, Young HF (1987) Contribution of CSF and vascular factors to elevation of ICP in severely head-injured patients. J Neurosurg 66(6):883–890
15. Marmarou A, Foda MA, Bandoh K et al (1996) Posttraumatic ventriculomegaly: hydrocephalus or atrophy? A new approach for diagnosis using CSF dynamics. J Neurosurg 85(6):1026–1035
16. Sliwka S (1980) A clinical system for the evaluation of selected dynamic properties of the intracranial system. Ph.D. thesis, Polish Academy of Sciences, Warsaw (in Polish)
17. Tisell M, Edsbagge M, Stephensen H et al (2002) Elastance correlates with outcome after endoscopic third ventriculostomy in adults with hydrocephalus caused by primary aqueductal stenosis. Neurosurgery 50:70–76

Ethical Considerations in Hydrocephalus Research That Involves Children and Adults

Michael A. Williams

Abstract Those who conduct clinical research in hydrocephalus face ethical challenges. Research subjects include infants, children, unborn fetuses, and adults with diminished decision-making capacity. The aim of clinical research is to acquire knowledge that will improve the health of future patients, and one of the goals of research ethics is to prevent the exploitation of research subjects.

The history of hydrocephalus treatment is marked by innovation. Surgical innovation should be followed by surgical research so that the innovation is proven to be better than existing treatments before it becomes accepted practice.

Because the long-term effects of genetic, pharmacologic, and stem cell therapies on the developing brain are unknown, researchers have an obligation to conduct short- and long-term research on children. Children should be asked for their assent or dissent. Assent is a child's affirmative agreement to participate in research. Absence of the child's objection is not sufficient; the child must say yes to participation in the research. A child's refusal to participate in research should be respected.

In disorders with dementia, such as normal pressure hydrocephalus, decision-making capacity of the research subject should be assessed. If the subject lacks decision-making capacity, a surrogate or guardian must provide consent. Assent to participate in research should also be obtained from adults with cognitive impairment.

Keywords Research ethics • Human experimentation • Human research subject protection • Research subjects • Hydrocephalus • Clinical trials, randomized

Introduction

The mission statement of the International Society for Hydrocephalus and Cerebrospinal Fluid Disorders (www.ishcsf.com) states that one of the Society's aims is "to support guidelines, standardized methods, and *ethically conducted clinical and basic research* in the hydrocephalus, CSF disorders, and related fields" [emphasis added]. Surprisingly, the topic of research ethics in the field of hydrocephalus has received little attention, especially considering that active clinical research in hydrocephalus has been conducted for over 50 years in infants, children, adolescents, adults, and the elderly. A PubMed search on May 15, 2010, of the terms *hydrocephalus* AND *research ethics* produced only six articles, none of which specifically addressed research ethics [Donnenfeld et al. Prenat Diagn 9:301–308, 1989; Guiney Eur J Pediatr Surg 4(Suppl 1):5–9, 1994; Rushton Am J Nurs 104:54–63, 2004; Stivaros et al. Radiology 252:825–832, 2009; Zahuranec Neurology 68:1651–1657, 2007; Zambelli et al. Childs Nerv Syst 23:123–126, 2007]. In addition, to the best of the author's knowledge and recollection, the topic of research ethics has never formally been discussed at any of the international hydrocephalus workshops or conferences held in the last decade. Considering that more clinical research in hydrocephalus is either underway or planned than at any other time in recent memory, it is imperative that we reflect on the important ethical considerations in clinical research.

The Challenge

Clinical research in the area of hydrocephalus faces many ethical challenges. We come from a tradition of surgical innovation in hydrocephalus, but we have not conducted as much research on novel surgical methods as we should have. Our research subjects include infants, children, unborn fetuses, and adults with cognitive impairment and diminished decision-making capacity. On the horizon is research involving implanted stem cells that have an as-yet-unknown

M.A. Williams
The Sandra and Malcolm Berman Brain & Spine Institute,
Adult Hydrocephalus Center, Sinai Hospital of Baltimore,
Baltimore, MD, USA
e-mail: michwill@lifebridgehealth.org

influence on the brain. If stem cell research is to be conducted in infants or children, not only could the potential benefit be long lasting — but so could any potential adverse effects. Biologics, pharmaceuticals, and stem cell treatments go beyond our usual research experience with surgical treatment and diagnostic modalities. Thus, we have new ethical considerations to contemplate.

Distinctions Between the Ethics of Clinical Care and Clinical Research

The aim of clinical care is to maximize the health and well-being of individual patients. Familiar ethical principles guide us: *beneficence* — maximizing benefit; *nonmaleficence* — minimizing harm; *respect for autonomy* — allowing patients, parents, or surrogates to accept or reject treatment recommendations (informed consent); and *justice* — fair distribution of resources [3]. In clinical care, our only duty is to the patient we are treating. Generally, treatment choices follow best practices, as supported by research, practice guidelines such as the 2005 idiopathic normal pressure hydrocephalus guidelines [17], or precedence ("accepted wisdom").

The aim of clinical research is to acquire clinically relevant knowledge that will improve the health of *future* patients. The beneficiary of research is society — not necessarily the human subjects who participate in the research. To phrase it candidly, research subjects are a means to the ends of clinical research. Researchers use research subjects to test hypotheses. One of the primary goals of research ethics, therefore, is to prevent the exploitation of research subjects, a problem that has regrettably occurred in many instances in many countries over many years [9, 10].

Some forms of ethically conducted research, such as phase I pharmaceutical studies, offer no benefit to research subjects but can expose them to harm. This kind of research is permissible as long as efforts to prevent harm are in place and subjects are informed of the risks. Despite these precautions, subjects are sometimes harmed. For example, in a 2006 phase I trial of the anti-CD28 monoclonal antibody TGN1412, six healthy volunteers became critically ill due to a rapid and unexpected "cytokine storm [22]." Fortunately, all survived.

A critical distinction exists between the ethics of clinical care and the ethics of clinical research. In clinical care, it is *ethically impermissible* to offer an intervention that has only risks and no expected benefit. In clinical research, it is *ethically permissible* to conduct research with a drug, biologic, or procedure that has only risks and no expected benefit, or that has risks and an unknown or unproven benefit, as long as safeguards are in place. Indeed, research could not occur if investigations were limited to only those treatments or interventions that have known benefit. The purpose of the research is to test the hypothesis that a new treatment has benefit.

The framework for research ethics is sufficiently different from the framework for clinical ethics that it bears explication. Emanuel and colleagues, in their 2000 *JAMA* article, provide a systematic and coherent framework with seven requirements for determining whether clinical research is ethical. Although most researchers are familiar with two of the requirements — independent review and informed consent — a research protocol should also have social or scientific value, scientific validity, fair subject selection, a favorable risk–benefit ratio, and respect for potential and enrolled subjects [10].

Innovation

When faced with unusual circumstances that carry risk of harm or death to the patient for which no intervention has been established, surgeons may attempt innovative approaches based on the principles of beneficence and informed consent, as applied to the clinical care of a specific patient. If the need for surgical innovation is encountered in mid-procedure, ideally, the family's consent should be sought; however, consent may be waived if the delay necessitated to obtain it would result in harm to the patient (principle of presumed consent for emergency treatment). Generally, innovation is needed in high-risk/high-reward scenarios. Innovation is not limited to surgical procedures. Intensivists and medical specialists can, and often do, innovate with off-label usage of medications, which is permissible under US law as long as the physician believes that the off-label use of the medication will benefit the patient.

The history of hydrocephalus treatment is marked by innovation. John Holter's invention of the first practical shunt inserted by neurosurgeon Eugene Spitz is a well-known example, as is Solomon Hakim's insertion of a shunt in the first few cases of normal pressure hydrocephalus (NPH) [2, 4]. The shunt for hydrocephalus in infants and children was so obviously life-saving that research to test its efficacy was not necessary. The same was thought to be true of shunt surgery for NPH; however, its use became so widespread that it was often performed on patients who, in retrospect, did not have NPH. The complication rate rose so high that the very existence of NPH and its responsiveness to shunting was questioned. The emergence of endoscopic third ventriculostomy (ETV) in the 1990s was also a result of innovation, but until recently, ETV was not compared head-to-head with shunt surgery. The question we must answer today is, when should surgical innovation be followed by surgical research so that the innovation is proven to be better than existing treatments before it becomes accepted practice?

The ethical rationale for requiring research on surgical innovations begins with the fact that medicine, as a profession, has an obligation to society to offer treatments that are proven to be safe and effective. To allow treatments to become the standard of care without randomized controlled trials (RCTs) is to risk promoting unsafe and ineffective treatments. Thus, we have a strong obligation to use RCTs or similarly valid research designs for new surgical interventions.

Research on new or innovative surgical procedures differs significantly from research on new drugs and biologics. Although no surgical equivalent of phase I trials exists for humans, new techniques can be evaluated in animal models. RCTs in surgery are rarely conducted because of the attendant challenges, including greater complexity than medical research protocols; variation in surgeon expertise and experience; necessity to involve the entire surgical team; difficulty in defining significant and meaningful outcomes; difficulty in ensuring that procedures are performed the same way for every subject; effective blinding of surgeons and subjects to prevent bias in outcome assessment; ensuring randomization to prevent allocation bias; and choosing the best comparator — e.g., placebo versus another procedure versus medical intervention [6, 11].

Most neurosurgical RCTs have involved implantation of complex devices, stem cells, or medication-releasing systems, such as in studies of deep-brain stimulation in parkinsonism, carmustine-impregnated polymer for glioblastoma multiforme [5], shunting in Alzheimer's disease [20], and comparison of shunting versus ETV for infants under 24 months with hydrocephalus [13].

Recent articles by Farrokhyar et al., Cook, and those in the *Oxford Textbook of Clinical Research Ethics* present excellent reviews on the challenges of surgical research [6, 9, 11].

Research Involving Children and Cognitively Impaired Adults

Because hydrocephalus affects children, and because the physiology of children is not the same as that of adults, it is both scientifically and ethically imperative that new interventions be investigated and validated in children. Aside from the use of innovation in dire circumstances, an argument can be made that it is unethical to use unproven treatments in children. Moreover, especially as the era of genetic, pharmacologic, and stem cell therapies for hydrocephalus is on the horizon and the long-term effects of these treatments on the developing brain are unknown, we have a strong obligation to conduct short- and long-term research on children.

The good news is that research involving children with hydrocephalus is increasing. The DRIFT trial of ventricular irrigation with fibrinolytic therapy has yielded provocative results, with fewer deaths or survivors with severe disability, compared with controls, despite the increased rate of intraventricular bleeding; Kulkarni's work on quality-of-life indicators for children with hydrocephalus provides tools for evaluating long-term outcomes; and the Hydrocephalus Clinical Research Network is at the leading edge of cooperative research design and best-practices design [1, 15, 25, 26]. Still, much more research in infants and children is needed.

Recent research in adults with hydrocephalus has yielded important scientific information but has also required significant research ethics considerations. Examples include (1) a blinded, placebo-controlled study of shunt surgery in a small cohort of elderly adults with extensive periventricular white matter disease and an average Mini-Mental State Examination score of 22.5 [23], which is a score low enough to be considered in the "gray zone" for ability to provide consent [14], and (2) nonbeneficial research on normal elderly human research subjects to determine reference values for CSF outflow resistance and intracranial pressure [16].

Consent and Assent for Children and Cognitively Challenged Adults

By law in most jurisdictions, children are presumed incompetent and unable to provide consent to research; thus, their parents must provide consent. Depending on their age and their experience with health and illness, children may be capable of providing assent to research. Generally, children older than age 7 years should be asked for their assent or dissent. Assent is a child's affirmative agreement to participate in research. Absence of the child's objection is not sufficient; the child must say yes to participation in the research. Assent procedures should be age and developmentally appropriate and, with institutional review board (IRB) approval, may sometimes be waived [7, 24].

A child's refusal to participate in research should be respected; it differs substantially from a child's refusal to have treatment or surgery as part of the standard of care for which the parents have provided consent. Children can be "forced" to have shunt surgery, despite their apparent refusal because the procedure is specifically intended to benefit their health; however, children cannot be "forced" to participate in research of an investigational treatment.

Adults with Cognitive Impairment

Adults with cognitive impairment are considered a vulnerable population in research and are afforded extra protections [18]. Especially in disorders with dementia, such as NPH, decision-making capacity should be assessed as part of the informed-consent process. If the potential research subject lacks decision-making capacity, a surrogate or guardian must provide consent. Further, a consensus is emerging that assent to participate in research should be obtained even from adults with cognitive impairment and that, as with children, adults' refusal to participate should be respected, except when an IRB has approved a waiver of assent such as in low-risk procedures (e.g., blood tests) for which any discomfort is minimal and temporary.

Although it might be tempting to suggest that the increased effort required to safeguard vulnerable subjects is reason enough to exclude them from research participation, children, cognitively impaired adults, and other vulnerable subjects have an interest in the outcome of research, as they could benefit from it. They also have an interest in research conducted on subjects who have the same disorders that they have. As part of respect for persons, we afford all subjects the opportunity to participate in research, unless a bona fide exclusion criterion exists.

Conclusion

Good research design and research ethics go hand in hand. We come from a tradition in which innovation sometimes becomes accepted wisdom and the standard of care without careful research to prove that the innovation is better. Only we can effect the change in our clinician-scientist culture to make scientifically and ethically designed studies a requirement. If we are committed to the goal of improving the care of and the outcomes for our patients with hydrocephalus, then we must summon the strength and the perseverance to design, fund, implement, and publish the best scientifically and ethically designed research. We should engage patients and families, funding agencies, and industry partners in achieving this goal.

If we remember that the aim of clinical research is to acquire clinically relevant knowledge that will improve the health of future patients, then our deference and respect for research ethics will earn us the respect and support that we need to conduct the research that will lead to proven and improved methods for treating hydrocephalus.

Conflicts of interest statement Dr. Williams's life partner holds stock in Medtronic.

References

1. http://www.hcrn.org/. Accessed 15 June 2010
2. Baru JS, Bloom DA, Muraszko K, Koop CE (2001) John Holter's shunt. J Am Coll Surg 192:79–85
3. Beauchamp TL, Childress JF (2009) Principles of biomedical ethics. Oxford University Press, New York
4. Boockvar JA, Loudon W, Sutton LN (2001) Development of the Spitz-Holter valve in Philadelphia. J Neurosurg 95:145–147
5. Brem H, Piantadosi S, Burger PC, Walker M, Selker R, Vick NA, Black K, Sisti M, Brem S, Mohr G et al (1995) Placebo-controlled trial of safety and efficacy of intraoperative controlled delivery by biodegradable polymers of chemotherapy for recurrent gliomas. The Polymer-brain Tumor Treatment Group. Lancet 345:1008–1012
6. Cook JA (2009) The challenges faced in the design, conduct, and analysis of surgical randomised controlled trials. Trials 10:9
7. Diekema DS (2006) Conducting ethical research in pediatrics: a brief historical overview and review of pediatric regulations. J Pediatr 149:S3–S11
8. Donnenfeld AE, Glazerman LR, Cutillo DM, Librizzi RJ, Weiner S (1989) Fetal exsanguination following intrauterine angiographic assessment and selective termination of a hydrocephalic, monozygotic co-twin. Prenat Diagn 9:301–308
9. Emanuel EJ, Grady C, Crouch RA, Lie R, Miller F (eds) (2008) The Oxford textbook of clinical research ethics. Oxford University Press, Oxford/New York
10. Emanuel EJ, Wendler D, Grady C (2000) What makes clinical research ethical? JAMA 283:2701–2711
11. Farrokhyar F, Karanicolas PJ, Thoma A, Simunovic M, Bhandari M, Devereaux PJ, Anvari M, Adili A, Guyatt G (2010) Randomized controlled trials of surgical interventions. Ann Surg 251:409–416
12. Guiney EJ (1994) Presidential address to the Society for Research into Spina Bifida and Hydrocephalus, at Hartford, Conn., USA. Eur J Pediatr Surg 4(Suppl 1):5–9
13. International infant hydrocephalus study: a multicenter, prospective, randomized study. Accessed at http://147.188.78.52/iihs/index.html. 15 June 2010
14. Karlawish J (2008) Measuring decision-making capacity in cognitively impaired individuals. Neurosignals 16:91–98
15. Kulkarni AV (2010) Quality of life in childhood hydrocephalus: a review. Childs Nerv Syst 26:737–743
16. Malm J, Jacobsson J, Birgander R, Eklund A (2011) Reference values for CSF outflow resistance and intracranial pressure in healthy elderly. Neurology 76:903–909
17. Marmarou A, Bergsneider M, Relkin N, Klinge P, Black PM (2005) Development of guidelines for idiopathic normal-pressure hydrocephalus: introduction. Neurosurgery 57:S1–S3; discussion ii–v
18. Rosenstein DL, Miller FG (2008) Research involving those at risk for impaired decision-making capacity. In: Emanuel EJ, Grady C, Crouch RA, Lie R, Miller F, Wendler D (eds) The Oxford textbook of clinical research ethics. Oxford University Press, Oxford/New York, pp 437–445
19. Rushton CH (2004) Ethics and palliative care in pediatrics. Am J Nurs 104:54–63
20. Silverberg GD, Mayo M, Saul T, Fellmann J, Carvalho J, McGuire D (2008) Continuous CSF drainage in AD: results of a double-blind, randomized, placebo-controlled study. Neurology 71:202–209
21. Stivaros SM, Sinclair D, Bromiley PA, Kim J, Thorne J, Jackson A (2009) Endoscopic third ventriculostomy: predicting outcome with phase-contrast MR imaging. Radiology 252:825–832
22. Suntharalingam G, Perry MR, Ward S, Brett SJ, Castello-Cortes A, Brunner MD, Panoskaltsis N (2006) Cytokine storm in a phase 1 trial of the anti-CD28 monoclonal antibody TGN1412. N Engl J Med 355:1018–1028

23. Tisell M, Tullberg M, Hellström P, Edsbagge M, Högfeldt M, Wikkelsö C (2011) Shunt surgery in patients with hydrocephalus and white matter changes. J Neurosurg 114(5):1432–1438. doi:10.3171/2010.11.JNS10967
24. Wendler D (2008) The assent requirement in pediatric research. In: Emanuel EJ, Grady C, Crouch RA, Lie R, Miller F, Wendler D (eds) The Oxford textbook of clinical research ethics. Oxford University Press, Oxford/New York, pp 661–671
25. Whitelaw A, Evans D, Carter M, Thoresen M, Wroblewska J, Mandera M, Swietlinski J, Simpson J, Hajivassiliou C, Hunt LP, Pople I (2007) Randomized clinical trial of prevention of hydrocephalus after intraventricular hemorrhage in preterm infants: brain-washing versus tapping fluid. Pediatrics 119:e1071–e1078
26. Whitelaw A, Jary S, Kmita G, Wroblewska J, Musialik-Swietlinska E, Mandera M, Hunt L, Carter M, Pople I (2010) Randomized trial of drainage, irrigation and fibrinolytic therapy for premature infants with posthemorrhagic ventricular dilatation: developmental outcome at 2 years. Pediatrics 125:e852–e858
27. Zahuranec DB, Brown DL, Lisabeth LD, Gonzales NR, Longwell PJ, Smith MA, Garcia NM, Morgenstern LB (2007) Early care limitations independently predict mortality after intracerebral hemorrhage. Neurology 68:1651–1657
28. Zambelli H, Barini R, Iscaife A, Cursino K, Braga Ade F, Marba S, Sbragia L (2007) Successful developmental outcome in intrauterine myelomeningocele repair. Childs Nerv Syst 23:123–126

Conservative Versus Surgical Management of Idiopathic Normal Pressure Hydrocephalus: A Prospective Double-Blind Randomized Controlled Trial: Study Protocol

Ahmed K. Toma, Marios C. Papadopoulos, Simon Stapleton, Neil D. Kitchen, and Laurence D. Watkins

Abstract There is no level I evidence to indicate whether placement of a shunt is effective in the management of idiopathic normal pressure hydrocephalus (INPH), because no trial has as yet compared the placement of a shunt versus no shunt in a randomized controlled manner. We started recruiting patients into a prospective double-blind randomized controlled study aiming to provide class I evidence supporting or refuting the role of surgical management in INPH. Inclusion criterion was the diagnosis of probable INPH plus objective improvement of walking speed following 72 h of extended lumbar drainage. Patients with concomitant Alzheimer's disease or vascular dementia were excluded. All patients included in the trial were to have a shunt placed with proGAV® adjustable valve. Patients were randomly assigned into two groups: group A was to have the shunt immediately adjusted to function, and group B was to have the shunt valve adjusted to the highest setting for 3 months then adjusted to function. Assessment of gait, cognitive function, and urinary symptoms were done before shunt insertion and at 3 months. Primary end point was to be an improvement in gait. Secondary end points were improvement in mental function or urinary function and incidence of complications. Final results are expected mid 2011.

Keywords Normal pressure hydrocephalus • Adjustable • Programmable • CSF shunt • Clinical trial

Introduction

Normal pressure hydrocephalus (NPH) was first described by Hakim and Adams in 1965 [9], yet despite 45 years of research and hundreds of peer-reviewed papers, its pathogenesis and natural history are still unknown [15].

Early clinical series reported a low rate of long-term significant improvement and a high rate of complications [10, 15]. Consequently, many physicians and even some neurosurgeons [3, 4, 15], are skeptical about the existence of NPH as a separate entity and have questioned the value of its surgical management.

A Cochrane review of shunting for NPH concluded that there is no evidence to indicate whether placement of a shunt is effective in the management of NPH [6].

Similarly the international guidelines for diagnosis and management of idiopathic normal pressure hydrocephalus (INPH) state that there is insufficient evidence to establish surgical management as a standard, since no trial has as yet compared the placement of a shunt versus no shunt in a randomized controlled manner. Surgical diversion of cerebrospinal fluid (CSF) is recommended as a guideline of management for patients in whom there is a favorable risk-to-benefit ratio [2, 14].

We live in an evidence-based medicine era; we realized the need for a randomized clinical trial for assessing the efficacy of shunting in the treatment of INPH. We set up this study; the aim is to provide class I evidence supporting or refuting the role of surgical management in INPH, and to answer the research question: Is there a role for surgical diversion of cerebrospinal fluid (CSF) in the management of INPH? Our goal is to present the trial protocol in this manuscript.

A.K. Toma (✉), N.D. Kitchen, and L.D. Watkins
Victor Horsley Department of Neurosurgery,
The National Hospital for Neurology and Neurosurgery,
London, UK
e-mail: ahmedktoma@yahoo.com

M.C. Papadopoulos and S. Stapleton
Academic Neurosurgery Unit,
St George's University of London,
London, UK

Methods

Inclusion Criteria

- Diagnosis of probable INPH [14]:
  - Clinical findings of gait/balance disturbance, plus at least one other area of impairment in cognition, urinary symptoms, or both.
  - No evidence of an antecedent event such as head trauma, intracerebral haemorrhage, meningitis, or other known causes of secondary hydrocephalus
  - No other neurological, psychiatric, or general medical condition that is sufficient to explain the presenting symptoms
  - A brain imaging study (CT or MRI) showing evidence of ventricular enlargement (Evans' index >0.3)
  - CSF opening pressure <18 mmHg.
- Objective improvement of walking speed following 72 h of extended lumbar drainage.

Exclusion Criteria

- Evidence of concomitant Alzheimer's disease or vascular dementia.

Trial Arms

All patients included in the trial will have a shunt insertion with proGAV® adjustable valve. All will have exactly the same management apart from the initial opening pressure of the valve for a set period of 3 months postoperatively. Patients will be randomly assigned into two groups. Patients will be blinded as to which group they are in.

- Group A: will have the shunt immediately adjusted to function, based on previous experience of using proGAV valve in an NPH population [16]. (shunt valve opening pressure of 5 cmH$_2$O).
- Group B: will have the shunt valve adjusted on the highest setting (20 cmH$_2$O) for 3 months then adjusted to function (shunt valve opening pressure of 5 cmH$_2$O).

This trial has been approved by the The National Hospital for Neurology and Neurosurgery and Institute of Neurology Joint Research Ethics Committee. Patients were provided with a comprehensive information sheet and asked to sign a consent form. Next of kin of cognitively impaired patients were provided with a separate information sheet and asked to sign an assent form in accordance with ethics committee standards. Randomization has been done using random blocks, and results kept in opaque envelopes as (open shunt) or (closed shunt). Envelopes will be opened prior to surgery when the patient consented to participate in the trial.

Baseline Measurements

Both groups were assessed prior to shunt insertion and at 3 months by an assessor who was blinded to the patient's group. Patients will be followed up at 6 months and 1 year, then annually following shunt insertion. Assessment was identical to that used in our unit for all NPH patients:

- Assessment of gait: 10-m timed walking test.
- Neuropsychological assessment: neuropsychological battery.
- Urinary function: grading scale for urinary continence.

End Points

Primary: Improvement in gait: as determined by the timed walking test.

Secondary:

- Improvement in mental function: as determined by neuropsychological testing
- Improvement in urinary function
- Incidence of complications.

Sample size calculations: Following the results obtained from a small pilot sample, we estimate that patients in group B (closed) will walk 10% faster (at most), while those in group A (open) will walk 50% faster (at least). To get a level of significance of 0.05 with 90% power, eight patients are needed in each arm.

Discussion

Simply comparing shunt insertion with no shunt insertion has the inherent limitation of possible placebo effect on patients and family, as well as inducing bias in outcome assessment and management. In addition, recruitment of a suspected INPH patient into a conservative arm might be difficult. Doing a sham (placebo) surgery or simply randomizing patients to ligated or open shunt tube groups is controversial from an ethical point of view, since patients with a nonfunctioning shunt will be subjected to unnecessary surgery, with its potential complications and with no personal benefit; again, recruitment into such a trial could prove to be a challenge [2, 5, 7, 8, 11, 13].

The ideal situation is to have a shunt valve system that can be opened and closed noninvasively; thus randomizing patients into open and closed shunt groups can be done with no added risk to the patient, with its advantages from an ethical and recruitment point of view.

The adjustable Miethke proGAV® shunt valve (Miethke GMBH & Co KG, Potsdam, Germany) has been in routine use in our unit for patients with INPH since 2007. It is composed of two units: an adjustable unit and a non-adjustable gravitational shunt assistant that protects against overdrainage. The adjustable unit uses a ball-in-cone valve system. The opening pressure of the proGAV® can be adjusted from 0 to 20 cmH$_2$O, in increments of 1 cmH$_2$O. The adjustment and verification instruments allow resetting noninvasively in an outpatient clinic setting, without having to expose the patient to X-ray radiation. The "Active-Lock" mechanism protects the proGAV® against accidental readjustment by external magnetic fields up to a 3-T MRI scanner [1, 12].

We considered a valve opening pressure of 20 cmH$_2$O as the nearest available option to a closed shunt that can be opened at the end of the study period noninvasively without adding risk or discomfort to the patient. One might argue that this will not be a really closed shunt; however, we routinely measure CSF opening pressure during lumbar drainage, and none of the patients included in the trial will have a pressure more than 20 cmH$_2$O. The proGAV® shunt valve pressure-flow performance curves, and operating, opening, and closing pressures were verified to fall within the limits specified by the manufacturer, The operating pressure increased when the shunt assistant was in the vertical position, as specified [1]. Recruitment started in July 2008 with an estimated time to finish the study by mid 2011.

Conclusion

The results of this prospective double-blind randomized controlled study should provide class I evidence supporting or refuting the role of surgical diversion of cerebrospinal fluid for the management of idiopathic normal pressure hydrocephalus.

Conflicts of interest statement A clinical research fellow post at the National Hospital for Neurology and Neurosurgery is supported by a grant from B. Braun Medical Ltd.

References

1. Allin DM, Czosnyka ZH, Czosnyka M, Richards HK, Pickard JD (2006) In vitro hydrodynamic properties of the Miethke proGAV hydrocephalus shunt. Cerebrospinal Fluid Res 3:9
2. Bergsneider M, Black PML, Klinge P, Marmarou A, Relkin N (2005) INPH guidelines, part IV: surgical management of idiopathic normal-pressure hydrocephalus. Neurosurgery 57:S2-29–S2-39
3. Bradshaw DY (2008) Lost to follow-up. Neurology 70:2081–2084
4. Brecknell JE, Brown JI (2004) Is idiopathic normal pressure hydrocephalus an independent entity? Acta Neurochir 146:1003–1006
5. Cohen PD, Herman L, Jedlinski S, Willocks P, Wittekind P (2007) Ethical issues in clinical neuroscience research: a patient's perspective. Neurotherapeutics 4:537–544
6. Esmonde T, Cooke S (2002) Shunting for normal pressure hydrocephalus (NPH). Cochrane Database Syst Rev (3): CD003157
7. Frank S, Kieburtz K, Holloway R, Kim SYH (2005) What is the risk of sham surgery in Parkinson disease clinical trials? A review of published reports. Neurology 65:1101–1103
8. Frank SA, Wilson R, Holloway RG, Zimmerman C, Peterson DR, Kieburtz K, Kim SYH (2008) Ethics of sham surgery: perspective of patients. Mov Disord 23:63–68
9. Hakim S, Adams R (1965) The special clinical problem of symptomatic hydrocephalus with normal cerebrospinal fluid pressure: observations on cerebrospinal fluid hydrodynamics. J Neurol Sci 2:307–327
10. Hebb AO, Cusimano MD, Mapstone TB, Cohen AR, McComb JG, Gjerris F, Bech-Azeddine R (2001) Idiopathic normal pressure hydrocephalus: a systematic review of diagnosis and outcome. Neurosurgery 49:1166–1186
11. Heckerling PS (2006) Placebo surgery research: a blinding imperative. J Clin Epidemiol 59:876–880
12. Meier U, Lemcke J (2006) First clinical experiences in patients with idiopathic normal-pressure hydrocephalus with the adjustable gravity valve manufactured by Aesculap (proGAV(Aesculap)). Acta Neurochir Suppl 96:368–372
13. Miller FG (2003) Sham surgery: an ethical analysis. Am J Bioeth 3:41–48
14. Relkin N, Marmarou A, Klinge P, Bergsneider M, Black PML (2005) Diagnosing idiopathic normal-pressure hydrocephalus. Neurosurgery 57:4–16
15. Stein SC, Burnett MG, Sonnad SS (2006) Shunts in normal-pressure hydrocephalus: do we place too many or too few? J Neurosurg 105:815–822
16. Toma AK, Tarnaris A, Kitchen ND, Watkins LD (2011) Use of proGAV® shunt valve in normal pressure hydrocephalus. Neurosurgery [Epub ahead of print]

Ten Years of Clinical Experience in the Use of Fixed-Pressure Versus Programmable Valves: A Retrospective Study of 159 Patients

Maria Mpakopoulou, Alexandros G. Brotis, Haralampos Gatos, Konstantinos Paterakis, and Kostas N. Fountas

Abstract *Aim*: The aim of this study was to present our 10-year experience with the use of fixed-pressure and programmable valves in the treatment of adult patients requiring cerebrospinal fluid (CSF) diversion.

Material and methods: Patients ($n=159$; 89 male and 70 female) suffering from hydrocephalus of various causes underwent CSF shunt implantation. Forty fixed-pressure and 119 programmable valves were initially implanted.

Results: The observed revision rate was 40% in patients with fixed-pressure valves. In 20% of these patients, a revision due to valve mechanism malfunction was undertaken, and the initial valve was replaced with a programmable one. The revision rate in the adjustable-pressure valve subgroup was 20%. The infection rate for the fixed-pressure and programmable valve subgroups were 3%, and 1.7%, respectively. Similarly, subdural fluid collections were noticed in 17% and 4% of patients with fixed-pressure valves and programmable valves, respectively.

Conclusions: The revision and over-drainage rates were significantly lower when using programmable valves, and thus, this type of valve is preferred whenever CSF has to be diverted.

Keywords Hydrocephalus • Outcome • Fixed-pressure valves • Programmable-pressure valves

M. Mpakopoulou, A.G. Brotis, H. Gatos, K. Paterakis, and K.N. Fountas (✉)
Department of Neurosurgery,
University Hospital of Larissa, Larissa, Greece
e-mail: knfountasmd@excite.com,
fountas@med.uth.gr

Introduction

Hydrocephalus has traditionally been defined as the excessive accumulation of cerebrospinal fluid (CSF) within the brain cavities, as a consequence of abnormal CSF production, flow, or absorption [12]. The estimated prevalence of hydrocephalus has been reported to be as high as 1–1.5% in the general population [6].

CSF diversion procedures and endoscopic third ventriculostomy are the two major surgical treatment options. Nowadays, a great variety of shunt mechanisms and diversion pathways are available [2, 6, 10]. Shunt implantation is considered a routine procedure in everyday neurosurgical practice, but the valve-related complications still remain a major problem for the neurosurgeon [2, 4-6]. The latter include, among others, undershunting or overshunting problems (subdural fluid collections, slit-ventricle syndrome), mechanical malfunctions, and infections [2, 3, 5, 6, 8, 12 13].

The goal of the present study is to review the use of adjustable valves in the treatment of hydrocephalus, as it permits a noninvasive management of many shunt- and valve-related complications [1–8, 15]. Toward this end, we collected data from adult patients who underwent CSF diversion in a teaching hospital serving central Greece during the last 10 years.

Materials and Methods

In a retrospective study, we reviewed 159 consecutive patients treated in our institute from 2001 to 2010. The patients were all adults, with a mean age of 58.2 years (range 23–78 years), among whom 89 were men (56%) and 70 women (44%). The indications for CSF-shunt implantation are shown in Table 1. All fixed-pressure valves were Codman Hakim valves (DePui, Warsaw, IN, USA). Regarding the programmable valves, 110 were Codman Hakim, 5 Miethke proGAV (Christoph Methike GMBH & CO KG, Potsdam, Germany), and 4 Sophysa (Sophysa, Orsay, France) (with an antisyphon device). A ventriculoatrial shunt was implanted in three cases,

Table 1 The description of the study groups

	Fixed-pressure valve group	Programmable-pressure valve group	Whole study sample
Number of patients	40	119	159
Age			
Mean years (range)	55.3 (23–73)	60.1 (35–78)	58.2 (23–78)
Sex			
Male	21 (52.5%)	57 (48%)	89 (56%)
Female	19 (47.5%)	62 (52%)	70 (44%)
Etiology			
Post-hemorrhagic hydrocephalus	8 (20%)	34 (28.5%)	42 (27%)
Posttraumatic hydrocephalus	8 (20%)	11 (9.24%)	19 (22%)
Space-occupying lesions	14 (35%)	32 (26.5%)	46 (28%)
INPH	10 (25%)	39 (32.7%)	49 (31%)
Pseudotumor cerebri	–	3 (2.5%)	3 (2%)

INPH idiopathic normal pressure hydrocephalus

lumboperitoneal in five cases, while in all other cases a ventriculoperitoneal shunt was initially inserted.

The decision for the selection of the opening pressure for each patient was based on the underlying diagnosis and the radiological findings, as these were demonstrated on computed tomography (CT) or magnetic resonance imaging (MRI). In the group of patients with idiopathic normal pressure hydrocephalus (INPH), a tap test was performed with drainage of 30 mL of CSF, and in some cases, the opening pressure was recorded during a lumbar infusion test, to determine which patients were likely to benefit from a shunt insertion [14]. Referring to the group of patients with adjustable-pressure valves, the determination of the initial pressure setting of the implanted valve was based on the intraoperative opening intracranial pressure. In uncertain cases, we preferred to arbitrarily adopt a median initial pressure of 120 mmH$_2$O, and then consequently modify it according to the clinical and imaging follow-up.

Patients were categorized into two groups according to the type of the implanted valve (fixed-pressure valves vs. programmable valves). All patients with CSF shunts implanted prior to 2004 received fixed-pressure valves, while those after that year carried programmable-pressure valves. The two groups were comparable in terms of age, sex, and etiology (Table 1).

The outcome of the CSF diversion was evaluated by assessing the patients' neurological examination, their Mini-Mental State Examination, and their imaging findings [6]. All patients received a postoperative CT within 48–72 h, to assure the proper placement of the ventricular catheter, and a shunt X-rays series. Clinical evaluation was obtained at 1, 3 6, 12, and 24 months, postoperatively. Radiological examination was required at 6 and 12 months or when there was a clinical deterioration. The minimum follow-up period was 12 months, while the mean follow-up time was 24 months.

Results

Fixed-Pressure Valve Group

In our cohort, 40 patients received fixed-pressure valves (Table 1). Catheter-related complications such as obstruction, kinking, migration, or disconnection were observed in three patients (7.5%). Surgical revision with replacement of the proximal or distal catheter was performed in these cases. The observed cumulative revision rate was 16/40 (40%), while the valve replacement rate was 13/40 (32.5%) (Tables 2 and 3). In addition, nine patients (22.5%) required replacement of their initially implanted valves due to undershunting or overshunting. Three patients underwent replacement of their initially implanted valve due to valve mechanism malfunction. One patient (2.5%) had his valve replaced because of an infection.

Programmable Valve Group

In our current series, 119 patients received programmable valves. One hundred and two patients required at least one adjustment of the initially programmed opening pressure. Pressure adjustment problems were encountered in one patient with a lumboperitoneal shunt, which was replaced by a ventriculoperitoneal one. Shunt-related subdural fluid collections were observed in five patients, while a symptomatic slit-ventricle syndrome occurred in one patient. In these cases, pressure adjustment was possible with consequent absorption of subdural effusions and resolution of the slit-ventricle-related symptoms, without any surgical interventions. Proximal or distal catheter-related malfunction requiring surgical revision, occurred in 19/119 patients (16%). The cumulative valve replacement rate was 5.5% caused by valve malfunctioning, pressure adjustment difficulties, and infections (Tables 2 and 3). Seventeen patients (15%) were never reprogrammed after the initial valve implantation, and their clinical and imaging examinations showed improvement of their condition.

Table 2 The complication type and rate of CSF shunting

Type of complication	Fixed-pressure valve group No. of patients (%)	Programmable-pressure valve group No. of patients (%)	Whole study sample No. of patients (%)
Valve-mechanism malfunction	3 (7.5%)	2 (1.7%)	5 (3%)
Catheter-related complications	3 (7.5%)	19 (16%)	22 (19%)
Adjustment difficulties	9 (22.5%)	1 (0.85%)	10 (6%)
Subdural collections	7 (17.5%)	5 (4%)	12 (7.5)
Infection	1 (2.5%)	2 (1.7%)	3 (2%)
Symptomatic slit-ventricle syndrome	0	1 (0.85%)	1 (0.6%)
Total	23 (57.5%)	30 (25.2%)	53 (33.3%)

CSF cerebrospinal fluid

Table 3 The cause of revisions

Indication for revision	Fixed-pressure valve group No. of patients (%)	Programmable-pressure valve group No. of patients (%)	Whole study sample No. of patients (%)
Valve mechanism malfunction	3 (7.5%)	2 (2%)	5 (3.14%)
Catheter-related complications	3 (7.5%)	19 (16%)	22 (13.8%)
Readjustment difficulties	9 (22.5%)	1 (0.84%)	10 (6.3%)
Infections	1 (2.5%)	2 (1.68%)	3 (1.9%)
Total	16 (40%)	24 (20.1%)	40 (25.1%)

Discussion

Treatment of hydrocephalus remains a controversial issue [1, 6, 9]. Despite the advances in CSF drainage techniques achieved in recent decades and the large number of different types of valves available nowadays, the optimal treatment of shunt-dependent patients still remains a problem.

Pollack et al. reported that the shunt system survival rate was 52% and 50% for the programmable and the fixed-pressure valves, respectively [11]. In contrast, we found that the shunt survival rate for the programmable valve group was 79.9%, while this percentage for the fixed-pressured valve group was only 60%. Interestingly, the single most common cause for surgical revision in the fixed-pressured group was the need for setting a different opening pressure, accounting for 56% of the revisions in this group. The respective percentage in our programmable valve group was only 0.8%.

Similarly, the complication rate was significantly lower in the programmable valve group in our study. The cumulative complication rate was 25.2% in the programmable-valve group, while the respective percentage in the fixed-valve group was 57.5%. The most common complication we encountered in the adjustable-pressure group was catheter-related problems in 16% of our patients, while adjustment difficulties (22.5%) and subdural collection formation (17.5%) were the most common complications in the fixed-valve group. The infection rates observed in both groups seem to be comparable, with slightly increased rates among patients with fixed-pressure valves (2.5% vs. 1.7%).

Programmable-pressure shunts seem to be superior to fixed-pressure systems, as they offer the ability to readjust the opening pressure and to avoid overdrainage and/or underdrainage [3, 8, 15]. Moreover, the use of a programmable valve seems to be an independent factor that predisposes to a longer survival time of the shunt, as it spares the patient from further surgical interventions, caused by mismatching between the opening pressure and the patient's CSF-flow dynamics [9, 11, 15].

Conclusion

Data presented in this study indicate a clear advantage in using programmable valves in the treatment of patients requiring CSF diversion. The use of programmable-pressure valves enables the clinician to modify noninvasively the valve's opening pressure, thus minimizing the overdrainage or underdrainage complications. More controlled modulation of CSF-distorted hydrodynamics leads to a significant improvement of the patient's clinical status by means of avoiding new surgical interventions and decreasing the days and the financial cost of hospitalization.

Conflicts of interest statement We declare that we have no conflict of interest.

References

1. Aschoff A, Kremer P, Benesch C et al (1995) Overdrainage and shunt technology. A critical comparison of programmable, hydrostatic and variable-resistance valves and flow-reducing devices. Childs Nerv Syst 11:193–202
2. Bergsneider M, Miller C, Vespa PM, Hu X (2008) Surgical management of adult hydrocephalus. Neurosurgery 62(Suppl 2):643–659; discussion 659–660
3. Carmel PW, Albright AL, Adelson PD et al (1999) Incidence and management of subdural hematoma/hygroma with variable- and

fixed-pressure differential valves: a randomized, controlled study of programmable compared with conventional valves. Neurosurg Focus 7:e7
4. Drake JM, Kestle JR, Tuli S (2000) CSF shunts 50 years on–past, present and future. Childs Nerv Syst 16:800–804
5. Ferguson SD, Michael N, Frim DM (2007) Observations regarding failure of cerebrospinal fluid shunts early after implantation. Neurosurg Focus 22:E7
6. Greenberg MS (2006) Hydrocephalus. In: Handbook of neurosurgery, 6th edn. Thieme, Stuttgard, pp 180–208
7. Hakim S, Adams RD (1965) The special clinical problem of symptomatic hydrocephalus with normal cerebrospinal fluid pressure. Observations on cerebrospinal fluid hydrodynamics. J Neurol Sci 2:307–327
8. Kamano S, Nakano Y, Imanishi T, Hattori M (1991) Management with a programmable pressure valve of subdural hematomas caused by a ventriculoperitoneal shunt: case report. Surg Neurol 35: 381–383
9. Kosteljanetz M (1986) CSF dynamics and pressure-volume relationships in communicating hydrocephalus. J Neurosurg 64:45–52
10. Nulsen FE, Spitz EB (1951) Treatment of hydrocephalus by direct shunt from ventricle to jugular vain. Surg Forum 399–403
11. Pollack IF, Albright AL, Adelson PD (1999) A randomized, controlled study of a programmable shunt valve versus a conventional valve for patients with hydrocephalus. Hakim-Medos Investigator Group. Neurosurgery 45:1399–1408; discussion 1408–1311
12. Pople IK (2002) Hydrocephalus and shunts: what the neurologist should know. J Neurol Neurosurg Psychiatry 73(Suppl 1):17–22
13. Sutcliffe JC, Battersby RD (1992) Do we need variable pressure shunts? Br J Neurosurg 6:67–70
14. Wikkelso C, Andersson H, Blomstrand C, Lindqvist G (1982) The clinical effect of lumbar puncture in normal pressure hydrocephalus. J Neurol Neurosurg Psychiatry 45:64–69
15. Zemack G, Romner B (2000) Seven years of clinical experience with the programmable Codman Hakim valve: a retrospective study of 583 patients. J Neurosurg 92:941–948

Changes of Fractional Anisotropy and Apparent Diffusion Coefficient in Patients with Idiopathic Normal Pressure Hydrocephalus

Koichiro Demura, Mitsuhito Mase, Tosiaki Miyati, Tomoshi Osawa, Manabu Hattori, Harumasa Kasai, Masaki Hara, Yuta Shibamoto, and Kazuo Yamada

Abstract Since ventricular dilation and periventricular abnormal intensities are commonly seen in patients with idiopathic normal pressure hydrocephalus (INPH) on magnetic resonance imaging (MRI), dysfunction of white matter may have an important role in the mechanism causing symptoms of INPH. To clarify the pathophysiology of INPH, we analyzed axonal water dynamics using diffusion tensor MRI. Thirty-six patients with possible INPH were included. Regional fractional anisotropy (FA) and apparent diffusion coefficient (ADC) were measured in several white matter regions before and 24 h after a cerebrospinal fluid tap test (CSF-TT). The patients were divided into two groups: patients who showed significant improvements in neurological status after the CSF-TT (positive, $n=17$) and those with no neurological improvement (negative, $n=19$). After CSF-TT, ADC values were significantly decreased in the frontal periventricular region and the body of the corpus callosum in the positive group ($p<0.05$), whereas no significant change was shown in the negative group. FA values were significantly increased in the body of the corpus callosum in both groups after CSF-TT ($p<0.05$). After CSF-TT, water molecules at the extracellular space could move to the intraventricular space, resulting in decreased ADC values. This suggests that changes of water dynamics in white matter may have a role in the mechanism causing symptoms of INPH.

Keywords Idiopathic normal pressure hydrocephalus • Diffusion tensor imaging • Fractional anisotropy • Apparent diffusion coefficient • Tap test

Introduction

The diagnosis of idiopathic normal pressure hydrocephalus (INPH) is sometimes difficult, and many patients are inaccurately diagnosed as suffering from Alzheimer's disease or Parkinson's disease. Recently, the cerebrospinal fluid tap test (CSF-TT) has come to be considered an essential diagnostic test because of its simplicity and high specificity to estimate shunt efficacy.

The diffusion tensor MR (magnetic resonance) imaging (DTI) technique is based on the characteristics of barriers, including the myelin sheath and cell membrane, which restrict diffusion of water into brain tissue. As a consequence, water molecules diffuse faster along axonal paths than across them. Fractional anisotropy (FA) is a measure of the directionality of diffusion. Isotropic diffusion of water in multiple directions is measured by the apparent diffusion coefficient (ADC). In general, measures of diffusivity, such as ADC, are inversely related to FA [8, 9].

In INPH patients, since ventricular dilation and periventricular abnormal intensities are commonly seen on MR images, dysfunction of white matter involving axonal fibers may have an important role in the causative mechanism of symptoms [5, 14]. But the mechanism of INPH symptoms remains unclear. To investigate the pathophysiology, we analyzed axonal water dynamics using DTI before and after CSF-TT.

Materials and Methods

Thirty-six patients with possible INPH who received a CSF-TT were included in this study. All examinations performed in this study were regular routine tests for the

K. Demura, M. Mase (✉), T. Osawa, and K. Yamada
Department of Neurosurgery, Nagoya City University Graduate School of Medical Sciences, Nagoya, Japan
e-mail: mitmase@med.nagoya-cu.ac.jp

T. Miyati
Faculty of Health Science, Institute of Medical, Pharmaceutical and Health Sciences, Kanazawa University, Kanazawa, Japan

M. Hattori
Department of Neurology, Nagoya City University Medical School, Nagoya, Japan

H. Kasai, M. Hara, and Y. Shibamoto
Department of Radiology, Nagoya City University Hospital, Nagoya, Japan

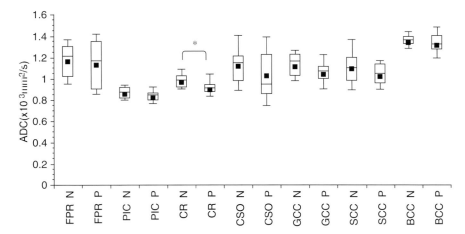

Fig. 1 Regions of interest (ROIs) analysis of apparent diffusion coefficient (ADC) values in each region between the tap test positive and negative groups before tap test. The pre-tap test ADC values in the corona radiata of the positive group were significantly lower than those of the negative group (*$p<0.05$). Mean pre-tap test ADC values of the positive group tended to be lower than those of the negative group, though the difference did not reach statistical significance. *FPR* frontal periventricular region, *PIC* posterior limb of the internal capsule, *CR* corona radiata, *CSO* centrum semiovale, *GCC* the genu of the corpus callosum, *SCC* the splenium of the corpus callosum, *BCC* the body of the corpus callosum, *N* negative group, *P* positive group

diagnosis of INPH except for MRI after the tap test. Informed consent was obtained to take part in this study from the patients or their family. Possible INPH was defined as having more than one of the clinical triad: gait disturbance, cognitive impairment, and urinary incontinence with ventricular dilation (Evans index >0.3). CSF-TT was performed until withdrawal of 30 mL of CSF or until CSF pressure reached 0 mmH$_2$O. All patients underwent neurological examinations and MRI before and 24 h after CSF-TT. Neurological conditions were estimated by Mini-Mental State Examination (MMSE), the Frontal Assessment Battery (FAB), the 3-m Timed Up-and-Go Test, and the Japanese Normal Pressure Hydrocephalus Grading Scale–Revised (JNPHGS-R) [7, 11]. Positive CSF-TT was defined as improvement of MMSE or FAB score of more than four points or improvement of time in the 3-m Timed Up-and-Go Test of more than 10%. Then, the 36 patients were divided into two groups: the CSF-TT positive group ($n=17$; mean age ± SD: 74.6 ± 6.31 years) and the CSF-TT negative group ($n=19$, 76.1 ± 5.20 years).

On a 1.5-T MRI system (Gyroscan Intera; Philips Medical Systems International, Best, The Netherlands), the DTI was obtained on the transverse plane using a multislice spin-echo single-shot echo planar imaging sequence with 15 axes diffusion gradients (b factor of 0 and 860 s/mm^2). Scan parameters used were 10150.5/90 ms (TR/TE), 2.7 mm slice thickness (0 mm gap), 256 × 256 mm FOV, 2.69 × 2.69 × 2.7 mm voxel size. ADC and FA maps were calculated, and regions of interest (ROIs) were manually set bilaterally in the frontal periventricular region (FPR), the posterior limb of the internal capsule (PIC), corona radiata (CR), and centrum semiovale (CSO). Location of FPR and PIC were determined on the axial image where pineal body was seen. Location of CR was determined as 15 mm above the previous image. Location of CSO was determined on the axial image where the top of the lateral ventricles were not visible. ROIs were round in shape and kept constant at about 60 mm^2. Each parameter was averaged from regions of both sides. In three segments of the corpus callosum (genu, body, and splenium), ROIs were determined on the sagittal image near the midline, which were round in shape and kept constant at about 20 mm^2.

Statistical analysis between the two groups was performed by Mann-Whitney's U test. ADC and FA analysis before and after the tap test in each group was performed by Wilcoxon signed-rank tests. Statistical significance was preset at $p<0.05$.

Results

The pre-CSF-TT ADC values in the CR of the positive group were significantly lower than those of the negative group. Mean pre-tap test ADC values of the positive group tended to be lower than those of the negative group, though the difference did not reach statistical significance ($p<0.05$) (Fig. 1). ADC values of the CSF-TT positive group were significantly decreased in the frontal periventricular region and the body of the corpus callosum after CSF-TT ($p<0.05$) (Fig. 2).

FA values in every region before CSF-TT were not significantly different between the two groups. FA values were significantly increased in the body of the corpus callosum of both groups after CSF-TT ($p<0.05$) (Fig. 3).

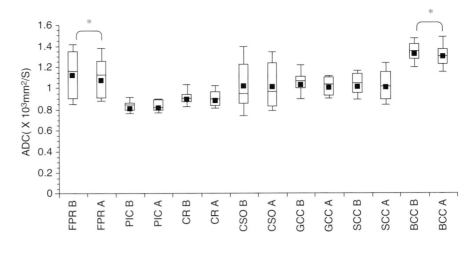

Fig. 2 Regions of interest (ROIs) analysis of apparent diffusion coefficient (ADC) values of the positive group. ADC values in the frontal periventricular region and the body of the corpus callosum were significantly decreased after tap test (*$p<0.05$). *B* before tap test, *A* after tap test

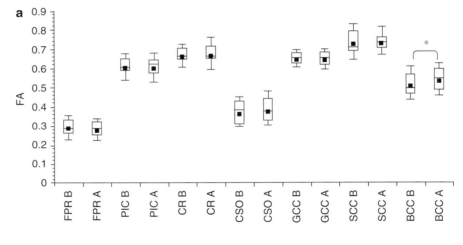

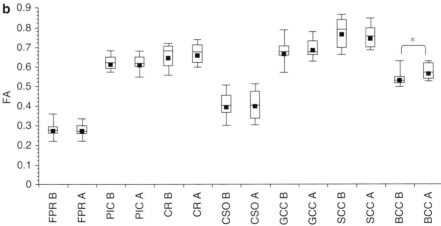

Fig. 3 Regions of interest (ROIs) analysis of pre-tap test fractional anisotropy (FA) values in the tap test negative group (**a**) and the positive group (**b**). FA values in the body of the corpus callosum of both groups were significantly increased after tap test (*$p<0.05$)

Discussion

In patients with INPH, extracellular water content in the periventricular regions is increased because of diffusion of water due to transependymal reabsorption of CSF [1]. Therefore, ADC values in patients with INPH are higher than in normal control cases. Also the age and duration of disease affect the ADC values [13]. Reduced ADC values in the periventricular region after shunt surgery or endoscopic third ventriculostomy has been reported [1], but not reported after CSF-TT.

In the present study, ADC values were significantly decreased after CSF-TT in the frontal periventricular region and the body of the corpus callosum in the positive group. It is supposed that water molecules in the extracellular space moved to the intraventricular space after CSF-TT, resulting in decreased ADC values. Extracellular water accumulation in brain tissue causes malfunction of nervous activity and of metabolism [4, 10]. Therefore, reduced extracellular water content might bring about neurological improvement after CSF-TT.

It is well known that FA shows a tendency to decline with age [8]. Neurodegenerative diseases such as multiple sclerosis, progressive supranuclear palsy, or brain edema in stroke also reduces FA values. Compression against axonal fibers does not always reduce FA values. For homogeneously aligned white matter fibers, mechanical pressure will cause higher packing of fibers and increased fiber density per unit area, resulting in increased FA values. Corpus callosum is the tissue most affected by the enlarged ventricles, because it is located just above them. In the literature, FA values of corpus callosum in patients with hydrocephalus were lower than those of normal control cases. This result suggests that strong compression perpendicular to axonal fibers reduces FA values [2, 3, 6, 12, 15].

In the present study, FA values were significantly increased in the body of the corpus callosum of both groups after CSF-TT. These results suggest that compression against axonal fibers in the body of the corpus callosum was relieved by reduction of the CSF, and FA values increased. But the reduction of the CSF after CSF-TT might be too little to change FA values in other regions. The correlation between neurological alteration and increased FA values was difficult to explain because of the same statistical changes in both groups. It might reflect morphological changes in the body of the corpus callosum.

Conclusion

After a tap test, ADC values in the periventricular regions reduced significantly, and neurological symptoms improved simultaneously. This suggests that changes of water dynamics in white matter may have a role in the mechanism causing symptoms of INPH.

Conflicts of interest statement We declare that we have no conflict of interest.

References

1. Anik Y, Demirci A, Anik I, Etus V, Arslan A (2008) Apparent diffusion coefficient and cerebrospinal fluid flow measurements in patients with hydrocephalus. J Comput Assist Tomogr 32:392–396
2. Assaf Y, Ben-Sira L, Constantini S, Chang LC, Beni-Adani L (2006) Diffusion tensor imaging in hydrocephalus: initial experience. AJNR Am J Neuroradiol 27:1717–1724
3. Commowick O, Fillard P, Clatz O, Warfield SK (2008) Detection of DTI white matter abnormalities in multiple sclerosis patients. Med Image Comput Comput Assist Interv 11:975–982
4. Go KG (1997) The normal and pathological physiology of brain water. Adv Tech Stand Neurosurg 23:47–142
5. Ishikawa M (2008) Idiopathic normal pressure hydrocephalus overviews and pathogenesis. Brain Nerve 60:211–217
6. Ito S, Makino T, Shirai W, Hattori T (2008) Diffusion tensor analysis of corpus callosum in progressive supranuclear palsy. Neuroradiology 50:981–985
7. Kubo Y, Kazui H, Yoshida T, Kito Y, Kimura N, Tokunaga H, Ogino A, Miyake H, Ishikawa M, Takeda M (2008) Validation of grading scale for evaluating symptoms of idiopathic normal pressure hydrocephalus. Dement Geriatr Cogn Disord 25:37–45
8. Lee CE, Danielian LE, Thomasson D, Baker EH (2009) Normal regional fractional anisotropy and apparent diffusion coefficient of the brain measured on a 3 T MR scanner. Neuroradiology 51:3–9
9. Malykhin N, Concha L, Seres P, Beaulieu C, Coupland NJ (2008) Diffusion tensor imaging tractography and reliability analysis for limbic and paralimbic white matter tracts. Psychiatry Res 164:132–142
10. Minamikawa J (1992) Experimental study on pathophysiology and treatment of congenital hydrocephalus evaluated by magnetic resonance imaging and magnetic resonance spectroscopy. Nippon Geka Hokan 61:35–61
11. Ravdin LD, Katzen HL, Jackson AE, Tsakanikas D, Assuras S, Relkin NR (2008) Features of gait most responsive to tap test in normal pressure hydrocephalus. Clin Neurol Neurosurg 110:455–461
12. Rovaris M, Agosta F, Pagani E, Filippi M (2009) Diffusion tensor MR imaging. Neuroimaging Clin N Am 19:37–43
13. Snook L, Paulson LA, Roy D, Phillips L, Beaulieu C (2005) Diffusion tensor imaging of neurodevelopment in children and yang adults. Neuroimage 26:1164–1173
14. Vacca V (2007) Diagnosis and treatment of idiopathic normal pressure hydrocephalus. J Neurosci Nurs 39:107–111
15. Wilde EA, McCauley SR, Chu Z, Hunter JV, Bigler ED, Yallampalli R, Wang ZJ, Hanten G, Li X, Romos MA, Sabir SH, Vasquez AC, Menefee D, Levin HS (2008) Diffusion tensor imaging of hemispheric asymmetries in the developing brain. J Clin Exp Neuropsychol 3:1–14

Virchow-Robin Spaces in Idiopathic Normal Pressure Hydrocephalus: A Surrogate Imaging Marker for Coexisting Microvascular Disease?

Andrew Tarnaris, J. Tamangani, O. Fayeye, D. Kombogiorgas, H. Murphy, Y.C. Gan, and G. Flint

Abstract *Background*: Virchow-Robin spaces (VRSs) surround perforating cerebral arteries and are reported to be found with increasing frequency with advancing age. In addition, some studies indicate an association between VRSs and vascular dementias. The present study examined the incidence of VRSs in patients with idiopathic normal pressure hydrocephalus (INPH) and considered their use as a potential surrogate imaging marker of coexisting microvascular disease in patients with this condition.

Methods: The MRI incidence of VRS in the centrum semiovale (CS), basal ganglia (BG), mesencephalon (MES), and the subinsular (SI) region was measured in 12 patients with INPH and in 12 control subjects, using the scoring system proposed by Patankar et al. (Am J Neuroradiology 26:1512, 2005). Historical control data were also used for further comparison.

Results: All 12 INPH patients had clearly visible VRSs, distributed in the CS (all 12), basal ganglia (11/12), SI region (9/12), and MES region (6/12). The mean Patankar scores of the INPH group were BG 2.25, CS 1.66, SI 0.91, and ME 0.5. The respective scores for our control group were 1.41, 1.5, 1.16, and 0.16, and for historical controls were 1.46, 0.51, 0.96, and 0.51. There were, however, no statistically significant differences between the INPH patients and either of the control groups. No correlation was found between age and the overall incidence of VRS.

Conclusion: This preliminary study suggests that there may be a higher incidence of VRSs in patients with INPH, when compared with normal patients of similar age, but our small numbers prevent us from demonstrating statistical significance, and larger studies are clearly required.

Keywords Normal Pressure Hydrocephalus • Virchow-Robin spaces • Imaging

Introduction

Various explanations have been proposed regarding the development of the syndrome of idiopathic normal pressure hydrocephalus (INPH), the most prevalent being chronic ischemia, disturbance of cerebrospinal fluid (CSF) dynamics [18], and, more recently, disturbance of neuronal metabolism [7]. None of the above is able to explain fully the development and progression of the syndrome. The relationship of INPH to vascular disease [3, 4, 8], cerebral blood flow [10, 12, 21], and ischemia [4, 5, 9] has been well documented, but, unfortunately, magnetic resonance (MR) imaging is not yet able to differentiate clearly between INPH and vascular dementia [20].

Virchow-Robin spaces (VRSs), first described in 1851 and 1859, are enlarged perivascular spaces accompanying penetrating intracerebral arteries [1]. Dilation of these spaces is usually perceived as being associated with aging and has been suggested as a potential indicator of cerebral microvascular disease [14]. Increased VRSs have certainly been linked with impaired cognitive function [11]. The aim of this study was to investigate the extent of VRSs in patients with INPH and to examine their potential use as a marker of coincident microvascular disease in these patients.

Materials and Methods

Twelve patients with INPH and with preoperative MR imaging were identified from the records of adult hydrocephalus patients treated in our unit. The 12 patients were selected from a larger cohort, because they had both

A. Tarnaris (✉), O. Fayeye, D. Kombogiorgas, H. Murphy
Y.C. Gan and G. Flint
Department of Neurosurgery, Queen Elizabeth Hospital,
Birmingham, UK
e-mail: andrewtarnaris@gmail.com

J. Tamangani
Department of Neuroradiology, Queen Elizabeth Hospital,
Birmingham, UK

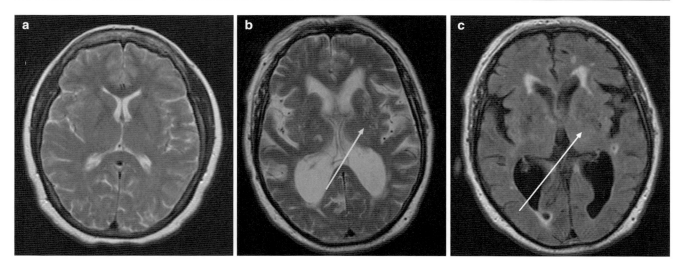

Fig. 1 (a) T2W MRI of basal ganglia of control subject: no Virchow-Robin spaces (VRSs) seen. (b, c) T2-weighted and FLAIR of idiopathic normal pressure hydrocephalus (INPH) patient: VRSs evident (*red arrows*)

preoperative imaging and lumbar infusion studies available. The diagnosis of INPH was based on history, examination, an Evans index >0.3, together with the demonstration of normal cerebrospinal fluid (CSF) pressure and increased CSF outflow resistance (R_{out}) during a lumbar infusion test (LIT). An R_{out} value larger than 15 mmHg/mL/min was considered pathological. Another 12 patients, who underwent imaging as part of screening for other, unrelated neurological disorders, or hearing loss, were selected as the control group. All control patients were found to be negative for any intracranial abnormality or neurological disorder. Vasculopathy risk factors were recorded for both groups.

The two groups were imaged with either a 1.5-Tesla (1.5 T) Siemens or 1.5 T GE machine, both using a dedicated head coil. The key sequences used to assess VRS were axial T1W, axial T2W, and either proton density or axial fluid attenuation inversion recovery (FLAIR) sequences. In a few patients, sagittal or coronal images were used in the analysis, if the axial images were not conclusive. As the analysis was retrospective, some imaging parameters (echo time, repetition time, and inversion time) were variable between different patients. However, slice thickness was constant at 5 mm for all sequences. Similarly, all images had a matrix of 256 × 256 and a field of view 230 × 230 mm. Images were viewed on dedicated GE PACS workstations and reviewed by a single neuroradiologist (J.T.) (Fig. 1).

The VRS scoring system proposed by Patankar et al. (Fig. 2) was applied to all patients [14]. In that study, the dementia patients and control subjects were imaged using a 1.5 T unit (Philips Medical Systems, Best, the Netherlands) and a birdcage head coil receiver. The imaging protocol included the following axial sequences: [1] fluid-attenuated inversion recovery (FLAIR, TR/TE/TI = 11,000/140/2600, section thickness 3.0 mm, no intersection gap) [2], T1-weighted inversion recovery (TR/TE/TI = 6850/18/300, section thickness 3.0 mm) [3], variable echo, fast spin echo (TR/TE1/TE2 = 5500/20/90, section thickness 3.0 mm), and [4] high-resolution 3D T1-weighted fast field-echo (TR/TE = 24/18, section thickness 0.89 mm, flip angle 30°). For all sequences, the matrix was 256 × 256, and the FOV was 230 × 230 mm. In brief, an ordinal score was given for each anatomical region examined: basal ganglia (BG), subinsular (SI) region, mesencephalon (MES), and centrum semiovale (CS) (Fig. 2). To qualify as VRSs, the identified features had to mirror the signal characteristics of CSF on all sequences, and there had to be an absence of gliotic changes and volume loss in association with the presumed perivascular spaces. High signal intensity regions were first identified within the four regions of interest on the axial T2W images. T1W and FLAIR (or proton density) sequences were then investigated to make sure the corresponding areas had the expected low signal intensity. Nonparametric tests (Mann–Whitney's U test and Spearman's rank correlation test) were used to assess for significant differences between our INPH and our control groups. The means and standard deviations were reported for numerical values. The level of significance was set at 0.05.

Results

Epidemiological characteristics and vascular comorbidities are presented in Table 1. Lumbar infusion studies in the INPH group revealed a mean opening pressure of 13.7 (±2.96) mmHg and mean Rout of 15.6 (± 9.15) mmHg/mL/min.

All 12 INPH patients had visible VRSs in the CS. Eleven out of 12 patients had VRSs in basal ganglia, 9 in the SI

Fig. 2 The grading system by Patankar et al. [14]. Basal ganglia (BG) scheme 1 was excluded from the assessment

VIRCHOW ROBIN SPACE CLASSIFICATION as presented by Patankar et al.

Centrum semiovale.
0 = none.
1 = less than 5 per slide.
2 = more than 5 on one or both slides.

Mesencephalon.
0 = absent.
1 = present.

Subinsular region lateral to lentiform nucleus.
0 = none.
1 = less than 5 per side.
2 = more than 5 on one or both sides.

Basal ganglia scheme 1:
0 = present only in the substantia innominata, and fewer than 5 on either side.
1 = more than 5 in the substantia innominata on either side or any VRS in the lentiform nucleus.
2 = VRS in the caudate nucleus on either side.

Basal ganglia scheme 2:
0 = present only in the substantia innominata, and fewer than 5 on either side.
1 = only in the substantia innominata or more than 5 dilated VRS on either side.
2 = less than 5 in the lentiform nucleus on either side.
3 = 5–10 VRS in the lentiform nucleus or fewer than 5 in the caudate nucleus on either side.
4 = more than 10 in the lentiform and less than 5 in the caudate nucleus on either side.
5 = more than 10 in the lentiform and less than 5 in the caudate nucleus on either side.

Table 1 Epidemiological characteristics of patient groups

	Control (n=12)	INPH (n=12)	p Value
Sex (M:F)	10:2	7:5	
Age	70.3 (3.7)	70 (7.4)	n.s.
Hypertension	5	8	n.s. (0.087)
Diabetes mellitus	4	1	n.s.
Transient ischemic attack	1	0	n.s.
Cerebrovascular accident	2	0	n.s.
Myocardial infarction	0	0	n.s.
Smoking	3	4	n.s.
Evans index	0.27	0.43	<0.001

INPH idiopathic normal pressure hydrocephalus, *n.s.* nonsignificant

Table 2 VRS scores by anatomical region

Region/ Patankar score	Control	Historical controls[a]	INPH	p Value
CS (0–2)	1.5?	0.51?	1.66	n.s.
SI region (0–1)	1.16	0.96	0.91	n.s.
BG (0–5)	1.41	1.46	2.25	n.s. (0.059)
MES (0–1)	0.16?	0.51?	0.5	n.s.

BG basal ganglia, *CS* centrum semiovale, *INPH* idiopathic normal pressure hydrocephalus, *MES* mesencephalon. *n.s.* nonsignificant, *SI* subinsular

[a]Historical group (n=35) as presented by Patankar et al. [14]

region, and 6 in the MES region. Table 2 shows the VRS scores of the study and control groups, together with the historical control group of Patankar et al. [14] (n=35, age 72.8±6.56 years). The INPH group had a higher score than the control and historical control in the CS and BG, a lower score than the control group in the SI region, and higher score than the control in the mesencephalon. The differences between our two study groups were not, however, statistically significant.

No correlation was found between age and VRS scores in either of the study groups. No correlation between VRS score and vascular risk factors was found in different anatomical regions. No correlation was found with Evans index, CSF opening pressure or Rout in the INPH group.

Discussion

It would appear that in this study the absence of any correlation with vascular risk factors does not support VRSs as an imaging marker for microvascular disease. There was no link with the degree of ventriculomegaly present nor was there any correlation with physiological measurements made during lumbar CSF infusion studies. The incidence of VRSs in our INPH patients was higher than in our control group in three out of four anatomical regions and in two out of four regions when comparison was made with historical controls, but none of these differences reached statistical significance, which clearly limits our ability to interpret the overall findings.

On the other hand, VRSs which contain interstitial fluid (ISF) are thought to be the main channels for bulk flow of ISF in grey matter [22]. It may be, therefore, that dilation of VRS in INPH results from disturbed bulk flow of brain ISF, in which case we might expect their size and incidence to correlate with INPH, rather than with vascular or other comorbidities. We know that there is continuity of ISF and CSF spaces, and that, when raised CSF pressure occurs, there is retrograde flow of CSF into the brain [6, 16]. Following perfusion of the ventriculocisternal space with horseradish peroxidase, Rennels et al. observed rapid periarterial flow of ISF, from CSF compartments into the brain [1, 17]. Proescholdt et al. have shown that an injection of [^{14}C]-inulin in awake rats, via chronically implanted cannulae into the lateral ventricles, leads to preferential downstream distribution throughout the ISF, especially within the hypothalamus and the brainstem [15]. Abnormal bulk flow of ISF along VRSs may therefore be a consequence of the underlying alteration of CSF dynamics in INPH. Even though CSF pressure is not constantly or pathologically raised in INPH, intermittently raised pressure in this group of patients does occur, especially at night [19]. The reduced compliance associated with INPH leads to increased arterial pulsations, which in turn result in increased perivascular shear stress [2] and which may, therefore, be the causative factor for the increased incidence of VRSs in INPH. It may be that the alteration in pulsatility in INPH leads to preferential bulk flow of ISF along routes of reduced resistance, i.e., perivascular spaces [13].

Conclusion

This preliminary study suggests that there may be a higher incidence of VRSs in patients with INPH, when compared with normal control patients and that regional anatomical differences exist, but the small numbers in our study prevent us from demonstrating statistical significance. A larger study is clearly needed to evaluate the clinical use of VRSs as surrogate markers of coexisting microvascular disease in INPH. Not only a larger study but also proper selection criteria for the study population and the utilization of identical tools (MRI imaging parameters) are necessary. At present, it remains unclear as to whether VRSs develop as a result of the microangiopathy known to coexist in many cases of INPH or whether they result from underlying disturbances of CSF dynamics. A larger study, with correlation of volumetric measurement of ischemic regions (DWMHs, PVHs) and regional pulsatility calculations, is also warranted.

Conflicts of interest statement We declare that we have no conflict of interest.

References

1. Abbott NJ (2004) Evidence for bulk flow of brain interstitial fluid: significance for physiology and pathology. Neurochem Int 45:545–552
2. Bateman G (2002) Pulse-wave encephalopathy: a comparative study of the hydrodynamics of leukoaraiosis and normal-pressure hydrocephalus. Neuroradiology 44:740–748
3. Boon AJ, Tans JT, Delwel EJ, Egeler-Peerdeman SM, Hanlo PW, Wurzer HA, Hermans J (1999) Dutch Normal-Pressure Hydrocephalus Study: the role of cerebrovascular disease. J Neurosurg 90:221–226
4. Bradley WG Jr, Whittemore AR, Watanabe AS, Davis SJ, Teresi LM, Homyak M (1991) Association of deep white matter infarction with chronic communicating hydrocephalus: implications regarding the possible origin of normal-pressure hydrocephalus. AJNR Am J Neuroradiol 12:31–39
5. Corkill RG, Garnett MR, Blamire AM, Rajagopalan B, Cadoux-Hudson TA, Styles P (2003) Multi-modal MRI in normal pressure hydrocephalus identifies pre-operative haemodynamic and diffusion coefficient changes in normal appearing white matter correlating with surgical outcome. Clin Neurol Neurosurg 105:193–202
6. Davson H (ed) (1956) Physiology of the ocular and cerebrospinal fluids. Churchill, London
7. Kondziella D, Sonnewald U, Tullberg M, Wikkelso C (2008) Brain metabolism in adult chronic hydrocephalus. J Neurochem 106: 1515–1524
8. Krauss JK, Droste DW, Vach W, Regel JP, Orszagh M, Borremans JJ, Tietz A, Seeger W (1996) Cerebrospinal fluid shunting in idiopathic normal-pressure hydrocephalus of the elderly: effect of periventricular and deep white matter lesions. Neurosurgery 39:292–299; discussion 299–300
9. Krauss JK, Regel JP, Vach W, Orszagh M, Jungling FD, Bohus M, Droste DW (1997) White matter lesions in patients with idiopathic normal pressure hydrocephalus and in an age-matched control group: a comparative study. Neurosurgery 40:491–495; discussion 495–496
10. Kristensen B, Malm J, Fagerland M, Hietala SO, Johansson B, Ekstedt J, Karlsson T (1996) Regional cerebral blood flow, white matter abnormalities, and cerebrospinal fluid hydrodynamics in patients with idiopathic adult hydrocephalus syndrome. J Neurol Neurosurg Psychiatry 60:282–288
11. MacLullich AMJ, Wardlaw JM, Ferguson KJ, Starr JM, Seckl JR, Deary IJ (2004) Enlarged perivascular spaces are associated with cognitive function in healthy elderly men. J Neurol Neurosurg Psychiatry 75:1519
12. Momjian S, Owler BK, Czosnyka Z, Czosnyka M, Pena A, Pickard JD (2004) Pattern of white matter regional cerebral blood flow and autoregulation in normal pressure hydrocephalus. Brain 127:965–972
13. Panczel G, Bönöczk P, Voko Z, Spiegel D, Nagy Z (2000) Impaired vasoreactivity of the basilar artery system in patients with brainstem lacunar infarcts. Cerebrovasc Dis 9:218–223
14. Patankar TF, Mitra D, Varma A, Snowden J, Neary D, Jackson A (2005) Dilatation of the Virchow-Robin space is a sensitive indicator of cerebral microvascular disease: study in elderly patients with dementia. AJNR Am J Neuroradiol 26:1512
15. Proescholdt MG, Hutto B, Brady LS, Herkenham M (1999) Studies of cerebrospinal fluid flow and penetration into brain following lateral ventricle and cisterna magna injections of the tracer [14C] inulin in rat. Neuroscience 95:577–592
16. Pullen RGL, Cserr HF (1984) Pressure dependent penetration of CSF into brain. Federation Proc 43:2521
17. Rennels ML, Blaumanis OR, Grady PA (1990) Rapid solute transport throughout the brain via paravascular fluid pathways. Adv Neurol 52:431

18. Silverberg GD (2004) Normal pressure hydrocephalus (NPH): ischaemia, CSF stagnation or both. Brain 127:947–948
19. Symon L, Dorsch NWC (1975) Use of long-term intracranial pressure measurement to assess hydrocephalic patients prior to shunt surgery. J Neurosurg 42:258–273
20. Tarnaris A, Toma AK, Kitchen ND, Watkins LD (2009) Ongoing search for diagnostic biomarkers in idiopathic normal pressure hydrocephalus. Biomarkers 3:787–805
21. Vorstrup S, Christensen J, Gjerris F, Sorensen PS, Thomsen AM, Paulson OB (1987) Cerebral blood flow in patients with normal-pressure hydrocephalus before and after shunting. J Neurosurg 66:379–387
22. Weller RO (1998) Pathology of cerebrospinal fluid and interstitial fluid of the CNS: significance for Alzheimer disease, prion disorders and multiple sclerosis. J Neuropathol Exp Neurol 57:885

Quantification of Normal CSF Flow Through the Aqueduct Using PC-Cine MRI at 3T

Eftychia Kapsalaki, Patricia Svolos, Ioannis Tsougos, Kyriaki Theodorou, Ioannis Fezoulidis, and Kostas N. Fountas

Abstract *Introduction*: Quantification of cerebrospinal fluid (CSF) flow through the cerebral aqueduct is of paramount importance in patients with hydrocephalus. The purpose of this study was to evaluate the normal CSF flow measurements at three different anatomical levels of the aqueduct utilizing 3-Tesla (3 T) magnetic resonance imaging.

Materials and methods: The CSF hydrodynamics in 22 healthy volunteers were evaluated. Phase-contrast cine MRI was performed on a 3 T General Electric MR system (GE Medical Systems, Milwaukee, WI, USA). A cardiac-gated, flow-compensated GRE sequence with flow encoding was used, and the aqueduct was visualized using a sagittal T1 FLAIR sequence. Velocity maps were acquired at three different anatomical levels. Region-of-interest (ROI) analysis was performed.

Results: CSF flow velocities were slightly increased at the upper in comparison with the lower part of the aqueduct. The mean values for the peak positive and negative velocity and the mean average flow were calculated for both ROIs.

Discussion/Conclusions: CSF peak positive velocity, peak negative velocity, and mean flow through the aqueduct were calculated in 22 young healthy volunteers performed at 3 T. Our measurements did not show significant difference compared with the reported measurements obtained at 1.5 T. Slight differences were observed in the CSF hydrodynamic measurements, depending on the anatomical level of the aqueduct; however, they did not vary significantly.

Keywords PC Cine MRI • CSF flow • Aqueduct • Hydrocephalus • Velocity • 3 T

Introduction

The mechanical coupling between the cerebral blood flow and the cerebrospinal fluid (CSF) flow throughout the cardiac cycle (CC) is of great importance. Cerebral blood volume variations, which are produced during the CC, cause the oscillatory movement of the CSF bidirectionally within the craniospinal axis. Phase-contrast (PC) cine magnetic resonance imaging (MRI) provides a noninvasive and rapid evaluation of CSF hydrodynamics. Using cardiac-gating, this technique is extremely sensitive in evaluating CSF flow dynamics and more accurate than conventional MRI to evaluate CSF flow [6, 7, 12, 14, 15]. MR images are sensitized to velocity changes in a specific direction, while signals from stationary protons and from motion in other directions are ruled out [13]. The utilization of higher field MR systems, such as 3 T, reinforces the potential dynamics of PC-cine MRI.

CSF flow measurements at the various parts of the aqueduct contribute to the diagnosis and therapeutic decisions of patients with hydrocephalus [3, 8]. However, the clinical application of CSF flow dynamics analysis has been restricted due to the fact that the normal CSF flow values measured in healthy volunteers have shown wide variation [5, 10].

Knowledge of normal CSF flow through the aqueduct is of paramount importance in differentiating those patients with hyperdynamic CSF flow and/or functional obstruction of the aqueduct. It has been previously postulated that normal pressure hydrocephalus patients with such characteristics may be good surgical candidates for shunting and benefit from such a procedure.

The purpose of our current study was to evaluate the normal CSF flow measurements in healthy volunteers, at three different anatomical levels of the aqueduct, on a 3 T MR System and compare these measurements with the results performed on 1.5 T. Moreover, estimation of user dependency with variation of region-of-interest (ROI) analysis was also performed.

E. Kapsalaki (✉) and I. Fezoulidis
Department of Radiology,
University of Thessaly, School of Medicine,
Larissa, Greece
e-mail: ekapsal@med.uth.gr

P. Svolos, I. Tsougos, and K. Theodorou
Department of Medical Physics, University of Thessaly,
Larissa, Greece

K.N. Fountas
Department of Neurosurgery, University of Thessaly,
Larissa, Greece

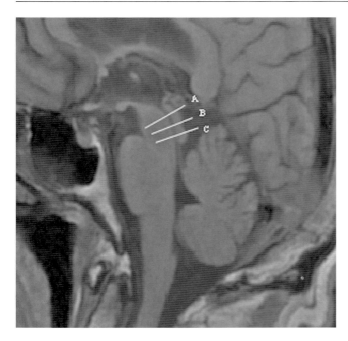

Fig. 1 Sagittal T1 FLAIR image showing the positioning of the localizers placed to measure cerebrospinal fluid (CSF) hydrodynamics at each anatomical level of the aqueduct (**a**) inlet, (**b**) ampulla, and (**c**) pars posterior

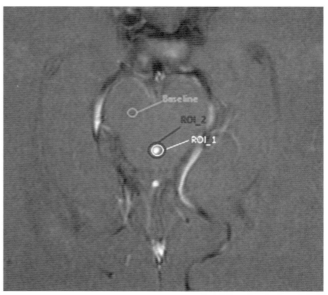

Fig. 2 Region-of-interest (ROI) analysis on the axial phase-contrast cine MR images. ROI_1 (*red*) placed exactly at the edge of the visualized aqueduct, ROI_2 (*blue*) concentrically placed around ROI_1, and Baseline ROI (*green*) placed at the level of the midbrain (zero flow)

Materials and Methods

Twenty-two healthy volunteers, aged 19–37 years (mean age 26.1), participated in this study. Two-dimensional phase-contrast cine MRI was performed on a 3 T whole-body MR system (GE Medical Systems, Milwaukee, WI, USA) using a neurovascular eight-channel coil. A sagittal T1 FLAIR sequence was used to visualize the aqueduct and to select the anatomical levels for flow quantification (Fig. 1). A cardiac-gated, flow-compensated, gradient echo sequence with flow encoding of 10 cm/s on the slice-selective direction was used with the following parameters: TR = 30 ms, TE = 8.8 ms, NEX = 1, flip angle = 20°, FOV = 16 × 16, slice thickness 4 mm, and acquisition time 3.5 min. Measurements were performed at three different anatomical levels of the aqueduct: the inlet, the ampulla, and the pars posterior. The total duration of the study was approximately 15 min.

Flow quantification was carried out using the software provided by the manufacturer (GE Report Card version 3.6) in CSF flow mode. In the latest version of this tool, the setting of a background to calculate flow velocity is not required, and therefore, no background subtraction was implemented.

ROI analysis was performed to measure the CSF hydrodynamics. In all cases, the ROI placement was performed independently by two of the authors (P.S., I.T.). The CSF parameters evaluated were the peak positive velocity (PPV) in cm/s, the peak negative velocity (PNV) in cm/s, and the average flow (AF) in ml/beat on the phase images. Each flow measurement, at the three different aqueductal levels, consisted of one ROI placed exactly at the edge of the aqueduct (ROI_1), and a second, slightly larger one (ROI_2), to evaluate user-dependent potential variations in the flow measurements. A background baseline ROI was set at the level of the midbrain to produce a distinct line (zero flow) separating the positive from the negative flow (Fig. 2). The mean value and the standard deviation for PPV, PNV, and AF were computed in the three different anatomical levels of the cerebral aqueduct using the SPSS 13.0 package. The results were evaluated depending on the anatomical location and compared with published measurements obtained by 1.5 T MR systems, respectively.

Results

During the CC the CSF flow curves showed a typical sinusoidal pattern in all of the healthy volunteers, representing the pulsatory CSF movement (Fig. 1). The mean values and standard deviations of the PPVs, PNVs, and AFs at the three different anatomical levels of the cerebral aqueduct are shown in Table 1. In the published literature, various studies performed on 1.5 T MRI units, present their results of measurements of CSF flow at various levels of the aqueduct. These measurements were used as a reference for our results performed at 3 T. Table 2 shows the mean values for Stroke Volume and Peak Velocities in healthy volunteers as reported in the literature.

Table 1 Mean average flow and mean peak positive and peak negative velocity at the different anatomical levels of the cerebral aqueduct

Anatomical level	ROI (mm²)	Mean AF (±SD) (mL/beat)	Mean PPV (±SD) (cm/s)	Mean PNV (±SD) (cm/s)	Mean ROI Area (±SD) (mm²)
Inlet	ROI_1	0.034±0.018	9.46±0.671	−8.24±2.011*	3.66±1.343
	ROI_2	0.055±0.022	9.46±0.671	−8.24±2.011	5.97±1.810
	Baseline	0.004±0.003	1.78±0.267	−0.01±0.014	0.53±0.286
Ampulla	ROI_1	0.036±0.010	8.71±1.134	−7.02±2.825	3.61±0.552
	ROI_2	0.055±0.016	8.71±1.134	−7.02±2.825	5.47±0.949
	Baseline	0.004±0.002	1.85±0.090	−0.00±0.00	0.42±0.186
Pars posterior	ROI_1	0.031±0.016	8.01±1.470	−5.54±2.915	4.33±1.802
	ROI_2	0.047±0.021	8.01±1.470	−5.54±2.915	6.68±2.647
	Baseline	0.003±0.002	1.57±0.274	−0.07±0.101	0.46±0.274

AF average flow, *PPV* peak positive velocity (diastolic), *PNV* peak negative velocity (systolic), *SD* standard deviation, *ROI_1* region of interest precisely on the edge of the aqueduct, *ROI_2* region of interest around ROI_1, *Baseline* region of interest at the midbrain (zero flow). *Minus (−) sign* indicates the direction of the flow (craniocaudal – systolic)

Table 2 Mean published stroke volume/flow and peak velocities values in healthy volunteers in various studies performed at 1.5 T

Author	SV/AF (±SD) (mL/beat)	PPV (±SD) (cm/s)	PNV (±SD) (cm/s)
Lee et al. 2004 [11]	0.02±0.0125 (inlet)	–	3.39±1.61 (inlet)
	0.03±0.0132 (ampulla)		3.65±1.59 (ampulla)
	0.02±0.0125 (pars posterior)		4.08±1.99 (pars posterior)
Stoquart-El Sankari et al. [16]	0.048±0.023 (ampulla)	–	–
Stoquart-El Sankari et al. [17]	0.044±0.025 (ampulla)	–	–
Abbey et al. [1]	0.017±0.010 (ampulla)	2.48±0.60	3.24±1.08
Algin et al. [2]	0.039±0.039 (ampulla)	–	4.78±2.48

SV stroke volume, *AF* average flow, *PPV* peak positive flow (diastolic), *PNV* peak negative velocity (systolic), *SD* standard deviation

Discussion

In our study, quantification of CSF hydrodynamic parameters using PC-cine MRI on a 3 T MRI system was conducted. The objectives of our study were to examine the potential user-dependency of the measurements of different ROI sizes, the variation of the measurements depending on the anatomic location of the aqueduct, and whether the velocity and flow values obtained on a 3 T MRI system differ from the ones acquired at 1.5 T

CSF flow may be evaluated qualitatively by using increased signal intensity at the level of the aqueduct. Qualitative measurement is dependent on many parameters that may alter normal signal intensity and thus limit the clinical significance of this method. On the other hand, quantitative CSF measurements are more accurate and reproducible, as long as several parameters are taken into consideration. Various studies have tried to evaluate the most appropriate location for measuring CSF flow through the aqueduct, which is most likely the middle part [1, 2, 4, 5, 9, 16, 17]. These studies were performed on 1.5 T MRI scanners. We performed our measurements at three anatomical levels of the aqueduct and not only the ampulla. An initial analysis of our results showed that the mean PPV and PNV were increased at the upper compared with the lower part of the aqueduct. However, comparing the mean PPV and mean PNV between ROI_1 and ROI_2 at the same anatomical level, and making the appropriate corrections for the different ROI sizes, no differences were actually observed. On the contrary, flow measurements were influenced by the area of the ROI being greater in ROI_2 than ROI_1, while the measured velocities were not. In quantitative measurement of CSF, the most important technical limitation is the accurate ROI placement exactly at the margins of the aqueduct.

Conclusion

CSF hydrodynamics can be quantitatively evaluated using phase-contrast cine MRI. It is of paramount importance to accurately define the normal range of flow parameters to diagnose pathological conditions and possibly identify patients, with dilated ventricular systems, who may or may not benefit from shunt placement.

Overall, our measurements performed on a 3 T MRI system did not vary significantly with the measurements obtained on 1.5 T MRI systems, and our results will be used as reference data in the evaluation of cases of obstructive and normal pressure hydrocephalus.

Conflicts of interest statement We declare that we have no conflict of interest.

References

1. Abbey P, Singh P, Khandelwal N, Mukherjee KK (2009) Shunt surgery effects on cerebrospinal fluid flow across the aqueduct of Sylvius in patients with communicating hydrocephalus. J Clin Neurosci 16(4):514–518
2. Algin O, Hakyemez B, Parlak M (2010) The efficiency of PC-MRI in diagnosis of normal pressure hydrocephalus and prediction of shunt response. Acad Radiol 17(2):181–187
3. Baledent O, Gondry-Jouet C, Stoquart-ElSankari S, Bouzerar R, Le Gars D, Meyer ME (2006) Value of phase contrast magnetic resonance imaging for investigation of cerebral hydrodynamics. J Neuroradiol 33(5):292–303
4. Baledent O, Henry-Feugeas MC, Idy-Peretti I (2001) Cerebrospinal fluid dynamics and relation with blood flow: a magnetic resonance study with semiautomated cerebrospinal fluid segmentation. Invest Radiol 36(7):368–377
5. Barkhof F, Kouwenhoven M, Scheltens P, Sprenger M, Algra P, Valk J (1994) Phase-contrast cine MR imaging of normal aqueductal CSF flow. Acta Radiol 35(2):123–130
6. Bhadelia RA, Bogdan AR, Kaplan RF et al (1997) Cerebrospinal fluid pulsation amplitude and its quantitative relationship to cerebral blood flow pulsations: a phase-contrast MR flow imaging study. Neuroradiology 39:258–264
7. Bhadelia RA, Bogdan AR, Wolpaert SM (1995) Analysis of cerebrospinal fluid flow waveforms with gated phase-contrast MR velocity measurements. AJNR Am J Neuroradiol 16:389–400
8. Bradley WG Jr, Scalzo D et al (1996) Normal-pressure hydrocephalus: evaluation with cerebrospinal fluid flow measurements at MR imaging. Radiology 198(2):523–529
9. Enzmann DR, Pelc NJ (1991) Normal flow patterns of intracranial and spinal cerebrospinal fluid defined with phase-contrast cine MR imaging. Radiology 178(2):467–474
10. Kolbitsch C, Schocke M, Lorenz IH, Kremser C, Zschiegner F, Pfeiffer KP et al (1999) Phase-contrast MRI measurement of systolic cerebrospinal fluid peak velocity (CSFV(peak)) in the aqueduct of Sylvius: a noninvasive tool for measurement of cerebral capacity. Anesthesiology 90(6):1546–1550
11. Lee JH, Lee HK, Kim JK, Kim HJ, Park JK, Choi CG. 2004 CSF flow quantification of the cerebral aqueduct in normal volunteers using phase contrast cine MR imaging. Korean J Radiol. Apr-Jun;5(2):81–6.
12. Levy LM, Di Chiro G (1990) MR phase imaging and cerebrospinal fluid flow in the head and spine. Neuroradiology 32(5):399–406
13. Naidich TP, Altman NR, Conzalez-Arias SM (1993) Phase contrast cine magnetic resonance imaging: normal cerebrospinal fluid oscillation and applications to hydrocephalus. Neurosurg Clin N Am 4(4):677–705
14. Nitz WR, Bradley WG Jr, Wantanabe AS, Lee R, Burgoyne B, O'Sullivan R, Herbst M (1992) Flow dynamics of cerebrospinal fluid: assessment with phase-contrast velocity MR imaging performed with retrospective cardiac gating. Radiology 183:395–405
15. Quencer RM, Post MJ, Hinks RS (1990) Cine MR in the evaluation of normal and abnormal CSF flow: intracranial and intraspinal studies. Neuroradiology 32:371–391
16. Stoquart-El Sankari S, Baledent O, Gondry-Jouet C, Makki M, Godefroy O, Meyer ME (2007) Aging effects on cerebral blood and cerebrospinal fluid flows. J Cereb Blood Flow Metab 27(9):1563–1572
17. Stoquart-El Sankari S, Lehmann P, Gondry-Jouet C, Fichten A, Godefroy O, Meyer ME, Baledent O (2009) Phase-contrast MR imaging support for the diagnosis of aqueductal stenosis. AJNR Am J Neuroradiol 30(1):209–214

Correlation Between Tap Test and CSF Aqueductal Stroke Volume in Idiopathic Normal Pressure Hydrocephalus

Souraya El Sankari, A. Fichten, C. Gondry-Jouet, M. Czosnyka, D. Legars, H. Deramond, and Olivier Balédent

Abstract *Introduction*: The diagnosis and management of idiopathic normal pressure hydrocephalus (INPH) remains unclear despite the development of guidelines. In addition, the role of cerebrospinal fluid (CSF) aqueductal stroke volume (ASV) remains unspecified.

Objectives: The aim of this study was to compare the results of the tap test (TT) and ASV in patients with possible INPH.

Materials and Methods: Among 21 patients investigated with both TT and phase-contrast (PC) MRI, we identified two groups, with either (1) a positive TT (PTT) or (2) a negative one (NTT), and we compared their ASV as measured by PC-MRI. ASV cutoff value was set at 70 µL/cardiac cycle (mean value +2 standard deviations in age-matched healthy subjects).

Results: In the PTT group ($n=9$), the mean ASV was 175 ± 71 µL. Among these patients, four were shunted, and improved after surgery. In the NTT group, two patients were finally diagnosed with aqueductal stenosis and excluded. Among the remaining patients ($n=10$), the mean ASV was 96 ± 93 µL ($p<0.05$). However, three of these patients presented with hyperdynamic ASV, and an associated neurodegenerative disorder was diagnosed. Two patients had ventriculoperitoneal shunting despite their NTT, and improved.

Discussion/Conclusions: In our patient population, the noninvasive measurement of hyperdynamic ASV correlated with PTT, suggesting PC-MRI could be utilized to select those patients who would benefit from shunting. ASV may therefore be an interesting supplemental diagnosis tool.

Keywords Idiopathic Normal Pressure Hydrocephalus • CSF removal test • Phase Contrast-MRI • Aqueductal Stroke Volume • Shunt responsiveness

S. El Sankari (✉)
Imaging and Biophysics Unit,
Amiens University Hospital,
Amiens, France,
TIDAM research unit, Jules Verne University of Picardy and Amiens University Hospital,
Amiens, France and
Neurology Department,
Amiens University Hospital, Amiens, France
e-mail: sorayaelsankari560@hotmail.com

A. Fichten and D. Legars
TIDAM research unit, Jules Verne University of Picardy and Amiens University Hospital, Amiens, France and
Neurosurgery Department,
Amiens University Hospital, Amiens, France

C. Gondry-Jouet and H. Deramond
TIDAM research unit, Jules Verne University of Picardy and Amiens University Hospital, Amiens, France and
Radiology Department,
Amiens University Hospital, Amiens, France

M. Czosnyka
Academic Neurosurgical Unit,
Department of Clinical Neurosciences,
University of Cambridge, Addenbroke's Hospital,
Cambridge, UK

O. Balédent
Imaging and Biophysics Unit,
Amiens University Hospital,
Amiens, France and
TIDAM research unit, Jules Verne University of Picardy and Amiens University Hospital,
Amiens, France
e-mail: olivier.baledent@chu-amiens.fr

Introduction

The diagnosis and management of idiopathic normal pressure hydrocephalus (INPH) remains problematic. Moreover, the value of supplemental tests in predicting the success of ventriculoperitoneal shunting remains unclear. The guidelines for diagnosis and management of INPH [5] tried to address these issues, and it was concluded that cerebrospinal fluid (CSF) tap test (TT) can reasonably be performed initially, because of its easiness, but should not be used as an exclusionary test, because of its low sensitivity (between 21% and 61%). Although they have greater sensitivity or positive predictive value, infusion test and external lumbar drainage (72 h) are less widely performed for different reasons (fear of complications, lack of personal experience, and costs of hospitalization). In contrast, phase-contrast MRI

(PC-MRI) presents an interesting noninvasive tool, but results concerning its efficiency in the evaluation of shunt responsiveness are controversial. Aqueductal CSF flow void [2] and aqueductal velocity measurements [3] have failed to prove any significant association with improvement after shunting. On the other hand, other studies have suggested that aqueductal CSF flow parameters could predict the shunt responsiveness [2, 4], but cutoff values were variable among studies, and further evidence was required.

In our institution, quantitative CSF flow measurements using PC-MRI are routinely performed and our aim was to compare these data with the CSF tap test results, and evaluate their support to shunt responsiveness prediction.

Materials and Methods

Patients

This retrospective study involved patients admitted to the Neurosurgery Department diagnosed for communicant hydrocephalus between June 2006 and April 2008. The inclusion criteria were the following: adults (1) aged over 60 years, (2) presenting with one or more symptoms of the classical triad (gait, urinary, or cognitive disorders), (3) with an insidious onset, (4) without any antecedent event such as head trauma, intracerebral hemorrhage, meningitis, or other known causes of secondary hydrocephalus, and (5) with ventricular enlargement on cerebral MRI (Evan's ratio >0.3), without macroscopic signs of obstruction to CSF flow. As the CSF opening pressure is not necessarily measured in our institution for chronic hydrocephalus, these patients were classified as "possible INPH" according to the published guidelines [5].

All patients in this study were investigated utilizing a CSF TT and phase-contrast MRI (PC-MRI) measurement of CSF dynamics. Patients were clinically evaluated by a senior neurosurgeon before and after the TT. The surgical option was considered on a clinical basis and on the positive response to TT. Among the nonresponders, the surgical option was considered if the clinical triad was present, with suggestive brain MRI, without associated neurodegenerative disorders. Postoperative follow-up was continued for 9–12 months, and improvement was clinically assessed, utilizing timed walking test and the Mini-Mental State Examination.

CSF Tap Test

CSF TT was performed on patients with a needle inserted in the lower lumbar region, and the removal of 40–50 mL of CSF. The clinical evaluation (timed walking test and Mini-Mental State Examination) was performed as usual before and 3–4 h after CSF removal, and the patients and their caregivers were asked to assess changes in clinical symptoms that occurred in this period. (To assess the change, a patient has to be evaluated before and after the TT. Did you utilize timed walking test and Mini-Mental State Examination before the tap test?) Any transient or long-lasting improvement was considered a positive TT. Patients were therefore divided into two groups: those with a positive TT (PTT) and those with a negative one (NTT).

Phase-Contrast MRI

All MRI exams were performed with a standardized imaging protocol, using a 3-Tesla (3 T) machine, and flow images were acquired with a 2D fast cine PC-MRI pulse sequence with retrospective peripheral gating, so that the 32 frames analyzed covered the entire cardiac cycle (CC). The MRI parameters were as described in previous publications [7]. Velocity (encoding) sensitization was set at 10 cm/s for the aqueduct (adjusted to 5 cm/s if no flow was detected, or increased to 20 cm/s if there was any aliasing) and 5 cm/s for the cervical subarachnoid spaces (SAS) and the prepontine cistern. Sections through these different levels for each flow series are represented on Fig. 1. The acquisition time for each flow series was about 1 min and 30 s on the 3 T machine, with a slight fluctuation that depended on the participant's heart rate.

Data were analyzed using an in-house image processing software [1] with an optimized CSF flows segmentation algorithm, which automatically extracts the region of interest (ROI) at each level.

Then, the CSF flow curves were generated versus the 32 segments of the CC, and the integration of this curve provided the CSF stroke volume, which represents the CSF volume displaced in both directions through the considered ROI at each level [1, 7].

Statistical Analysis

Demographic and clinical data were retrospectively collected for all patients. We also reported if a surgical procedure was performed, and its outcome. All clinical and PC-MRI results were compared between groups (PTT and NTT), using the t-test or Mann–Whitney test, for parametric and nonparametric data, retrospectively. The level for statistical significance was set at 0.05.

Fig. 1 Phase-contrast (PC) MRI acquisition. Sagittal scout view was used as localizer to select the anatomical levels for flow quantification. The acquisition planes were selected perpendicular to the presumed direction of the flow, and acquired at the aqueductal (1), prepontine cistern (2), and intracerebral subarachnoidian (3) cerebrospinal fluid (CSF) levels

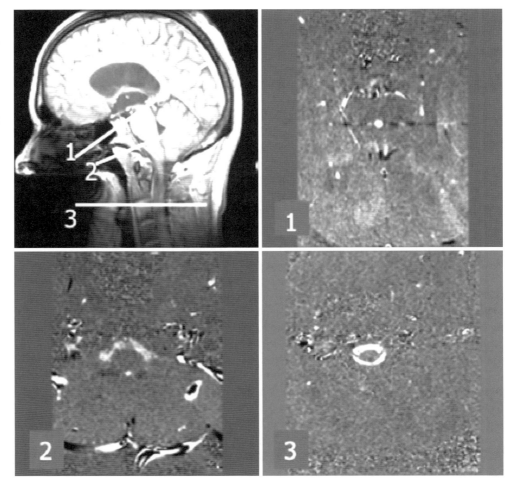

Results

Clinical and PC-MRI results were summarized in Table 1. The aqueductal stroke volumes (ASV) ranged from 72 to 286 µL in patients with PTT. These values were greater than the cutoff value considered as the mean value in a healthy age-matched population [7], which equalled 70 µL. Among these nine patients with PTT, four were shunted and had a positive outcome (survey of 9–12 months). The remaining five patients did not undergo surgery, due to general conditions (myasthenia, respiratory or cardiac contraindications) or associated vascular dementia.

Among 12 patients with a NTT, two had a final diagnosis of aqueductal stenosis, as their aqueductal SV was null. They were therefore excluded from the analysis. They underwent an endoscopic third ventriculostomy and improved after surgery. Four patients with NTT had an ASV ranging from 34 to 56 µL, and their diagnosis was frontotemporal dementia, based on the clinical and imaging investigation. Two patients had highly increased ASV (152 and 297 µL), and thus, although their TT was negative, they were shunted, and their medical assessment at 6 and 24 months showed clinical

Table 1 Clinical and phase-contrast MRI results are represented in the negative tap test (NTT) and positive TT (PTT) groups

	Negative TT (n=10)	Positive TT (n=9)	p value
Age (mean ± SD)	75 ± 8	71 ± 3	NS
Sex ratio: females	7 (70%)	1 (11%)	<0.01
Gait	8 (80%)	9 (100%)	NS
Cognitive	8 (80%)	9 (100%)	NS
Bladder	6 (60%)	7 (78%)	NS
One of triad	2 (20%)	1 (11%)	NS
Two of triad	4 (40%)	2 (22%)	NS
Complete triad	4 (40%)	7 (78%)	<0.05
Aqueductal CSF SV	96 ± 93 µL	175 ± 71 µL	<0.05
Cervical CSF SV	390 ± 137 µL	468 ± 153 µL	NS
Prepontine CSF SV	269 ± 134 µL	262 ± 171 µL	NS

SD standard deviation, *CSF* cerebrospinal fluid, *SV* stroke volume, *NS* nonsignificant

improvement. Finally, despite clinically possible INPH and increased ASV, four patients with NTT were not operated on. Three of them had associated neurodegenerative diseases

(Alzheimer's [AD], Parkinson's, or vascular disease), and one had severe dementia.

Discussion

Our study is limited due to the small size of the patient population and the low proportion of shunted patients (6 among 21), which prevents reliable calculation of sensitivity/specificity and predictive values. However, this retrospective study suggests that PC-MRI is a useful tool, which can supplement CSF TT in selecting those patients who would benefit from ventriculoperitoneal shunting.

In addition, although normally considered as differential diagnoses, INPH and other nonsurgical neurodegenerative diseases (such as AD or Parkinson's disease) may coexist. Moreover, they share common risk factors, such as hypertension, identified both in INPH and vascular dementia [6]. In addition, MRI may fail to distinguish the underlying reasons which cause white matter abnormalities in these patient populations [8].

In some patients presenting with symptoms of both diseases, the decision to shunt may be restrained because of associated dementia due to AD; for instance, high ASV may tempt neurosurgeons to conduct surgery to improve clinical symptoms related to INPH on the one hand, and on the other hand to hamper the deterioration due of AD symptoms related to its association with INPH.

Finally, we stress the importance of predefined cutoff values, based on normal SV measured in healthy age-matched controls, as has been investigated in a previous work [7]. Actually, discrepancies regarding the accurate support of ASV in predicting shunt responsiveness are mainly due to heterogeneous thresholds in the literature. We believe that identifying the definition of normal cutoff values in each center according to the type of scanning machine, the sequence parameters, and the protocol used is a mandatory requisite.

Conclusion

According to the INPH guidelines [5], "to date, a single standard for the prognostic evaluation is lacking." PC-MRI presents the advantages of being a rapid (5-min) and noninvasive complementary tool. Further prospective studies are needed in larger populations with a greater proportion of shunted patients, to compare the prognostic value of CSF TT with PC-MRI data. Moreover, ASV should be evaluated in presurgical and postsurgical assessments, to better apprehend the mechanisms of improvement in CSF dynamics after shunting in INPH.

Acknowledgments This work was supported by European Community Grant Interreg (Inter-regional cooperation between University Hospital of Amiens and the University of Cambridge).

Conflicts of interest statement We declare that we have no conflict of interest.

References

1. Balédent O, Henry-Feugeas MC, Idy-Peretti I (2001) Cerebrospinal fluid dynamics and relation with blood flow: a magnetic resonance study with semiautomated cerebrospinal fluid segmentation. Invest Radiol 36(7):368–377
2. Bradley WG, Scalzo D, Queralt J, Nitz WN, Atkinson DJ, Wong P (1996) Normal-pressure hydrocephalus: evaluation with cerebrospinal fluid flow measurements at MR imaging. Radiology 198(2): 523–529
3. Dixon GR, Friedman JA, Luetmer PH, Quast LM, McClelland RL, Petersen RC, Maher CO, Ebersold MJ (2002) Use of cerebrospinal fluid flow rates measured by phase-contrast MR to predict outcome of ventriculoperitoneal shunting for idiopathic normal-pressure hydrocephalus. Mayo Clin Proc 77(6):509–514
4. Luetmer PH, Huston J, Friedman JA, Dixon GR, Petersen RC, Jack CR, McClelland RL, Ebersold MJ (2002) Measurement of cerebrospinal fluid flow at the cerebral aqueduct by use of phase-contrast magnetic resonance imaging: technique validation and utility in diagnosing idiopathic normal pressure hydrocephalus. Neurosurgery 50(3):534–543
5. Marmarou A, Bergsneider M, Klinge P, Relkin N, Black PM (2005) The value of supplemental prognostic tests for the preoperative assessment of idiopathic normal-pressure hydrocephalus. Neurosurgery 57(3 Suppl):S17–S28
6. Stivaros SM, Jackson A (2007) Changing concepts of cerebrospinal fluid hydrodynamics: role of phase-contrast magnetic resonance imaging and implications for cerebral microvascular disease. Neurotherapeutics 4(3):511–522
7. Stoquart-ElSankari S, Balédent O, Gondry-Jouet C, Makki M, Godefroy O, Meyer ME (2007) Aging effects on cerebral blood and cerebrospinal fluid flows. J Cereb Blood Flow Metab 27(9): 1563–1572
8. Tullberg M, Hultin L, Ekholm S, Mansson JE, Fredman P, Wikkelso C (2002) White matter changes in normal pressure hydrocephalus and Binswanger disease: specificity, predictive value and correlations to axonal degeneration and demyelination. Acta Neurol Scand 105(6): 417–426

Overview of the CSF Dual Outflow System

Michael Pollay

Abstract It was firmly established in the mid-twentieth century that the arachnoid villi represented an open pathway between the subarachnoid space and the dural venous sinuses. Intracellular and extracellular pathways within the villous structure provided the conduit for cerebrospinal fluid (CSF) and particulate matter. The importance of the lymphatic system was established by the demonstration of CSF tracers entering the nasal lymphatic system via the perineural subarachnoid space enveloping the olfactory nerve rootlets. It appears that because of the late development of the arachnoid villus (AV) system, the lymphatic outflow system is the more dominant one in the young animal, but in the mature animal the importance of both systems appears equal. In general, the lymphatic system in lower animals appears dominant, but in the case of primates, this may not be the case. The global outflow system has a definite opening pressure of ca. 50–70 mm of water, and the balance between production of CSF and absorption occurs at a resting pressure of ca. 115 mm water. The bicompartmental CSF outflow curves obtained from hydrocephalic patients support the presence of a dual outflow system utilized in normal CSF drainage.

Keywords CSF dual outflow systems • Arachnoid villi • Nasal perineural CSF drainage • CSF drainage dynamics • CSF outflow obstruction

In the Beginning

Historically the two important studies in the evolution of our understanding of the two systems responsible for cerebrospinal fluid (CSF) drainage are the original observations of Pacchioni in 1705 and the observed dual outflow of CSF tracer as described in 1875 by Key and Retzius.

The former was able to visualize the arachnoid granulations in relationship to the superior sagittal sinus, while the latter observed the penetration of a colored tracer into both the lacuna lateralis and the nasal lymphatic system.

The Cranial and Spinal Arachnoid Villi

The original view of Weed was that the arachnoid villus was a blind semipermeable diverticulum though which CSF passed into cerebral venous blood due to both a hydrostatic and osmotic gradient. This was later refuted by Davson and Segal who observed that the outflow of CSF was not greatly affected when CSF and plasma protein concentration were equal and the 3–5 mmHg hydrostatic gradient between the CSF and venous blood was responsible for normal CSF outflow [5]. The modern era began with the findings of Welch and colleagues that the primate arachnoid villi (AV) consisted of open endothelial tubes that collapsed when the hydrostatic gradient between the subarachnoid CSF was reversed [17]. Flow occurred at a definitive opening pressure (OP) as the hydrostatic gradient was established. Using the AV laden wall of the green monkey as an occluding membrane in a perfusion chamber, they demonstrated an OP of between 30 and 50 cm H_2O and an outflow curve (CSF to sinus) that increased with perfusion pressure. Flow in the reverse direction was markedly restricted. Particulate matter passed with some ease across the villi laden membrane. The particle size up to 7.5 μm appeared to pass with ease. Grzybowski and her associates demonstrated, using human AV in an in vitro and ex vivo perfusion system, a similar asymmetry of fluid movement with a definitive OP and open flow utilizing normal hydrostatic gradients with the ability to

M. Pollay
Emeritus Chairman and Professor of Neurosurgery,
University of Oklahoma College of Medicine
e-mail: m0325@aol.com
Sun City West, AZ, USA

pass particulate matter [9]. The anatomical basis for the open pathway AV system revealed differences between primates and lower animals [16]. In primates, trans villus flow was demonstrated to be primarily intracellular via both paracellular and intracellular (primarily via vacuoles) mechanisms, which became apparent by both transmission and scanning electron microscopy with tissue fixed under pressure [5, 15]. While both intracellular and paracellular mechanisms were observed in lower animals, the intracellular mechanism was primarily by pinocytosis [16].

The spinal AV have demonstrated similar properties as the cranial villi. They are sporadically found in the subarachnoid projections along the dorsal root adjacent to the dorsal root ganglion [18]. In primates they are more commonly found in the lower spinal areas. Some actually penetrate the dura to enter directly into the spinal veins, although most end in the extradural space, often in relation to lymphatic and venous structures. Clusters of arachnoidal cells are also seen within the subarachnoid space at the blind end near the dorsal root ganglion. The outflow of CSF from the spinal compartment has been reported to be 15 and 25% of total CSF outflow, although a study in healthy individuals reported it be considerably higher. It appears that greater percentages of outflow from the spinal compartment are noted primarily in humans [2, 6].

Functional Morphology of the Lymphatic Outflow System

Early CSF tracer studies, in a variety of animal species, demonstrated significant accumulation in the nasal and cervical lymphatics. It has also been shown that the nasal lymphatic pathways are important for CSF drainage and as pathways for the cerebral immune response to antigens [3]. Although a perineural subarachnoid space is found along many of the cranial nerves, the projections with the olfactory rootlets are the most important.

The more recent studies on the role of the lymphatic system in CSF drainage have firmly established the structural anatomy and the functional capability of this outflow system. In a variety of animals, the egress of microfil into the lymphatic system is via the olfactory nerve rootlets with direct communication with the lymphatic vessels. In a series of studies in sheep, the Toronto group measured the volumetric capacity not only of the nasal lymphatic outflow system, but by physical isolation, that of the cranial and spinal AV outflow systems [1, 2]. At 22 h, the recovery from the lymphatic and AV outflow was 25.1% and 20.8%, respectively [1]. After increasing the intracranial pressure 10 cm of water above the OP, the clearance from the CSF was nearly equal for the lymphatic and AV drainage systems [2]. Obstructing the nasal lymphatic outflow was also noted to significantly lead to an increase in outflow resistance in the sheep model. A higher pressure was required to reach normal flow, which suggests that the cranial and spinal AV drainage pathways represented a high-pressure outflow system. Eliminating the spinal compartment further increased outflow resistance with an associated fall in the rate of CSF drainage. It was also noted in these studies that the global drainage of CSF is almost the same in fetal, neonatal, and adult sheep. The overall conclusion from these studies on sheep is that the lymphatic system is dominant in early life with an increase in utilization of the AV outflow system in the maturing animal.

Alternate Sites for CSF Absorption

The choroid plexus has been suggested as a possible site for CSF absorption. There is no evidence, either anatomical or physiological, to support this view. Direct observation of the exposed surface of the arachnoid membrane gives no evidence of net CSF movement over the entire membrane but only at the AV structures themselves. It has been recently shown that the dural membrane is very vascular and contains fluid channels, which might offer in the immature AV system an alternate CSF drainage pathway [14]. This is an interesting possibility but needs to be further clarified. The question of the role of the blood–brain barrier (cerebral capillary endothelium) is not settled, although water transport has been associated with the glucose and protein cotransporters at this interface. It is also not clear what role aquaporin 4 at the adjacent glial end feet may have in transendothelial water movement, but the proximity to the capillary wall suggests a possible role in blood–brain barrier water transport [11]. In the case of hydrocephalus, the aquaporins and the cotransporters are upgraded.

Consequences of Morphologic Changes in CSF Outflow Structures

The congenital absence or paucity of AV in association with hydrocephalus has been reported in humans. Similarly, anatomical abnormalities of the olfactory nasal lymphatic system in malformations of the bony skull base have also been associated with hydrocephalus, but the intactness of the total CSF outflow systems was not evaluated. It has been reported that following cranial base surgery, some 8% of patients develop hydrocephalus. It is assumed this is due to the obstructing or severing of the olfactory nerve rootlet CSF pathways, although entry of blood and other contaminants into the subarachnoid space may also affect other elements of the global outflow systems. My experience has been that traumatic injuries of the anterior fossa and removal of tumors in this region have rarely resulted in hydrocephalus. The mucopolysaccharide accumulation in the AV secondary to dietary deficiency of vitamin A in rabbits, calves, and infants (secondary to cystic fibrosis) is also associated with the development of hydrocephalus.

Hydrocephalus may be the consequence of meningitis and subarachnoid hemorrhage, but it is hard to separate the individual changes in the various components comprising the total CSF outflow system. In general, defining the relative role of the AV, lymphatic outflow system, and subarachnoid space is not possible, since each site is not evaluated at the same time.

Some evidence for a dual system has been derived from studies in the total CSF drainage system in humans with hydrocephalus. Sokolowski constructed in normal and hydrocephalic patients, outflow curves using the bolus injection method [13]. The configuration of the semilogarithmic plots of volume versus time, in which the peak pressure represents primarily compliance and the outflow is a measure of CSF absorption. In normal patients, the relationship is mostly linear, while in hydrocephalic patients, the break in the curve suggests two separate compartments. In another study in hydrocephalic patients, using a ventricular perfusion method, two types of outflow patterns were observed [10]. The type 1 absorption defect consisted of an elevated OP >160 mm CSF pressure but a normal rate of fluid absorption of 0.0069 mL/min/mm. The type 2 absorption defect had a normal OP but a decreased rate of fluid absorption of 0.0026 mL/min/mm. These two studies might indicate a dual system with only one of the systems affected [10, 13]. The perceived high and low outflow system suggested from these studies appears to agree with studies in sheep after separating the nasal lymphatic outflow system from the cranial and spinal compartments

Dynamics of the Total CSF Drainage System

The relationship between CSF formation and drainage has been studied in humans. At a rate of 0.37 mL/min for CSF formation, the intercept of flow and rate of absorption occurs at a normal resting pressure of ca. 112 mm CSF pressure [4]. Over a wide range of pressures seen clinically, the CSF pressure relationship with that of the venous pressure in the sagittal sinus remains stable. In a series of curves representing increasing rate of ventricular perfusion, a steady state can be reached between CSF pressure and time when the rate of perfusion is at or below 1.0 mL/min [12]. After that point, there is no steady state reached between volume and time, post injection. Presumably the CSF pressure at this rate of infusion leads to collapse of the cranial venous system and loss of the CSF-venous pressure differential with cessation of absorption. The pressure at this rate of infusion reached >900 mmH$_2$O. Ekstedt found the relationship between CSF outflow and pressure to be rectilinear up to a CSF pressure of ca. 6 kPa (61 cmH$_2$O), after reaching a CSF pressure of ca. 60 mmH$_2$O required to initiate CSF outflow [8]. This suggested to him that the AV once opened are not further distended by pressure. It is apparent now that the outflow resistance and conductance that he measured in humans represents both the outflow via the cranial and spinal AV and the olfactory lymphatic outflow system. This suggests that the values for the total system outflow resistance (R_o) and absorptive capacity may represent a combined average value for both pathways. The maximum capacity of the CSF drainage systems to handle the volume of CSF produced before developing ventriculomegaly has not been fully defined. The response of the CSF system to elevated rates of CSF formation (overproduction) has been studied in a child with hydrocephalus associated with a choroid plexus papilloma, using a ventriculolumbar perfusion system [7]. In this patient, the rate of CSF formation was four times (1.43 mL/min) that seen normally in children (normal ~ 0.35 mL/min). The rate of absorption (V_a) in this case was measured at 130 mmH$_2$O and found to be 0.59 mL/min, which is almost equal to that found in normal children with an unobstructed pathway (V_a = 0.61 mL/min). Following the removal of the choroid plexus tumor, the intracranial pressure in the child returned to normal, and the head size fell to the 50th percentile for age.

Conclusion

It can be concluded from this study that even with an intact outflow system, there is a maximum level of absorptive capacity with excess fluid formation, but the level after which a steady state between pressure and flow is not obtainable has not been established in humans. The perfusion studies by Mann and colleagues in the dog demonstrated that the ability of the CSF system to reach a new steady state is exceeded when the infusion into the CSF space is ≥1.0 mL/min [12].

Conflicts of interest statement We declare that we have no conflict of interest.

References

1. Boulton M, Amstrong D, Flessner M, Hay J, Szalai JP, Johnston M (1998) Raised intracranial pressure increases cerebrospinal fluid drainage through arachnoid villi and extra cranial lymphatics. Am J Physiol 275:R889–R896
2. Bozanovic-Sosic R, Mollanji R, Johnston M (2001) Spinal and cranial contributions to total cerebrospinal fluid transport. Am J Physiol Regul Integr Comp Physiol 281:R909–R916

3. Cserr HF, Harling-Berg CJ KPM (1992) Drainage of brain extracellular fluid into blood and deep cervical lymphatics and its immunological significance. Brain Pathol 4:269–276
4. Cutler RWP, Page L, Galicih J, Watters GV (1968) Formation and absorption of cerebrospinal fluid. Brain 91:707–720
5. Davson H, Segal MB (1984) Physiology of the cerebrospinal fluid and blood-brain barriers, 1st edn. CRC Press, London, pp 489–523
6. Edsbagge M, Tissel M, Jacobsson L, Wikkelso C (2004) Spinal cerebrospinal fluid absorption in healthy individuals. Am J Physiol Regul Integr Comp Physiol 287:R1450–R1455
7. Eisenberg HM, Mcomb JG, Lorenzo AV (1974) Cerebrospinal fluid overproduction and hydrocephalus associated with choroid plexus papilloma. J Neurosurg 40:381–385
8. Eksted J (1977) Cerebrospinal fluid hydrodynamic studies in man. J Neurol Neurosurg Psychiatry 40:105–119
9. Grzybowski DM, Holman DW, Katz SE, Lubow M (2006) In vitro model of cerebrospinal fluid outflow through human arachnoid granulations. Invest Ophthamol Vis Sci 47:3664–3672
10. Lorenzo AV, Page LK, Watters GV (1970) Relationship between cerebrospinal fluid formation, absorption, and pressure in human hydrocephalus. Brain 93:679–690
11. MacAulay N, Zeuthen T Water transport between CNS compartments: contributions of aquaporins and cotransporters. Neuroscience. (2010) 168(4):941–56
12. Mann JD, Maffeo CJ, Rosenthal JD, Johnson RN, Butler AB, Bass NH (1976) Regulation of intracranial pressure in rat, dog and man: manometric assessment of cerebrospinal fluid dynamics using a constant flow system. Trans Am Neurol Assoc 101:182–185
13. Sokolowski SJ (1976) Bolus injection test for measurement of cerebrospinal fluid absorption. J Neurol Sci 28:491–504
14. Squier W, Lindberg E, Mack J, Darby S (2009) Demonstration of fluid channels in human dura and their relationship to age and intradural bleeding. Childs Nerv Syst 25:925–931
15. Tripathi BJ, Tripathi RC (1974) Vacuolar trans cellular channel as a drainage pathway for cerebrospinal fluid. J Physiol 239:195–206
16. Upton ML, Weller RO (1985) The morphology of cerebrospinal fluid drainage pathways in human arachnoid granulations. J Neurosurg 63:867–875
17. Welch K, Friedman V (1960) The cerebrospinal fluid valves. Brain 83:454–469
18. Welch K, Pollay M (1963) The spinal arachnoid villi of monkeys Ceropithe aethopis and Macaca irus. Anat Rec 145:43–48

Hydrocephalus and Aquaporins: The Role of Aquaporin-1

M.Y.S. Kalani, A.S. Filippidis, and H.L. Rekate

Abstract *Introduction*: Aquaporins (AQPs) are membrane proteins that facilitate water and small solute movement in tissues. Hydrocephalus is a major central nervous system disorder associated with defective cerebrospinal fluid (CSF) turnover. Aquaporin-1 (AQP1) is a water channel located mainly at the choroid plexus epithelium and plays an active role in CSF production. The aim of this study is to review the pertinent literature concerning the role of aquaporin-1 in the pathophysiology of hydrocephalus.

Methods: We performed a MEDLINE search using the terms *aquaporin* AND *hydrocephalus*. The results of the search were further refined to exclude studies not related to aquaporin-1.

Results: Five studies were identified. Three of these studies utilized an animal model, while only two studies referred to a few human cases of hydrocephalus. Most of the studies indicate that there is a down-regulation of AQP1 expression in choroid plexus in models of hydrocephalus. A small series of human choroid plexus tumors showed that AQP1 expression is up-regulated. In cases of human choroid plexus tumors, there are indications that AQP1 may have alternative physiologic roles, but it is not clear whether this is associated with a specific type of hydrocephalus or the genetic burden of the tumor.

Conclusion: There has been a paucity of research on the link between aquaporins and hydrocephalus. Most studies have relied on animal models. An adaptive and protective role of AQP1 as a regulator of CSF production is proposed in the pathophysiology of hydrocephalus. Further research is needed to clarify if this association exists in humans.

Keywords Aquaporin • AQP1 • Cerebrospinal fluid (CSF) • Hydrocephalus • Water channel

M.Y.S. Kalani, and A.S. Filippidis
Division of Neurological Surgery, Barrow Neurological Institute,
St. Joseph's Hospital and Medical Center,
Phoenix, AZ, USA

H.L. Rekate (✉)
The Chiari Institute, Hofstra,
Northshore LIJ College of Medicine,
865 Northern Boulevard, 11021 Great Neck NY, USA
e-mail: haroldrekate@gmail.com

Introduction

The pathophysiology of hydrocephalus relies mainly on the delicate equilibrium between the production, the absorption, and the circulation of cerebrospinal fluid (CSF). CSF consists mostly of water. Water homeostasis is significant in the physiology of the central nervous system [6]. Aquaporins (AQPs) are transmembrane proteins that regulate the movement of water and small solutes through the cell membrane, contributing to water homeostasis [1, 22, 23]. AQP1 and AQP4 are expressed in abundance in the central nervous system, while AQP4 shows the highest expression pattern of any member of the AQP family [23]. The presence of AQPs in the central nervous system and especially the high expression of AQP1 at the ventricular side of the choroid plexus epithelium [12, 13, 18] is stimulating research in the field of CSF and water turnover hydrocephalus [2, 23].

The aim of this study is to review the pertinent literature concerning the role of AQP1 in cerebrospinal fluid turnover and the pathophysiology of hydrocephalus. The information obtained from this process will be used to clarify any potential association between AQP1 and hydrocephalus.

Methods

We performed a MEDLINE search using the terms *aquaporin* AND *hydrocephalus*. The results of the search were further refined to exclude studies not related to AQP1. The studies were divided according to the species and models used.

Results

The expression of the AQP1 water channel at the ventricular side of the choroid plexus, as the literature indicates, led Oshio and colleagues to study the CSF production and intracranial pressure (ICP) in mice lacking AQP1 expression (AQP1 knockout) and wild-type mice [14, 15] (Table 1).

Table 1 Studies concerning hydrocephalus and aquaporin-1

Studies	Species	Method	AQPs studied	Results
Mao et al. [9]	Rats	Kaolin inj.	AQPs 1,4,9	AQP1 w/o a significant change in HCP
Paul et al. [16]	Rats	H-Tx, choroid plexus culture	AQPs 1,4	AQP1 low /AQP4 high
Oshio et al. [15]	Mice	AQP1-KO	AQP1	Lower ICP, lower CSF production
Smith et al. [20]	Humans	Choroid plexus hyperplasia, case report	AQP1	Down-regulated
Longatti et al. [7]	Humans	Choroid plexus tumors series	AQP1	Mostly strong expression in tumors with hydrocephalus

AQP aquaporin, *HCP* hydrocephalus, *obstr* obstructive, *AQP4-KO* aquaporin-4 knockout mice, *H-Tx* congenital hydrocephalic rats, *ICP* intracranial pressure

The production of CSF was reduced by 20–25% in AQP1-knockout mice. ICP was also 56% reduced in AQP1-knockout compared with wild-type mice. The osmotic water permeability of the choroid epithelium cells was reduced fivefold. The authors also pointed out that the systemic effects of loss of AQP1 expression in the kidneys in AQP1-knockout mice were responsible for the lower central venous pressure in this group. The lower central venous pressure in AQP1-knockout mice was the major contributor to reduction of CSF production and ICP, although the loss of AQP1 from the choroid plexus also made a significant contribution [14, 15].

Paul and colleagues studied the expression of AQP1 and AQP4 in congenital hydrocephalic H-Tx rats with polymerase chain reaction (quantitative RT-PCR), Western blot, immunohistochemistry, and ELISA [16]. They also found that AQP1 expression was significantly decreased in choroid plexus of H-Tx rats, while AQP4 expression was increased in the whole brain and cortex and slightly decreased in the choroid plexus.

Longatti and colleagues, Mobasheri and Marples, as well as Praetorius and Nielsen confirmed the presence of AQP1 at the ventricular side of the choroid plexus in humans [8, 12, 18]. Interestingly, some reports indicate that AQP1 expression is down-regulated in hydrocephalus. Smith et al. report a case of a 15-month-old girl with choroid plexus hyperplasia. Choroid plexus hyperplasia is a rare case of nonobstructive hydrocephalus related to CSF hyperproduction by choroid plexuses [20]. The choroid plexus was excised, and immunohistochemistry revealed a dramatic decrease in immunoreactivity of AQP1 of the specimen compared with controls.

Longatti et al. reported a series of nine patients with choroid plexus tumors. The observed expression levels of AQP1 were not homogenous in cases with a choroid plexus tumor and hydrocephalus. AQP1 showed a strong expression in four cases of choroid plexus papillomas with hydrocephalus (obstructive in three and communicating in one), while weak expression was observed in one case of choroid plexus carcinoma complicated by obstructive hydrocephalus [7, 20].

Discussion

AQP1 is highly expressed at the ventricular surface of the choroid plexus epithelium in mice, rats, humans, and other species [2, 8, 12, 13, 18, 21]. AQP1 expression has also been reported at the basolateral (blood side) of the choroid plexus epithelium in rodents and humans but shows a weaker pattern [12, 13]. The higher ventricular expression of AQP1 is thought to play a significant role in transcellular transport of water molecules for the production of CSF [2, 8, 12, 13, 18, 21]. The weak basolateral expression of AQP1 at the choroid plexus could explain how water molecules enter the choroid plexus cells and are subsequently filtered into the ventricle to produce CSF [3, 5, 8, 17, 18, 21]. The polarized expression of AQP1 at the choroid plexus has been confirmed in humans [8, 12, 18]. Since AQP1 distribution is dominant in choroid plexus, and it demonstrates a specific localization at the ventricular side facing CSF, its role in the production of CSF was highly suspect and gave rise to studies of AQP1 and hydrocephalus.

Few studies concerning AQP1 and hydrocephalus exist. Most of these studies rely on animal models such as congenital hydrocephalic rats (H-Tx rats), kaolin-induced hydrocephalus in rats or AQP1-knockout mice. Human studies are based on few observations in cases of hydrocephalus associated with choroid plexus hyperplasia or choroid plexus tumors. Few studies show that AQP1 expression is down-regulated in hydrocephalus or that the loss of AQP1 lowers SF production and ICP [14–16, 20]. One study was not able to identify any changes [9], while one human study by Longatti et al. [7] indicated mostly a strong expression in choroid plexus tumors with hydrocephalus. Currently, the patterns of expression of AQP1 in hydrocephalus are not clear in the literature. Thus, the results concerning the expression of AQP1 in hydrocephalus or its contribution to CSF production and ICP should be interpreted with caution and used only as indications of the role of AQP1 in hydrocephalus and not as facts.

Although further research should be conducted, these preliminary data indicate that AQP1 is usually down-regulated in cases of hydrocephalus [16, 20]. It is possible that a feedback mechanism exists, and this is the proposed explanation. This mechanism should regulate the expression of AQP1 in choroid plexus in the presence of hydrocephalus as an adaptation process. Adaptive feedback mechanisms exist and regulate the expression of AQP1 in the choroid plexus under specific circumstances – e.g., low gravity reduces the amount of AQP1 in the choroid plexus [10]. In addition, AQP1 expression is down-regulated in cases of compromised cerebral perfusion [4, 10, 11], while Silverberg et al. demonstrated that CSF production is reduced in patients with chronic hydrocephalus [19]. AQP1 down-regulation in the choroid plexus in cases of hydrocephalus could be an adaptive protective mechanism to lower the production of CSF and reduce the increased ICP. This effect was observed in AQP1-knockout mice in a study by Oshio et al. [14, 15] AQP1 loss could lead to reduction of CSF production and ICP. Interestingly, the results in the study of Oshio et al. indicated that systemic effects on the kidneys, where AQP1 is normally present, and reduction of central venous pressure could also contribute to this phenomenon apart from the loss of AQP1 at the choroid plexus [14, 15].

Other studies did not identify the down-regulation of AQP1 in hydrocephalus. The study of Mao et al. used a kaolin-induced hydrocephalus model in rats [9]. There were no significant changes in AQP1 expression after the induction of hydrocephalus. Longatti et al. in a series of human choroid plexus tumors found mixed expression patterns of AQP1 in cases complicated by hydrocephalus [7]. AQP1 showed strong expression in four cases of choroid plexus papillomas with hydrocephalus (obstructive in three and communicating in one) while weak expression was observed in one case of choroid plexus carcinoma complicated by obstructive hydrocephalus. It is not clear whether this is associated with a specific type of hydrocephalus or the genetic burden of the tumor. The small number of human cases reported, the heterogeneous expression of AQP1 in these cases, and the use of immunohistochemistry (a qualitative method) not accompanied by quantitative methods such as immunofluorescence, Western blot, or RT-PCR protocols cannot reveal the real patterns of expression of AQP1 in humans with hydrocephalus at present.

Conclusion

In summary, aquaporins, and especially AQP1 could possibly play a significant role in hydrocephalus as this is indicated in AQP1 expression studies in animal models of hydrocephalus and a few human case reports. Most of these studies show a down-regulation of AQP1 expression in hydrocephalus suggesting an adaptive feedback mechanism that acts to lower the production of CSF and ICP. Other studies failed to confirm these observations. Further research studies should be conducted to provide a clear picture of the role of AQP1 in hydrocephalus subtypes, validate the observations in humans, and provide the background for translational research strategies.

Conflicts of interest statement We declare that we have no conflict of interest.

References

1. Agre P, King LS, Yasui M, Guggino WB, Ottersen OP, Fujiyoshi Y, Engel A, Nielsen S (2002) Aquaporin water channels–from atomic structure to clinical medicine. J Physiol 542:3–16
2. Badaut J, Lasbennes F, Magistretti PJ, Regli L (2002) Aquaporins in brain: distribution, physiology, and pathophysiology. J Cereb Blood Flow Metab 22:367–378
3. Brown PD, Davies SL, Speake T, Millar ID (2004) Molecular mechanisms of cerebrospinal fluid production. Neuroscience 129:957–970
4. Edwards RJ, Dombrowski SM, Luciano MG, Pople IK (2004) Chronic hydrocephalus in adults. Brain Pathol 14:325–336
5. Johansson PA, Dziegielewska KM, Ek CJ, Habgood MD, Møllgård K, Potter A, Schuliga M, Saunders NR (2005) Aquaporin-1 in the choroid plexuses of developing mammalian brain. Cell Tissue Res 322:353–364
6. Kimelberg HK (2004) Water homeostasis in the brain: basic concepts. Neuroscience 129:851–860
7. Longatti P, Basaldella L, Orvieto E, Dei Tos A, Martinuzzi A (2006) Aquaporin(s) expression in choroid plexus tumours. Pediatr Neurosurg 42:228–233
8. Longatti PL, Basaldella L, Orvieto E, Fiorindi A, Carteri A (2004) Choroid plexus and aquaporin-1: a novel explanation of cerebrospinal fluid production. Pediatr Neurosurg 40:277–283
9. Mao X, Enno TL, Del Bigio MR (2006) Aquaporin 4 changes in rat brain with severe hydrocephalus. Eur J Neurosci 23:2929–2936
10. Masseguin C, Corcoran M, Carcenac C, Daunton NG, Güell A, Verkman AS, Gabrion J (2000) Altered gravity downregulates aquaporin-1 protein expression in choroid plexus. J Appl Physiol 88:843–850
11. Masseguin C, Mani-Ponset L, Herbuté S, Tixier-Vidal A, Gabrion J (2001) Persistence of tight junctions and changes in apical structures and protein expression in choroid plexus epithelium of rats after short-term head-down tilt. J Neurocytol 30:365–377
12. Mobasheri A, Marples D (2004) Expression of the AQP-1 water channel in normal human tissues: a semiquantitative study using tissue microarray technology. Am J Physiol Cell Physiol 286: C529–C537
13. Nielsen S, Smith BL, Christensen EI, Agre P (1993) Distribution of the aquaporin CHIP in secretory and resorptive epithelia and capillary endothelia. Proc Natl Acad Sci USA 90:7275–7279
14. Oshio K, Song Y, Verkman AS, Manley GT (2003) Aquaporin-1 deletion reduces osmotic water permeability and cerebrospinal fluid production. Acta Neurochir Suppl 86:525–528
15. Oshio K, Watanabe H, Song Y, Verkman AS, Manley GT (2005) Reduced cerebrospinal fluid production and intracranial pressure in mice lacking choroid plexus water channel Aquaporin-1. FASEB J 19:76–78

16. Paul L, Madan M, Rammling M, Behman B, Pattisapu JV (2009) The altered expression of aquaporin 1 and 4 in choroid plexus of congenital hydrocephalus. Cerebrospinal Fluid Res 6:S7
17. Praetorius J (2007) Water and solute secretion by the choroid plexus. Pflugers Arch 454:1–18
18. Praetorius J, Nielsen S (2006) Distribution of sodium transporters and aquaporin-1 in the human choroid plexus. Am J Physiol Cell Physiol 291:C59–C67
19. Silverberg GD, Huhn S, Jaffe RA, Chang SD, Saul T, Heit G, Von Essen A, Rubenstein E (2002) Downregulation of cerebrospinal fluid production in patients with chronic hydrocephalus. J Neurosurg 97:1271–1275
20. Smith ZA, Moftakhar P, Malkasian D, Xiong Z, Vinters HV, Lazareff JA (2007) Choroid plexus hyperplasia: surgical treatment and immunohistochemical results. Case report. J Neurosurg 107:255–262
21. Speake T, Freeman LJ, Brown PD (2003) Expression of aquaporin 1 and aquaporin 4 water channels in rat choroid plexus. Biochim Biophys Acta 1609:80–86
22. Tait MJ, Saadoun S, Bell BA, Papadopoulos MC (2008) Water movements in the brain: role of aquaporins. Trends Neurosci 31:37–43
23. Verkman AS (2009) Aquaporins: translating bench research to human disease. J Exp Biol 212:1707–1715

Hydrocephalus and Aquaporins: The Role of Aquaporin-4

A.S. Filippidis, M.Y.S. Kalani, and H.L. Rekate

Abstract *Introduction*: Aquaporins (AQPs) are membrane proteins that facilitate water and small solute movement in tissues. Hydrocephalus is the major central nervous system disorder associated with defective cerebrospinal fluid turnover. Aquaporin-4 (AQP4) is a water channel located mainly at the blood–brain barrier (BBB) and blood–cerebrospinal fluid (CSF) interfaces and is associated with the elimination of cerebral edema via these routes. The aim of this study is to review the pertinent literature concerning the role of AQP4 in the pathophysiology of hydrocephalus.

Methods: We performed a MEDLINE search using the terms *aquaporin* AND *hydrocephalus*. The results of the search were further refined to exclude studies not related to aquaporin-4.

Results: Six studies were identified. All studies utilized an animal model such as AQP4-knockout mice, H-Tx rats, and kaolin and L-α-lysophosphatidylcholine (LPC) stearoyl injection models of hydrocephalus. Most studies indicate that there is an up-regulation of AQP4 expression at the BBB and blood–CSF interfaces in cases of hydrocephalus. One study, reported sporadic cases of obstructive hydrocephalus in a subgroup of AQP4-knockout mice.

Conclusions: Few publications have studied the association between aquaporins and hydrocephalus. Currently, all the existing studies rely on animal models. An adaptive and protective role of AQP4 to increase the resolution of the "hydrocephalic" edema at the BBB and blood–CSF interfaces is proposed in the pathophysiology of hydrocephalus. Further research is needed to clarify if this association exists in humans.

Keywords Aquaporin • AQP4 • Cerebrospinal fluid (CSF) • Hydrocephalus • Water channel

A.S. Filippidis, and M.Y.S. Kalani
Division of Neurological Surgery, Barrow Neurological Institute,
St. Joseph's Hospital and Medical Center,
Phoenix, AZ, USA

H.L. Rekate (✉)
The Chiari Institute, Hofstra,
Northshore LIJ College of Medicine,
865 Northern Boulevard, 11021 Great Neck NY, USA
e-mail: haroldrekate@gmail.com

Introduction

The pathophysiology of hydrocephalus relies mainly on the delicate equilibrium between production, absorption, and circulation of cerebrospinal fluid (CSF). Cerebrospinal fluid consists mostly of water. Water homeostasis is significant in the physiology of the central nervous system [9]. Aquaporins (AQPs) are transmembrane proteins that regulate the movement of water and small solutes through the cell membrane, contributing to water homeostasis [1, 25, 28]. AQP1 and AQP4 are expressed in abundance in the central nervous system, while AQP4 shows the highest expression pattern of any other member of the AQP family [28]. The presence of AQPs in the central nervous system provides a background and a trigger for research in the field of CSF and water turnover especially in brain edema and hydrocephalus [4, 14, 28].

The aim of this study is to review the pertinent literature concerning the role of AQP4 in cerebrospinal fluid turnover and pathophysiology of hydrocephalus. The information obtained from this process will be used to clarify any potential association between AQP4 and hydrocephalus, define further experimental approaches, and focus on key pathophysiological steps as candidates for pharmacological treatment.

Methods

We performed a MEDLINE search using the terms *aquaporin* AND *hydrocephalus*. The results of the search were further refined to exclude studies not related to AQP4. Animal studies were identified and categorized according to species and models used.

Results

Six studies were identified. The animal models used were AQP4-knockout mice, H-Tx rats, and kaolin and L-α-lysophosphatidylcholine (LPC) stearoyl injection models of hydrocephalus.

Bloch and colleagues, used AQP4-knockout mice and wild-type mice and reproduced obstructive hydrocephalus with kaolin injection in the cisterna magna [5]. Significant ventriculomegaly, and increased intracranial pressure (ICP) and brain water content (increased by 2–3%) were observed in the AQP4-knockout mice group [5]. The increased brain water content in AQP4-knockout mice indicated the existence of "hydrocephalic edema." A 5-day survival study revealed that 84% of the wild-type mice survived compared with 66% of AQP4-knockout mice, indicating that hydrocephalus induced by kaolin injection was much more severe in mice that do not express AQP4. The authors also used a computational model to reconfirm the observations obtained and predicted that the severity of hydrocephalus will be much more reduced when AQP4 expression increases. A protective role of AQP4 concerning hydrocephalus was suggested [5].

Mao and colleagues also used a kaolin injection hydrocephalus model to study AQP4 changes in normal rat brains that finally developed severe hydrocephalus [13]. Kaolin injection resulted in up-regulation of AQP4 expression 3–4 weeks later. High expression areas of AQP4 were identified in perivascular areas, parietal cerebrum and hippocampus, ependymal lining and glia limitans. AQP4 levels do not increase significantly until rats become 7 weeks old, while elevated expression can be observed for up to 9 months indicating a time-sensitive and pressure or extracellular fluid (due to transparenchymal flow of CSF in hydrocephalus) adaptive mechanism. The white matter demonstrated significant edema and showed evidence of fragmentation in the youngest group of hydrocephalic rats, while it was atrophic in the older group [13].

The congenital hydrocephalic rat (H-Tx rat) is an established animal model of hydrocephalus. Paul et al. and Shen et al. studied the expression of AQP4 in this animal model [21, 24]. Areas of AQP4 overexpression were identified. AQP4 was highly expressed at the ependymal lining, the end-feet processes of pericapillary astrocytes, and the subpial zone in H-Tx rats and indicated an adaptive mechanism. Shen et al. further discussed the role of AQP4 in the pathophysiology of a subset H-Tx rat group with "arrested hydrocephalus" [24]. This interpretation and the definition of "arrested hydrocephalus" were mainly based on the higher survival of animals expressing more AQP4, without providing any evidence about the severity of ventriculomegaly [15].

Communicating inflammatory hydrocephalus was modeled in rats using L-α-lysophosphatidylcholine (LPC) stearoyl injections. Tourdias et al. studied the AQP4 expression in this model [27]. AQP4 was also up-regulated at the blood–CSF and blood–brain barrier interfaces in hydrocephalic rat brains compared with controls [27]. Magnetic resonance studies in these rats revealed a significantly bigger apparent diffusion coefficient (APC) and larger CSF volumes, which were correlated with elevated expression of AQP4.

Table 1 Studies concerning aquaporin-4 and hydrocephalus

Studies	Species	Method	AQPs studied	Results
Shen et al. [24]	Rats	H-Tx	AQP4	Upregulated
Mao et al. [13]	Rats	Kaolin injected	AQPs 1,4,9	AQP4 upregulated
Tourdias et al. [27]	Rats	LPC injected inflammatory HCP	AQP4	Upregulated
Paul et al. [21]	Rats	H-Tx, choroid plexus culture	AQPs 1,4	AQP1 low/ AQP4 high
Bloch et al. [5]	Mice	AQP4-KO, kaolin injected	AQP4	Higher ICP, CSF volume, lower survival in AQP4-KO
Feng et al. [7]	Mice	AQP4-KO	AQP4	Sporadic obstr HCP

AQP aquaporin, *HCP* hydrocephalus, *obstr* obstructive, *AQP4-KO* aquaporin-4 knockout mice, *H-Tx* congenital hydrocephalic rats, *ICP* intracranial pressure, *LPC* L-α-lysophosphatidylcholine stearoyl

Feng and colleagues published an interesting observation concerning AQP4-knockout mice [7]. In a series of 612 AQP4-knockout mice, a percentage of 9.6% demonstrated obstructive hydrocephalus. The level of cerebral aqueduct was identified as the site of obstruction, leading to aqueductal stenosis. Marked ependymal disorganization was present at the site of stenosis. The authors attributed the presence of sporadic obstructive hydrocephalus in a subset of AQP4-knockout mice, to AQP4 polymorphisms that could contribute to the development of aqueductal stenosis [7, 28].

Discussion

Hydrocephalus is a disease of the central nervous system with a pathophysiology associated with the disruption of the delicate equilibrium between CSF production, absorption, and circulation. CSF physiology is linked to water circulation and distribution in the central nervous system, since CSF consists mostly of water. Aquaporins are water channels with a significant role in water homeostasis in various systems as well as the central nervous system [9]. Currently there are no studies concerning hydrocephalus and AQP4 in humans. The association between aquaporins and hydrocephalus is demonstrated in studies (Table 1) based mainly in animal models like AQP4-knockout mice, kaolin- or LPC-induced hydrocephalus in rats, and congenitally hydrocephalic rats (H-Tx rats). Thus, the knowledge concerning the role of AQP4 in hydrocephalus derives mainly from the laboratory. Whether the results obtained can be revalidated in humans is not known.

Most hydrocephalus studies show that AQP4 expression is up-regulated in the blood–CSF and blood–brain barriers [13, 21, 24, 27]. Whether this up-regulation is linked to the cause of hydrocephalus or depicts an adaptive feedback mechanism that tries to resolve the hydrocephalic changes needs further clarification. Few clues exist that could help us understand the pathophysiology underlying AQP4 up-regulation in hydrocephalus models. In the study of Bloch et al. [5], AQP4-knockout mice survived for a shorter time than wild-type mice when hydrocephalus was induced by kaolin injection in the cisterna magna. This observation indicates that the presence of AQP4 could act protectively in this context. The significant role of AQP4 in the clearance of excess brain water and specifically vasogenic brain edema has been documented in multiple other studies [2, 3, 8, 12, 14, 17–20, 23, 26]. These studies provide us with clues about the potential role of AQP4 in hydrocephalus as an adaptive mechanism that is up-regulated to aid the resolution of excess brain water termed "hydrocephalic edema" by Klatzo et al. [10]. This type of interstitial brain edema is subsequent to impaired CSF turnover and increased ICP. It is observed as transependymal CSF flow in neuroimaging studies of hydrocephalus [10, 25]. The role of AQPs in relation to the resolution of the "hydrocephalic edema" could be significant and shed more light on the pathophysiology and treatment of hydrocephalus.

An interesting perspective is the identification of the sites of "hydrocephalic edema" clearance related to AQP4 contribution. Aquaporins are highly expressed at known sites of CSF production and absorption such as the choroid plexus and extrachoroidal sites and ependymal cells, glia limitans interna, and CSF circulation at the cortical subarachnoid space such as in the glia limitans externa, subpial zone, and meninges. In addition, AQP4 is highly expressed at the endfeet of the astrocyte processes that are part of the blood–brain barrier [4, 6, 11, 16, 22, 25, 28]. In the studies of AQP4 and brain edema, three brain edema clearance pathways have been identified [25]. The first one is the brain parenchyma-ventricular pathway, which drives excess water in the ventricles. The second one is the brain parenchyma–brain cortex–subarachnoid space pathway driving excess water to the subarachnoid space, and the last is the brain parenchyma–astrocyte endfeet processes–brain capillaries pathway driving excess water from the brain to the systemic circulation. The pathway that is used to resolve the "hydrocephalic edema" via an AQP4-mediated route is currently unknown.

Conclusion

The results obtained from animal studies indicate that AQP4 plays a distinct role in hydrocephalus. An adaptive feedback mechanism is proposed. Indications exist about the up-regulation of AQP4, which acts protectively in cases of hydrocephalus and provides a pathway for "hydrocephalic edema" clearance. The results should be revalidated in human studies to provide a useful armamentarium in the treatment of hydrocephalus and aid in the design of a new class of drugs that deal with the regulation of AQPs in hydrocephalus.

Conflicts of interest statement We declare that we have no conflict of interest.

References

1. Agre P, King LS, Yasui M, Guggino WB, Ottersen OP, Fujiyoshi Y, Engel A, Nielsen S (2002) Aquaporin water channels–from atomic structure to clinical medicine. J Physiol 542:3–16
2. Agre P, Kozono D (2003) Aquaporin water channels: molecular mechanisms for human diseases. FEBS Lett 555:72–78
3. Badaut J, Brunet JF, Grollimund L, Hamou MF, Magistretti PJ, Villemure JG, Regli L (2003) Aquaporin 1 and aquaporin 4 expression in human brain after subarachnoid hemorrhage and in peritumoral tissue. Acta Neurochir Suppl 86:495–498
4. Badaut J, Lasbennes F, Magistretti PJ, Regli L (2002) Aquaporins in brain: distribution, physiology, and pathophysiology. J Cereb Blood Flow Metab 22:367–378
5. Bloch O, Auguste KI, Manley GT, Verkman AS (2006) Accelerated progression of kaolin-induced hydrocephalus in aquaporin-4-deficient mice. J Cereb Blood Flow Metab 26:1527–1537
6. Cserr HF (1971) Physiology of the choroid plexus. Physiol Rev 51:273–311
7. Feng X, Papadopoulos MC, Liu J, Li L, Zhang D, Zhang H, Verkman AS, Ma T (2009) Sporadic obstructive hydrocephalus in Aqp4 null mice. J Neurosci Res 87:1150–1155
8. Hirt L, Ternon B, Price M, Mastour N, Brunet J-F, Badaut J (2009) Protective role of early aquaporin 4 induction against postischemic edema formation. J Cereb Blood Flow Metab 29:423–433
9. Kimelberg HK (2004) Water homeostasis in the brain: basic concepts. Neuroscience 129:851–860
10. Klatzo I (1994) Evolution of brain edema concepts. Acta Neurochir Suppl 60:3–6
11. Macaulay N, Zeuthen T (2010) Water transport between CNS compartments: contributions of aquaporins and cotransporters. Neuroscience 168:941–956
12. Manley GT, Binder DK, Papadopoulos MC, Verkman AS (2004) New insights into water transport and edema in the central nervous system from phenotype analysis of aquaporin-4 null mice. Neuroscience 129:983–991
13. Mao X, Enno TL, Del Bigio MR (2006) Aquaporin 4 changes in rat brain with severe hydrocephalus. Eur J Neurosci 23:2929–2936
14. Marmarou A (2007) A review of progress in understanding the pathophysiology and treatment of brain edema. Neurosurg Focus 22:E1
15. Mcallister JP, Miller JM (2006) Aquaporin 4 and hydrocephalus. J Neurosurg 105:457–458; discussion 458
16. Mobasheri A, Marples D (2004) Expression of the AQP-1 water channel in normal human tissues: a semiquantitative study using tissue microarray technology. Am J Physiol Cell Physiol 286:C529–C537
17. Nico B, Mangieri D, Tamma R, Longo V, Annese T, Crivellato E, Pollo B, Maderna E, Ribatti D, Salmaggi A (2009) Aquaporin-4 contributes to the resolution of peritumoural brain oedema in human glioblastoma multiforme after combined chemotherapy and radiotherapy. Eur J Cancer 45:3315–3325

18. Papadopoulos MC, Manley GT, Krishna S, Verkman AS (2004) Aquaporin-4 facilitates reabsorption of excess fluid in vasogenic brain edema. FASEB J 18:1291–1293
19. Papadopoulos MC, Saadoun S, Binder DK, Manley GT, Krishna S, Verkman AS (2004) Molecular mechanisms of brain tumor edema. Neuroscience 129:1011–1020
20. Papadopoulos MC, Verkman AS (2007) Aquaporin-4 and brain edema. Pediatr Nephrol 22:778–784
21. Paul L, Madan M, Rammling M, Behman B, Pattisapu JV (2009) The altered expression of aquaporin 1 and 4 in choroid plexus of congenital hydrocephalus. Cerebrospinal Fluid Res 6:S7
22. Praetorius J, Nielsen S (2006) Distribution of sodium transporters and aquaporin-1 in the human choroid plexus. Am J Physiol Cell Physiol 291:C59–C67
23. Saadoun S, Papadopoulos M, Bell B, Krishna S, Davies D (2002) The aquaporin-4 water channel and brain tumour oedema. J Anat 200:528
24. Shen XQ, Miyajima M, Ogino I, Arai H (2006) Expression of the water-channel protein aquaporin 4 in the H-Tx rat: possible compensatory role in spontaneously arrested hydrocephalus. J Neurosurg 105:459–464
25. Tait MJ, Saadoun S, Bell BA, Papadopoulos MC (2008) Water movements in the brain: role of aquaporins. Trends Neurosci 31:37–43
26. Tait MJ, Saadoun S, Bell BA, Verkman AS, Papadopoulos MC (2010) Increased brain edema in aqp4-null mice in an experimental model of subarachnoid hemorrhage. Neuroscience 167:60–67
27. Tourdias T, Dragonu I, Fushimi Y, Deloire MSA, Boiziau C, Brochet B, Moonen C, Petry KG, Dousset V (2009) Aquaporin 4 correlates with apparent diffusion coefficient and hydrocephalus severity in the rat brain: a combined MRI-histological study. Neuroimage 47:659–666
28. Verkman AS (2009) Aquaporins: translating bench research to human disease. J Exp Biol 212:1707–1715

Effect of Acetazolamide on Aquaporin-1 and Fluid Flow in Cultured Choroid Plexus

Pouya A. Ameli, Meenu Madan, Srinivasulu Chigurupati, Amin Yu, Sic L. Chan, and Jogi V. Pattisapu

Abstract Acetazolamide (AZA), used in treatment of early or infantile hydrocephalus, is effective in some cases, while its effect on the choroid plexus (CP) remains ill-defined. The drug reversibly inhibits aquaporin-4 (AQP4), the most ubiquitous "water pore" in the brain, and perhaps modulation of AQP1 (located apically on CP cells) by AZA may reduce cerebrospinal fluid (CSF) production. We sought to elucidate the effect of AZA on AQP1 and fluid flow in CP cell cultures.

CP tissue culture from 10-day Sprague–Dawley rats and a TRCSF-B cell line were grown on Transwell permeable supports and treated with 100 μM AZA. Fluid assays to assess direction and extent of fluid flow, and AQP1 expression patterns by immunoblot, Immuncytochemistry (ICC), and quantitative reverse transcriptase polymerase chain reaction (qRT-PCR) were performed.

Immunoblots and ICC analyses showed a decrease in AQP1 protein shortly after AZA treatment (lowest at 12 h), with transient AQP1 reduction mediated by mRNA expression (lowest at 6 h). Transwell fluid assays indicated a fluid shift at 2 h, before significant changes in AQP1 mRNA or protein levels.

Timing of AZA effect on AQP1 suggests the drug alters protein transcription, while affecting fluid flow by a concomitant method. It is plausible that other mechanisms account for these phenomena, as the processes may occur independently.

Keywords Acetazolamide • Aquaporin-1 • Hydrocephalus • Choroid plexus • TRCSF-B • Cerebrospinal fluid

Introduction

Hydrocephalus is a disorder caused by an excessive accumulation of cerebrospinal fluid (CSF) within the cranial cavity, often causing developmental and functional deficits in the pediatric age group. Recent literature suggests that hydrocephalus accounts for 1.8% of days in children's hospitals (0.6% of admissions) and 3.1% of all pediatric hospital charges [26].

Acetazolamide (AZA) is a carbonic anhydrase (CA) inhibitor used as an initial treatment in certain cases of early or infantile hydrocephalus, glaucoma, idiopathic intracranial hypertension, and seizures [3, 4, 12, 31]. Understanding the role of choroid plexus (CP) in CSF production or absorption is necessary to effectively treat hydrocephalus, and elucidating the effects of AZA on this structure may provide future therapeutic targets for such fluid disorders [7].

Aquaporins (AQPs) are ubiquitously expressed cellular pores capable of transporting water, ions, and small non-polar molecules [1, 2]. The brain expresses 6 aquaporin isoforms (AQP1, AQP3, AQP4, AQP5, AQP8, and AQP9) [2, 14, 22, 32, 34], of which three have been significantly characterized (AQP1, AQP4, AQP9). AQP4 is predominant in the brain, while AQP1 is of particular interest for its abundance in CP cells [9, 36]. The high expression levels of AQP1 in the apical layer of CP cells implies a role in CSF production, fluid flow, and injury response [21, 37]. Interestingly, the role of AQP1 in these mechanisms is controversial, since AZA also decreases CSF production in AQP1-null mice [25].

Our goal was to determine the relationships between AZA, AQP1, and fluid flow, and we postulated that AZA alters active AQP1 levels in CP cells (via alterations in expression and/or function), by a mechanism unrelated to changes in fluid flow.

P.A. Ameli, M. Madan, S. Chigurupati, A. Yu, S. Chan, and J.V. Pattisapu (✉)
Burnett School of Biomedical Sciences, College of Medicine, University of Central Florida, Orlando, FL, USA
e-mail: jogi.pattisapu@UCF.edu

Methods

All protocols were approved by the Institutional Animal Care Committee at our institution.

Tissue Culture

CP tissue was harvested from lateral and fourth ventricles and digested in 0.25% trypsin. The solution was passed through a 100 μm cell strainer and stored in culture medium [6, 8]. Cells were maintained at 37°C, 5% CO_2 on laminin-coated cultureware, and the medium was changed every 24–48 h. Primary cultures were grown in DMEM:F12 with 10% FBS, 4 mM glutamine, 5 μg/mL insulin, 10U/mL Penicillin, 0.1 mg/mL streptomycin, 10 ng/mL EGF, 5 μg/mL Insulin, 5 μg/mL transferrin, and 5 ng/mL sodium selenite. For the first 96 h of culture, 4uM cytosine arabinoside was supplemented to reduce fibroblast contamination. The immortalized CP cell line (TRCSF-B) cell line was grown according to published guidelines, and the medium was changed every 24–48 h [28].

Reverse Transcriptase Polymerase Chain Reaction (RT-PCR)

CP primary culture was treated with either 1× fluid assay buffer (FAB) alone or with 100 μM AZA (A6011; Sigma). Baseline wells treated with vehicle were harvested at 24 h. RNA was harvested with RLT buffer (Qiagen) and the RNeasy kit (Qiagen, Germantown, MD, USA) at 1, 3, 6, 12, and 24 h. cDNA was prepared with the iScript kit (Bio-Rad). Analysis of AQP1 mRNA via qRT-PCR utilized primers described below, with 18S as an internal control.

AQP1 F: CCCTCTTCGTCTTCATCAGC	18S F: GTAACCCGTTGAACCCCATT
AQP1 R: GTTGAGGTGAGCACCACTGA	18S R: CCATCCAATCGGTAGTAGCG

Immunoblot

Cells were treated with fetal bovine serum (FBS) media, FAB (baseline), or 100 μM AZA in FAB for 6, 12, and 24 h, and lysed with Laemlli buffer. Blocking was done with 5% milk/PBS-T/0.05% Tween-20 and probed with anti-AQP1 Ab (AQP11-A; Alpha Diagnostics) and goat anti-rabbit 1:5,000 secondary Ab (sc-2004; Santa Cruz Biotechnology). Anti-β-Actin (A1978; Sigma, Saint Louis, MO, USA) and goat anti-mouse (sc-2020; Santa Cruz Biotechnology) were also used.

Fluid Assay

Monolayer confluence was assessed by Lucifer Yellow passage assay and trans-epithelial electrical resistance (TEER) (EVOm2 machine; World Precision Instruments). Ten percent FBS medium was exchanged for 0.5% FBS medium 1 day prior to assay. Fluid assay was done in FAB (15 mM NaHCO3, 15 mM HEPES, 0.5 mM Na_2HPO_4, 0.5 mM NaH_2PO_4, 17.5 mM glucose, 122 mM NaCl, 4 mM KCl, 1 mM $CaCl_2$, 1 mM $MgCl_2$, 5 μg/mL insulin, pH 7.3) following Hakvoort et al. [8]. Apical and basolateral fluids were harvested at 2, 6, 12, and 24 h. Baseline wells were harvested at 2 h. All measures were in triplicate and averaged. The follow equation for fluid flow was used: $V_{sec} = [(CFD_i - CFD_a) \div CFD_i] \times V_0$. Where V_{sec} = volume secreted (μL/h); CFD_i = initial fluorescent reading; CFD_a = final fluorescent reading; V_0 = initial volume of fluid applied to transwell membrane (350 μL).

Immunocytochemistry

Transwell membranes were fixed at 4% PFA and blocked with 10% goat serum/0.1% Triton X-100 prior to incubation with 1:200 primary Ab (AQP1, AQP11-A; Alpha Diagnostics; Kir 7.1, sc-22440; Santa Cruz Biotechnology). Incubation with 1:200 secondary Ab (Goat Anti-Rabbit Alexa Fluor 488 or Goat Anti-Mouse Alexa Fluor 568), and nuclear staining with Hoescht 33362 was done. Membranes were mounted with fluorsave (345789; Calbiochem).

Results

Immunoblots revealed that treated cells displayed a decrease and subsequent return of AQP1 protein expression, as compared with baseline, when harvested at 2, 6, 12, and 24 h. This trend implies a relationship between AZA and AQP1 expression mechanisms (Fig. 1). Immunoblots correlated with the immunocytochemistry images, which revealed initial decrease and subsequent punctate resurgence of AQP1 protein (Fig. 2).

RT-PCR using AQP1 primers and 18S (loading control) illustrated a trend in mRNA expression similar to that seen in the immunoblot and immunocytochemistry, suggesting that previously observed alterations in protein expression were mediated by AQP1 mRNA levels. It appears AZA affects AQP1 expression via a mechanism that decreases AQP1 mRNA (Fig. 1).

Fluid assay with AZA was performed on confluent transwells seeded with CP primary culture or TRCSF-B cell line. Both primary culture and cell line showed immediate shift in fluid transport away from the apical chamber. The fluid shift occurs earlier than the decrease in AQP1 expression, indicating that the shift in fluid flow after AZA treatment is minimally related to AQP1 levels (Fig. 3).

Fig. 1 Aquaporin-1 (AQP1) protein and mRNA expression levels in acetazolamide (AZA)-treated choroid plexus (CP) primary culture (**a**) Immunoblot of AQP1 expression, normalized to β-actin. (**b**) Densitometric analysis of AQP1 immunoblot. Decrease of AQP1 protein at 12 h is significant. (**c**) RT-PCR of AQP1 mRNA levels, normalized to 18S (*Veh* Vehicle, *NT* Nontreated) (*p<0.05, **p<0.01, ***p<0.001)

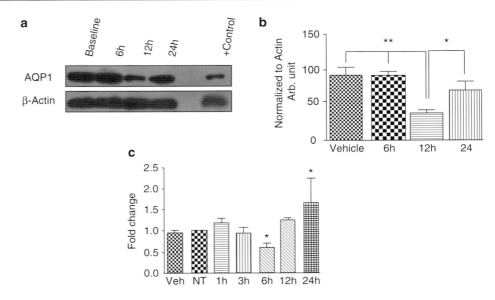

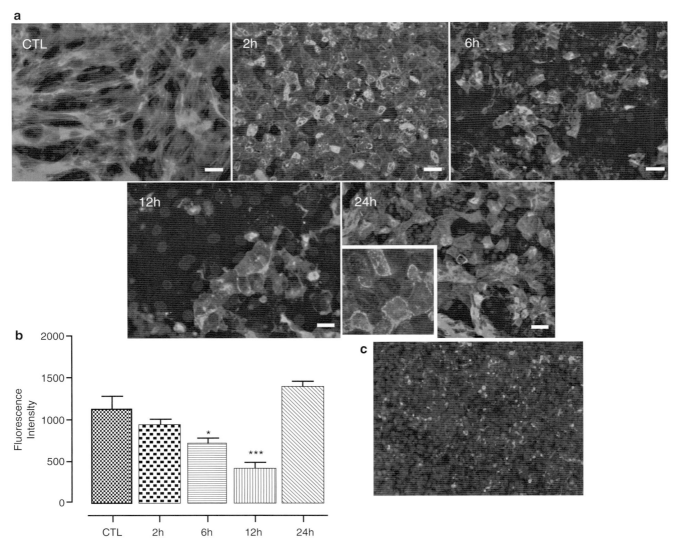

Fig. 2 Immunocytochemistry of choroid plexus (CP) primary cultures. (**a**) Aquaporin-1 (AQP1) levels shown (*green*) along with Hoescht nuclear stain (*blue*). Gradual decrease and return of AQP1 protein is observed. Insert of 24-h time point displays punctate AQP1 with strong localization to cell membranes. (**b**) Quantification of AQP1 fluorescent intensity in ICC. Decreases in AQP1 at 6 and 12 h are significant. (**c**) ICC of Kir 7.1 CP marker in primary culture shows sufficient enrichment of CP cells. *Scale bar* 20 μm (*p<0.05, **p<0.01, ***p<0.001)

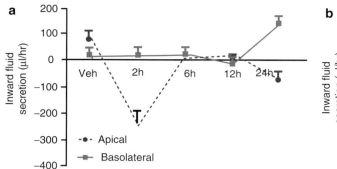

Fig. 3 TRITC-Dextran fluid assay of acetazolamide (AZA)-treated confluent monolayers. (**a**) Fluid assay of choroid plexus (CP) primary culture shows an AZA-induced decrease in apical fluid flow at 2 h. (**b**) Fluid assay of TRCSF-B cell line culture displays a similar trend to that seen in primary culture

Discussion

Aquaporins play a key role in several neurologic disorders and understanding their physiology is important for effective medical management [15, 24, 25, 35]. The majority of the brain's AQP1 is located at the apical membrane of the CSF-producing CP, which is of particular interest in hydrocephalus [11, 23]. Decreased AQP1 expression levels in rat CP have been correlated with reduced CSF production, and AQP1-null mice display a 25% reduction in CSF production [20, 24, 25].

A diuretic which inhibits CA, AZA is used in the treatment of multiple fluid disorders [3, 12]. The drug inhibits AQP4, and in hydrocephalic states, AZA possibly reduces CSF production by inhibiting AQP1 [5, 17]. Although it has a negligible effect on purified AQP1 protein, CSF production is decreased in AQP1-null mice receiving the drug, raising questions about its mechanism of action [25, 27]. The relationship between AZA, AQP1, and CSF production is controversial, and this study was undertaken to further elucidate these relationships.

Immunoblots and ICC of AZA-treated CP cells revealed a continual decrease in AQP1 protein over 12 h, before return to baseline levels at 24 h (Figs. 1 and 2). Interestingly, a rebound phenomenon was seen at 24 h with a notable increase in mRNA levels and a modest increase in protein, similar to prior rodent studies [20].

At later time points, ICC images showed an increase in punctate AQP1 within the cell, suggesting AZA regulation of AQP1 may occur at the level of transcription (Fig. 2). RT-PCR results demonstrate a maximum decrease in AQP1 mRNA levels at 6 h that corresponds temporally to the illustrated decreases in AQP1 protein at 12 h (Fig. 1). This would imply that the effect of AZA on AQP1 does not involve direct interaction of drug with protein, corresponding to previous reports of AZA inability to inhibit purified AQP1 [27].

Primary CP cells grown in transwells identified AZA-induced fluid flow change at 2 h (Fig. 3). This decrease in apical flow suggests less CSF production, but occurs earlier than the decreases in both AQP1 mRNA and protein expression. Notably, the apical fluid flow was decreased at 2 h without corresponding increase in basolateral fluid flow, suggesting retention of fluid by CP cells during AZA treatment. This is consistent with the changes in cell morphology (large, round cells seen in immunocytochemistry) (Fig. 2). AZA has previously been shown to increase cell volume and water retention [10].

The TRCSF-B cell line expressed very low levels of AQP1 protein, and was therefore used as a negative control for AQP1-rich CP primary culture cells. Transwell studies of confluent TRCSF-B cells demonstrated similar fluid flow characteristics (as seen in primary culture) despite the lack of AQP1 protein (Fig. 3).

Initial changes in AQP1 expression appear unrelated to fluid flow alterations as observed by the timing of these events. Previous data are contradictory regarding AZA–AQP1 interactions, and these findings may be partially reconciled with our data suggesting AZA alters fluid flow early, with delayed effect on AQP1 expression [5, 17, 25]. To our knowledge, we are the first to show that AZA treatment affects AQP1 levels in a manner unrelated to fluid flow.

In recent studies, soluble adenylyl cyclase (sAC) is activated by the presence of bicarbonate ion [30]. Interestingly, it has also been shown that increases in Protein Kinase A (PKA) activity increases AQP1 levels [18, 19, 29]. In the lung, PKA-mediated thyroid transcription factor-1 (TTF-1) phosphorylation is activated by cAMP [16]. TTF-1 is coexpressed with AQP1 in rat CP, which enhances transcription of the aquaporin [13]. Thus, it is possible for AZA (a known inhibitor of CA) to modulate adenylyl cyclase and affect AQP1 expression in a manner independent of fluid flow [12]. These pathways offer a potential reason for the delayed overexpression of AQP1 observed in these experiments.

Acetazolamide treatment of CP monolayers decreases the apical fluid flow and leads to an associated fall and subsequent resurgence in the levels of AQP1 at both the protein and RNA levels. This drug-induced change in AQP1 expression may be mediated by adenylyl cyclase, cAMP, PKA, and TTF-1, perhaps causing the observed rebound increase in the water channel protein.

Conclusion

AZA affects CP fluid flow via a mechanism initially independent of AQP1 expression, and future studies should focus on the relationship between AZA and AQP1 as well as AZA and apical fluid flow. Improved understanding of such mechanisms will facilitate drug development for treating brain fluid disorders (including hydrocephalus) [7, 33].

Acknowledgements We would like to thank Mr. Larry Phillips and Codman DePuy, a Johnson & Johnson company for funding this project, Erica Lankenau for her role in preparation of experimental materials, and Prof. Tetsuya Terasaki for providing the TRCSF-B cell line.

Conflicts of interest statement We declare that we have no conflict of interest.

References

1. Agre P (1998) Aquaporin null phenotypes: the importance of classical physiology. Proc Natl Acad Sci USA 95:9061–9063
2. Agre P, King LS, Yasui M, Guggino WB, Ottersen OP, Fujiyoshi Y, Engel A, Nielsen S (2002) Aquaporin water channels–from atomic structure to clinical medicine. J Physiol 542:3–16
3. Celebisoy N, Gokcay F, Sirin H, Akyurekli O (2007) Treatment of idiopathic intracranial hypertension: topiramate vs acetazolamide, an open-label study. Acta Neurol Scand 116:322–327
4. Custer JW, Rau RE (eds) (2009) The Harriet Lane handbook. Elsevier Mosby, Philadelphia
5. Gao J, Wang X, Chang Y, Zhang J, Song Q, Yu H, Li X (2006) Acetazolamide inhibits osmotic water permeability by interaction with aquaporin-1. Anal Biochem 350:165–170
6. Gath U, Hakvoort A, Wegener J, Decker S, Galla HJ (1997) Porcine choroid plexus cells in culture: expression of polarized phenotype, maintenance of barrier properties and apical secretion of CSF-components. Eur J Cell Biol 74:68–78
7. Haddoub R, Rutzler M, Robin A, Flitsch SL (2009) Design, synthesis and assaying of potential aquaporin inhibitors. Handb Exp Pharmacol 190: 385–402
8. Hakvoort A, Haselbach M, Galla HJ (1998) Active transport properties of porcine choroid plexus cells in culture. Brain Res 795:247–256
9. Johanson CE, Duncan JA 3rd, Klinge PM, Brinker T, Stopa EG, Silverberg GD (2008) Multiplicity of cerebrospinal fluid functions: new challenges in health and disease. Cerebrospinal Fluid Res 5:10
10. Johanson CE, Murphy VA (1990) Acetazolamide and insulin alter choroid plexus epithelial cell [Na+], pH, and volume. Am J Physiol 258:F1538–F1546
11. Johansson PA, Dziegielewska KM, Ek CJ, Habgood MD, Mollgard K, Potter A, Schuliga M, Saunders NR (2005) Aquaporin-1 in the choroid plexuses of developing mammalian brain. Cell Tissue Res 322:353–364
12. Kaur IP, Smitha R, Aggarwal D, Kapil M (2002) Acetazolamide: future perspective in topical glaucoma therapeutics. Int J Pharm 248:1–14
13. Kim JG, Son YJ, Yun CH, Kim YI, Nam-Goong IS, Park JH, Park SK, Ojeda SR, D'Elia AV, Damante G, Lee BJ (2007) Thyroid transcription factor-1 facilitates cerebrospinal fluid formation by regulating aquaporin-1 synthesis in the brain. J Biol Chem 282:14923–14931
14. King LS, Kozono D, Agre P (2004) From structure to disease: the evolving tale of aquaporin biology. Nat Rev Mol Cell Biol 5:687–698
15. Kleffner I, Bungeroth M, Schiffbauer H, Schabitz WR, Ringelstein EB, Kuhlenbaumer G (2008) The role of aquaporin-4 polymorphisms in the development of brain edema after middle cerebral artery occlusion. Stroke 39:1333–1335
16. Li J, Gao E, Mendelson CR (1998) Cyclic AMP-responsive expression of the surfactant protein-A gene is mediated by increased DNA binding and transcriptional activity of thyroid transcription factor-1. J Biol Chem 273:4592–4600
17. Ma B, Xiang Y, Mu SM, Li T, Yu HM, Li XJ (2004) Effects of acetazolamide and anordiol on osmotic water permeability in AQP1-cRNA injected Xenopus oocyte. Acta Pharmacol Sin 25:90–97
18. Marinelli RA, Pham L, Agre P, LaRusso NF (1997) Secretin promotes osmotic water transport in rat cholangiocytes by increasing aquaporin-1 water channels in plasma membrane. Evidence for a secretin-induced vesicular translocation of aquaporin-1. J Biol Chem 272:12984–12988
19. Marinelli RA, Tietz PS, Pham LD, Rueckert L, Agre P, LaRusso NF (1999) Secretin induces the apical insertion of aquaporin-1 water channels in rat cholangiocytes. Am J Physiol 276:G280–G286
20. Masseguin C, Corcoran M, Carcenac C, Daunton NG, Guell A, Verkman AS, Gabrion J (2000) Altered gravity downregulates aquaporin-1 protein expression in choroid plexus. J Appl Physiol 88:843–850
21. McCoy E, Sontheimer H (2010) MAPK induces AQP1 expression in astrocytes following injury. Glia 58:209–217
22. Morishita Y, Sakube Y, Sasaki S, Ishibashi K (2004) Molecular mechanisms and drug development in aquaporin water channel diseases: aquaporin superfamily (superaquaporins): expansion of aquaporins restricted to multicellular organisms. J Pharmacol Sci 96:276–279
23. Nielsen S, Smith BL, Christensen EI, Agre P (1993) Distribution of the aquaporin CHIP in secretory and resorptive epithelia and capillary endothelia. Proc Natl Acad Sci USA 90:7275–7279
24. Oshio K, Song Y, Verkman AS, Manley GT (2003) Aquaporin-1 deletion reduces osmotic water permeability and cerebrospinal fluid production. Acta Neurochir Suppl 86:525–528
25. Oshio K, Watanabe H, Song Y, Verkman AS, Manley GT (2005) Reduced cerebrospinal fluid production and intracranial pressure in mice lacking choroid plexus water channel Aquaporin-1. FASEB J 19:76–78
26. Simon TD, Lamb S, Murphy NA, Hom B, Walker ML, Clark EB (2009) Who will care for me next? Transitioning to adulthood with hydrocephalus. Pediatrics 124:1431–1437
27. Tanimura Y, Hiroaki Y, Fujiyoshi Y (2009) Acetazolamide reversibly inhibits water conduction by aquaporin-4. J Struct Biol 166:16–21
28. Terasaki T, Hosoya K (2001) Conditionally immortalized cell lines as a new in vitro model for the study of barrier functions. Biol Pharm Bull 24:111–118
29. Tietz PS, Marinelli RA, Chen XM, Huang B, Cohn J, Kole J, McNiven MA, Alper S, LaRusso NF (2003) Agonist-induced coordinated trafficking of functionally related transport proteins for water and ions in cholangiocytes. J Biol Chem 278:20413–20419
30. Tresguerres M, Parks SK, Salazar E, Levin LR, Goss GG, Buck J (2010) Bicarbonate-sensing soluble adenylyl cyclase is an essential sensor for acid/base homeostasis. Proc Natl Acad Sci USA 107:442–447
31. Vagal AS, Leach JL, Fernandez-Ulloa M, Zuccarello M (2009) The acetazolamide challenge: techniques and applications in the evaluation of chronic cerebral ischemia. AJNR Am J Neuroradiol 30:876–884

32. Verkman AS (2005) Novel roles of aquaporins revealed by phenotype analysis of knockout mice. Rev Physiol Biochem Pharmacol 155:31–55
33. Wolburg H, Paulus W (2010) Choroid plexus: biology and pathology. Acta Neuropathol 119:75–88
34. Yamamoto N, Yoneda K, Asai K, Sobue K, Tada T, Fujita Y, Katsuya H, Fujita M, Aihara N, Mase M, Yamada K, Miura Y, Kato T (2001) Alterations in the expression of the AQP family in cultured rat astrocytes during hypoxia and reoxygenation. Brain Res Mol Brain Res 90:26–38
35. Zador Z, Stiver S, Wang V, Manley GT (2009) Role of aquaporin-4 in cerebral edema and stroke. Handb Exp Pharmacol 190: 159–170
36. Zelenina M (2010) Regulation of brain aquaporins. Neurochem Int 190:468–488
37. Zhang D, Vetrivel L, Verkman AS (2002) Aquaporin deletion in mice reduces intraocular pressure and aqueous fluid production. J Gen Physiol 119:561–569

Physical Phantom of Craniospinal Hydrodynamics

R. Bouzerar, M. Czosnyka, Z. Czosnyka, and Olivier Balédent

Abstract *Introduction*: Inside the craniospinal system, blood, and cerebrospinal fluid (CSF) interactions occurring through volume exchanges are still not well understood. We built a physical model of this global hydrodynamic system. The main objective was to study, in controlled conditions, CSF–blood interactions to better understand the phenomenon underlying pathogenesis of hydrocephalus.

Materials and methods: A structure representing the cranium is connected to the spinal channel. The cranium is divided into compartments mimicking anatomical regions such as ventricles or aqueduct cerebri. Resistive and compliant characteristics of blood and CSF compartments can be assessed or measured using pressure and flow sensors incorporated in the model. An arterial blood flow input is generated by a programmable pump. Flows and pressures inside the system are simultaneously recorded.

Results: Preliminary results show that the model can mimic venous and CSF flows in response to arterial pressure input. Pulse waveforms and volume flows were measured and confirmed that they partially replicated the data previously obtained with phase-contrast magnetic resonance imaging. The phantom shows that CSF oscillations directly result from arteriovenous flow, and intracranial pressure measurements show that the model obeys an exponential relationship between pressure and intracranial volume expansion.

Conclusion: The phantom will be useful to investigate the hydrodynamic hypotheses underlying development of hydrocephalus.

Keywords Cranio spinal hydrodynamics • CSF flow • Blood flow • Physical model

R. Bouzerar and O. Balédent (✉)
Imaging and Biophysics Unit, Amiens University Hospital, Amiens, France
e-mail: olivier.baledent@chu-amiens.fr

M. Czosnyka and Z. Czosnyka
Academic Neurosurgical Unit, Department of clinical Neurosciences, University of Cambridge, Addenbroke's Hospital, Cambridge, UK

Introduction

The craniospinal system consists of a rigid cranial box and a compliant spinal compartment. Arterial blood flow, which is not constant but pulsatile during the cardiac cycle, is not instantaneously compensated by venous outflow. This instantaneous difference between arterial and venous flows leads to an intracranial blood volume change during a cardiac cycle [6]. To compensate for this temporal blood volume expansion, cerebrospinal fluid (CSF) volume flushes into the spinal compartment during systole and returns to the cranium during diastole [4, 8, 14].

Marmarou and colleagues established an exponential relationship [18] between cerebral volume increase and intracranial pressure (ICP). Infusion tests and cerebral pressure monitoring are still using this approach. Different studies have tried to simulate ICP, blood, and CSF interactions using lumped parameter, pressure volume, mathematical, or computational fluid dynamic (CFD) models [1, 3, 10, 16, 18, 20, 21, 24]. These approaches have led to significant insights into interactions between fluid, tissue, and pressure inside the craniospinal system.

These interactions between the considered fluids and structures are actually so complex that numerical approaches can hardly apprehend the system in its complexity. Electrical analog models are restrictive and limited because they do not take into account the actual fluid mechanical principles. At present, engineers still have difficulties linking a CFD approach with boundary deformation of vessels or tissues. It is likely that we will have to wait a few years before obtaining a global CFD model of craniospinal hydrodynamics.

Using phase-contrast magnetic resonance imaging (PC-MRI), noninvasive direct measurements of CSF and cerebral blood flows are feasible [11–13, 19]. Many studies have established normal values of cerebral flows in healthy populations [6, 22, 23] and have shown alterations of these flows in pathological conditions such as hydrocephalus [5, 7, 9, 17].

The objective of this work was to design a physical, "realistic phantom" of the global craniospinal fluid dynamics and to study, in strictly controlled conditions, its feasibility using the dynamic response of CSF to arterial input flow.

Materials and Methods

Based on the anatomy of the craniospinal system, we have developed a phantom (Fig. 1). A polycarbonate structure representing the cranium (cranial volume = 2,000 mL) is connected to the spinal channel (spinal volume = 200 mL) ending in a calibrated compliance. The cranium is divided into various compartments, mimicking the simplified anatomical regions such as ventricles and aqueduct cerebri.

The ventricular volume was 50 mL and the brain volume nearly 500 mL. Deformable parts are represented by rubber-like hyperelastic materials. Realistic cerebral arterial blood flow is generated by a numerically accurate programmable pump. Flows and pressures inside the system are simultaneously recorded. Resistances and compliances of blood and CSF compartments can be assessed or measured separately using the pressure and flow sensors incorporated in the model. The sensors were plugged into a data acquisition interface, and measurements were recorded on a computer. The temporal resolution of the measurements system was 1 ms.

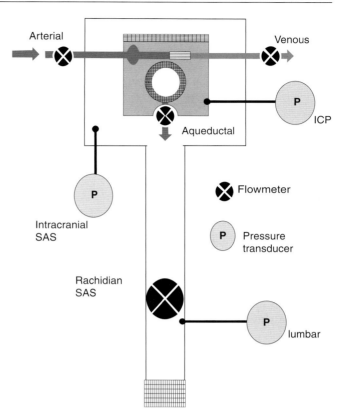

Fig. 1 Schematic drawing of the physical model. Measurement locations for flow and pressure are indicated. Compliant parts are also pointed out

Results

Measurements of compliance in stand-alone compartments showed an exponential behaviour of pressure as a function of infused volume as described by Marmarou et al. [18] in humans.

The curves depicted in Fig. 2 represent the comparison between CSF and blood flows measured inside the phantom (continuous lines) with PC-MRI reference data (dashed lines). These results show that cerebral arterial flow is accurately generated by the pump and that the venous outflow response generated by the phantom is in good agreement with PC-MRI measurements. Ventricular CSF flow (aqueduct) oscillates, and the curve correlates with the physiological PC-MRI curve. Spinal CSF flow amplitudes are also in the normal range but present additional oscillations during the diastolic phase of the cardiac cycle.

We have made measurements using horizontal and upright positions of the phantom. Pressure and flow curves are represented in the spinal and cerebral compartments during two cardiac cycles for each configuration (Fig. 3). For the horizontal position, ICP and spinal pressures were equivalent.

As in humans, aqueductal CSF flow presented a temporal delay compared with cervical CSF flow. For the vertical position, owing to gravity, the phantom showed elevated spinal pressure in comparison with ICP. In addition, CSF oscillation amplitudes in the aqueduct were significantly increased (40%), mainly during the flushing period. The change of pressure distribution also markedly modified the shape of the spinal flow curve.

We have also studied the influence of the cardiac frequency ($N_1 = 0.8$ Hz and $N_2 = 1.25$ Hz). The main consequence of the frequency increase affected the spinal compartment where CSF flow and pressure amplitudes were markedly increased, whereas all the other curves were not significantly affected.

Discussion

We have built a realistic physical model of the global craniospinal hydrodynamics that takes the major features of cerebral dynamics into account.

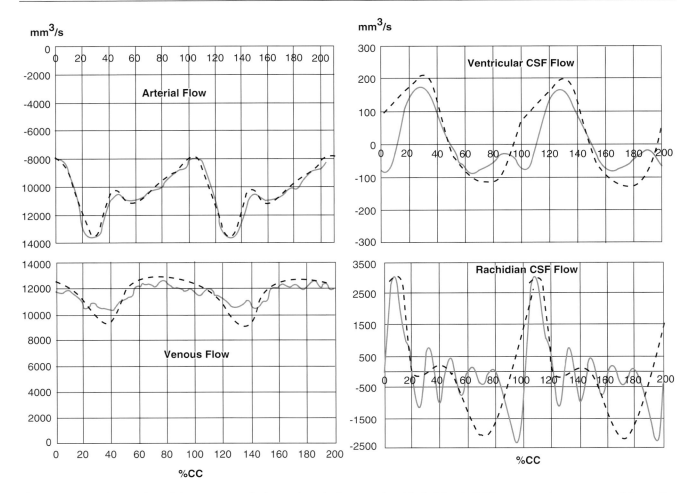

Fig. 2 Measured signals of arterial, venous, ventricular cerebrospinal fluid (*CSF*), and spinal CSF flows throughout two cycles. Measured data (*continuous lines*) are compared with phase-contrast MRI reference data (*dashed lines*). %CC represents the percentage of the cardiac cycle duration, whereas flows are given in mm³/s

Using a generated physiological arterial input flow, preliminary results have shown that the phantom was able to replicate CSF oscillations and venous outflows in agreement with PC-MRI measurements in adults. The influence of body position as well as cardiac heart rate on the measured parameters was significant. This strengthens the conclusion that our model is sensitive enough to detect variations of the dynamical parameters governing cerebral dynamics. The changes observed after switching from horizontal to vertical posture were in complete agreement with the observations of Alperin et al. [2] and Kim et al. [15] in human experiments. Indeed, Alperin et al. [2] showed that measured spinal CSF flow as well as a modeled mean ICP value decreased from one posture to another. The measured ICP waveform in patients also decreased according to Kim et al. [15]. In addition, we also showed that aqueductal flow increased concomitantly with the previous observations.

Conclusion

After this feasibility study, much remains to be done to fully mimic human cerebral fluid–tissue interactions. Nevertheless, we strongly believe that this physical model will help us to explain and understand the impact of hydrodynamics in hydrocephalus. We also think that this should be helpful to study cerebral infusion and shunt material behaviour under pulsatile conditions by quantifying the relationship between flow dynamics and pressure waves inside the system.

In the future, this MRI-compatible phantom will be used to explore the opportunity to develop PC-MRI as a noninvasive tool for ICP measurements and to explore new ways of understanding the mechanisms underlying cerebral pathologies.

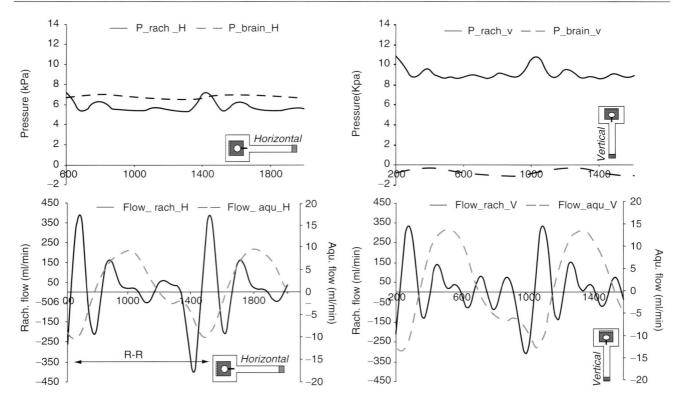

Fig. 3 The flow and pressure measurements in the cerebral and spinal compartments using horizontal (*left side*) and upright positions (*right side*). Pressure and flow curves represented during two cardiac cycles for each configuration. *H and V suffix* represent horizontal and upright positions, respectively. *P_rach* spinal pressure, *P_brain* brain pressure (ICP), *Flow_rach* spinal flow, *Flow_aqu* aqueductal flow

Acknowledgements This work was supported by European Community Grant Interreg (inter-regional cooperation between university hospitals of Amiens and Cambridge).

Conflicts of interest statement We declare that we have no conflict of interest.

References

1. Agarwal GC, Berman BM, Stark L (1969) A lumped parameter model of the cerebrospinal fluid system. IEEE Trans Biomed Eng 16(1):45–53
2. Alperin N, Hushek SG, Lee SH, Sivaramakrishnan A, Lichtor T (2005) MRI study of cerebral blood flow and CSF flow dynamics in an upright posture: the effect of posture on the intracranial compliance and pressure. Acta Neurochir Suppl 95:177–181
3. Ambarki K, Baledent O, Kongolo G, Bouzerar R, Fall S, Meyer ME (2007) A new lumped-parameter model of cerebrospinal hydrodynamics during the cardiac cycle in healthy volunteers. IEEE Trans Biomed Eng 54(3):483–491
4. Baledent O, Fin L, Khuoy L, Ambarki K, Gauvin AC, Gondry-Jouet C, Meyer ME (2006) Brain hydrodynamics study by phase-contrast magnetic resonance imaging and transcranial color Doppler. J Magn Reson Imaging 24(5):995–1004
5. Baledent O, Gondry-Jouet C, Meyer ME, De Marco G, Le Gars D, Henry-Feugeas MC, Idy-Peretti I (2004) Relationship between cerebrospinal fluid and blood dynamics in healthy volunteers and patients with communicating hydrocephalus. Invest Radiol 39(1):45–55
6. Baledent O, Henry-Feugeas MC, Idy-Peretti I (2001) Cerebrospinal fluid dynamics and relation with blood flow: a magnetic resonance study with semiautomated cerebrospinal fluid segmentation. Invest Radiol 36(7):368–377
7. Bateman GA (2009) Cerebral blood flow and hydrocephalus. J Neurosurg Pediatr 3(3):244
8. Bateman GA, Loiselle AM (2007) Can MR measurement of intracranial hydrodynamics and compliance differentiate which patient with idiopathic normal pressure hydrocephalus will improve following shunt insertion? Acta Neurochir (Wien) 149(5):455–462
9. Bradley WG Jr, Scalzo D, Queralt J, Nitz WN, Atkinson DJ, Wong P (1996) Normal-pressure hydrocephalus: evaluation with cerebrospinal fluid flow measurements at MR imaging. Radiology 198(2):523–529
10. Egnor M, Rosiello A, Zheng L (2001) A model of intracranial pulsations. Pediatr Neurosurg 35(6):284–298
11. Enzmann DR, Pelc NJ (1991) Normal flow patterns of intracranial and spinal cerebrospinal fluid defined with phase-contrast cine MR imaging. Radiology 178(2):467–474
12. Feinberg DA, Mark AS (1987) Human brain motion and cerebrospinal fluid circulation demonstrated with MR velocity imaging. Radiology 163(3):793–799
13. Greitz D, Wirestam R, Franck A, Nordell B, Thomsen C, Stahlberg F (1992) Pulsatile brain movement and associated hydrodynamics studied by magnetic resonance phase imaging. The Monro-Kellie doctrine revisited. Neuroradiology 34(5):370–380
14. Henry-Feugeas MC, Idy-Peretti I, Baledent O, Poncelet-Didon A, Zannoli G, Bittoun J, Schouman-Claeys E (2000) Origin of subarachnoid cerebrospinal fluid pulsations: a phase-contrast MR analysis. Magn Reson Imaging 18(4):387–395
15. Kim DJ, Czosnyka Z, Keong N, Radolovich DK, Smielewski P, Sutcliffe MP, Pickard JD, Czosnyka M (2009) Index of cerebrospinal

compensatory reserve in hydrocephalus. Neurosurgery 64(3): 494–501
16. Linninger AA, Xenos M, Sweetman B, Ponkshe S, Guo X, Penn R (2009) A mathematical model of blood, cerebrospinal fluid and brain dynamics. J Math Biol 59(6):729–759
17. Luetmer PH, Huston J, Friedman JA, Dixon GR, Petersen RC, Jack CR, McClelland RL, Ebersold MJ (2002) Measurement of cerebrospinal fluid flow at the cerebral aqueduct by use of phase-contrast magnetic resonance imaging: technique validation and utility in diagnosing idiopathic normal pressure hydrocephalus. Neurosurgery 50(3):534–543
18. Marmarou A, Shulman K, LaMorgese J (1975) Compartmental analysis of compliance and outflow resistance of the cerebrospinal fluid system. J Neurosurg 43(5):523–534
19. Nitz WR, Bradley WG Jr, Watanabe AS, Lee RR, Burgoyne B, O'Sullivan RM, Herbst MD (1992) Flow dynamics of cerebrospinal fluid: assessment with phase-contrast velocity MR imaging performed with retrospective cardiac gating. Radiology 183(2):395–405
20. Piechnik SK, Czosnyka M, Harris NG, Minhas PS, Pickard JD (2001) A model of the cerebral and cerebrospinal fluid circulations to examine asymmetry in cerebrovascular reactivity. J Cereb Blood Flow Metab 21(2):182–192
21. Rekate HL, Brodkey JA, Chizeck HJ, el Sakka W, Ko WH (1988) Ventricular volume regulation: a mathematical model and computer simulation. Pediatr Neurosci 14(2):77–84
22. Stoquart-ElSankari S, Baledent O, Gondry-Jouet C, Makki M, Godefroy O, Meyer ME (2007) Aging effects on cerebral blood and cerebrospinal fluid flows. J Cereb Blood Flow Metab 27(9):1563–1572
23. Stoquart-Elsankari S, Lehmann P, Villette A, Czosnyka M, Meyer ME, Deramond H, Baledent O (2009) A phase-contrast MRI study of physiologic cerebral venous flow. J Cereb Blood Flow Metab 29(6):1208–1215
24. Ursino M, Lodi CA (1997) A simple mathematical model of the interaction between intracranial pressure and cerebral hemodynamics. J Appl Physiol 82(4):1256–1269

Programmable Shunt Assistant Tested in Cambridge Shunt Evaluation Laboratory

Marek Czosnyka, Zofia Czosnyka, and John D. Pickard

Abstract *Objective*: The programmable Shunt Assistant (capped!) (ProSA) shunt system has recently been introduced into clinical use. The system can be in vivo adjusted magnetically, and this adjustability is supposed to affect CSF drainage only in the vertical body position.

Materials and methods: We tested a combination of ProSA with fixed differential pressure valve designed to drain cerebrospinal fluid (CSF) from the brain ventricles into the peritoneal cavity.

Results: The ProSA showed good mechanical durability and stability of hydrodynamic performance over a 60-day period. The flow-pressure performance curves and operating pressures were stable, fell within the limits specified by the manufacturer, and changed according to the programmed performance levels. The ProSA system has higher than usual hydrodynamic resistance (around 8.8 mmHg/(mL/min)) in the vertical position. Operating pressure in the vertical position reacted repeatedly to changes of settings within the limits 0–40 cmH$_2$O and was reduced gradually when the axis of the valve declined from vertical to horizontal. External programming proved to be reliable. Strong magnetic fields (3-T MRI) were not able to change the programming of ProSA.

Conclusion: ProSA works in the horizontal position as differential fixed pressure low hydrodynamic resistance and in the vertical position as an adjustable, normal hydrodynamic resistance valve. It is able to compensate for posture-related overdrainage

Keywords Shunt • Hydrocephalus • Cerebrospinal fluid

M. Czosnyka (✉)
Department of Clinical Neurosciences,
University of Cambridge, Cambridge, UK and
Neurosurgery Unit, Addenbrooke's Hospital,
Cambridge, UK
e-mail: mc141@medschl.cam.ac.uk

Z. Czosnyka and J.D. Pickard
Department of Clinical Neurosciences,
University of Cambridge, Cambridge, UK

Introduction

An ideal shunt should restore the normal circulation of cerebrospinal fluid (CSF) and the normal pattern of extrachoroidal fluid flow within the brain, prevent excessive build-up of intracranial pressure, and encourage restitution of physiological cerebral blood flow in white matter [3].

The long-term stability of a valve's behaviour is tested in a laboratory environment that mimics, at least in part, conditions within the human body [1, 2]. The tests are able to demonstrate whether the shunt is susceptible to alteration in CSF drainage caused by postural changes, external pressure, change in ambient temperature, and the presence of a pulsating pattern in inlet pressure. Results of such an evaluation also proved to be helpful in post-implantation shunt testing performed in patients to assess functioning of their shunts [4].

Material

The programmable shunt assistant (ProSA) is a gravitational overdrainage compensating device which can be magnetically adjusted after implantation using a special magnetic tool. It is intended to work together with CSF valve-adjustable or fixed pressure.

In this evaluation study, we tested the ProSA combined with fixed pressure MiniNAV valve, referring to the whole system (valve and Shunt Assistant) as the ProSA System.

The role of the ProSA is to control CSF flow in the upright body position. In classic differential pressure ventriculoperitoneal valves, flow is accelerated by the gravity force of a fluid filling a long tube connecting ventricles and abdomen. A classic (nonadjustable) shunt assistant works on the principle of additional weight increasing opening pressure of the 'ball in cone' inlet controlling CSF flow. One disadvantage of the very popular Shunt Assistant was that the weight was fixed. In cases of paediatric hydrocephalus, with growing, requirements for siphon control become stronger in time. Therefore the programmable shunt assistant was designed to allow external adjustment of the weight to new conditions.

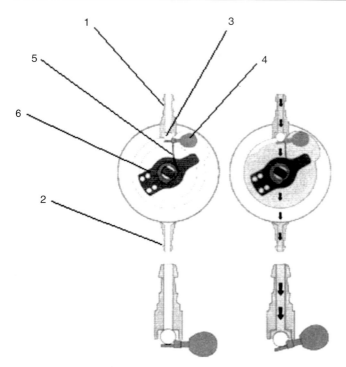

Fig. 1 Schematic diagram of construction of the ProSA (figure copied from the manufacturer's Web page). Labels indicate (*1*) inlet connector, (*2*) outlet connector, (*3*) sapphire ball, (*4*) weight, (*5*) bow spring, (*6*) rotor with micro magnets

ProSA works as a programmable valve activated only in the vertical body position. Horizontally it is nonprogrammable. Therefore in conjunction with a programmable valve, it may optimise conditions to CSF drainage both in horizontal and vertical positions. In conjunction with a fixed-pressure valve, it is just intended to prevent posture-related overdrainage in variable conditions.

The general scheme of the Shunt Assistant is presented in Fig. 1 (copied from the manufacturer's Web page). Inlet (1) and outlet (2) allow connection of standard silicone tubing (1.2 mm internal diameter tubing is recommended by the manufacturer). A sapphire ball sitting in an inlet cone (3) controls the CSF flow. The weight (4) is supporting the sapphire ball and its cantilevering its movement in cone. The cantilever force is adjusted by a bow spring (5). Tension of the spring is controlled by the profiled rotor (6). Greater tension increases the performance pressure of ProSA by decreasing the gravitational force of the effective weight acting on the sapphire ball. In the horizontal position, the effective force of the weight is zero, and the ProSA remains open. In intermediate positions, the force is gradually reduced by a factor proportional to the sine of the angle of inclination. The rotor may be moved after implantation of the shunt system with a special programmer (provided by the manufacturer). In this way, the operating pressure of the valve can be changed within the range from 0 to 40 cmH$_2$O. Additional pressing against the casing releases a mechanical 'brake' and allows movement of the rotor; in that way the ProSA is secured against an accidental change of setting by an external magnetic field (up to 3-T MRI scanner). Both the ProSA and MiniNAV have hard titanium cases.

The ProSA should be implanted together with the valve (programmable or fixed), controlling the operating pressure in horizontal position and preventing reflux. In this evaluation program, we analysed a system consisting of ProSA and fixed pressure MiniNAV valve operating at 5 cmH$_2$O.

Methods

The shunt testing rig has been described before [2]. The shunt under test is submerged in a water bath at a constant temperature at a defined depth (h).

The working fluid (deionised and deaerated water) is supplied by the fluid container or infusion pump. A pulse pressure of controlled amplitude created by the pulse pressure generator can be added to the static pressure. The viscosity and specific gravity of water reflect the physical properties of CSF under normal conditions.

In hydrocephalus, the patient's own resistance to CSF outflow is usually increased but finite. A model of resistance to CSF outflow can be added before the shunt to study the shunt's performance in conditions mimicking the in vivo environment. Pressure before the shunt is measured with a pressure transducer. Fluid flowing through the shunt is collected in a container placed on the electronic balance.

Measurement is controlled by a standard IBM-compatible personal computer that reads and zeroes the balance periodically (every 15 s) to calculate the flow rate. This enables us to measure the weight of the outflowing fluid incrementally, which cancels the influence of fluid vaporisation from the outlet container. The computer analyses the pressure waveform from the pressure transducer and controls the rate of the infusion pump. The effect of changes in atmospheric pressure is compensated by using the reference barometer.

The shunt and pressure transducer are placed on the same level. The water column in the fluid container (*H*), the degree of the shunt submersion (*h*), and the level of the outlet tubing (*O*) may be changed according to the test protocol.

The shunt is tested under two different regimes: (1) when the differential pressure is measured while flow through the shunt is controlled (flow-pressure) and (2) when flow through the shunt is measured while the differential pressure across the shunt is controlled (pressure-flow).

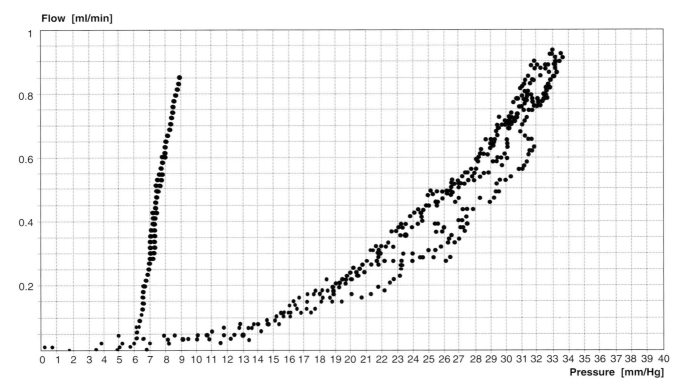

Fig. 2 Flow pressure curves in vertical (wider, more nonlinear) and horizontal (steeper, more linear) positions

Statistical Methods

Mean values, standard deviations, and maximal-minimal values are used to express average parameters and their spread.

To evaluate fluctuations of parameters in altered conditions a paired *t*-test for parameters at a baseline and in altered conditions is used. The *t*-test is used to evaluate sample-related differences in parameters.

Analysis of variance (ANOVA), with time as the independent factor, is used to evaluate the stability of parameters with time.

Results

ProSA Parameters Under Normal Conditions: Pressure Set for 30 cmH$_2$O

The typical pressure-flow curve (with pressure plotted along the x-axis and flow along the y-axis) for a valve is presented in Fig. 2. The valve without a distal catheter had slightly non linear, exponential characteristics. Its gradient was equivalent to the inverse of the hydrodynamic static resistance. In horizontal position the pressure-flow curve is much steeper and more linear.

The hydrodynamic resistance in vertical position was 8.8 ± 0.72 mmHg/mL/min (for the valve permanently open, i.e. flow rate 0.5–1.5 mL/min). Due to the nonlinear characteristic of the valve for the low flow, resistance over a range of flow from 0.05 to 0.15 mL/min was 16.3 + 4.1 mmHg/(mL/min). In horizontal orientation, hydrodynamic resistance was 3.2 mmHg/(mL/min).

Operating pressure was very stable and convergent; mean value was 22.1 mmHg, range from 17.1 to 24.5 mmHg (95% confidence interval, 20.2–23 mmHg).

Valve Performance Under Altered Conditions (Setting 30 cmH$_2$O)

A pulse pressure with an amplitude changing from 1 to about 60 mmHg produced a significant decrease in operating pressure. However, this decrease was observed above the peak-to-peak amplitude of 14 mmHg. In normal conditions, average intracranial pressure (ICP) peak-to-peak amplitude is lower (around 2–5 mmHg); 14 mmHg is seen very rarely and only in extreme conditions.

None of the parameters (operating pressure and resistance) were altered by a temperature change from 30°C to 40°C. Therefore we would not expect a change in CSF drainage even during a high fever or when ambient temperature is low.

The ProSA increases CSF drainage rate when applying negative outflow pressure. Formally in the testing rig, with shunt system open, when decreasing outlet level by 40 cmH$_2$O, flow increases by around 3 mL/min. However, this does not simulate real conditions well when the patient with an implanted shunt changes body position from horizontal to vertical. Let us presume normal ICP in horizontal position to be around 10 cmH$_2$O, the distance from ventricles to abdomen around 60 cm, and initial fall of ICP in upright position to -10 cmH$_2$O. Presuming abdominal pressure 0 cmH$_2$O, the addition to the shunt system opening pressure of 5 cmH$_2$O produced by the ProSA unit will be +30 cmH$_2$O. Therefore the initial drainage rate will be 15 cmH$_2$O divided by shunt resistance – i.e. around 1.2 mL/min. If the ProSA setting in this case is 40 cmH$_2$O, the drainage rate will be around 0.5 mL/min, only a fraction greater than normal production of CSF, unlikely to produce any clinically relevant overdrainage.

External pressures did not have any influence on shunt performance

None of the parameters were altered by residual resistance to CSF outflow. Changes in the patient's own reabsorption capacity with time should not change drainage characteristics.

Programming

Programming of the ProSA has been checked using flow-pressure tests. Good agreement of the pressure-flow curves with the nominal data has been recorded.

A family of flow-pressure curves for different settings of ProSA is presented in Fig. 3a.

Operating pressures (for flow 0.3 mL/min) and 95% confidence limits are presented in graphical form in Fig. 3b.

Verification of the settings of ProSA unit and readjustments are very easy and reliable. Rotation of the valve under the skin may theoretically constitute a problem; however, the big bottom surface of the shunt should minimise such a risk

Operating pressure of the valve depends additionally on an angle of inclination from horizontal (0°) to vertical (90°) – see Fig. 1.

Other Properties

Operating pressure displayed very limited variations during all the tests. The changes were not systematically time-related. When the valve was unpacked and filled for the first time with testing fluid, it started to work normally almost immediately (providing that all air bubbles had been removed). The hydrodynamic resistance and operating pressure did not exhibit any time-related trends during the 3 months of testing.

No significant ($p > 0.05$) differences in measured parameters were found between the three ProSA samples tested. All the values of operating pressures were measured within the tolerance limits given by the manufacturer.

The ProSA did not show any reflux when tested according to the ISO standard. Valves did not exhibit reversal of flow for an outlet-inlet differential pressure of up to 200 mmHg.

The valve cannot be reprogrammed by an external magnetic field up to 3 T (MRI magnet). Therefore the ProSA seems to be safe in a 3 T MRI magnet. It does not heat up. Maximal translational force was measured as 0.001N, the values considered as safe after implantation.

Distortion of the MRI scan is considerable (GE: 201 cm^3 and T1: 11 cm^3); however, it is a little bit smaller than in the PrGAV Valve.

Assembled junctions did not break when a test specimen was subjected to a load of 1 kgf for 1 min. All junctions remained free from leakage when the water pressure was increased to 3 kPa (about 25 mmHg).

Discussion

The ProSA is the first adjustable gravitational device, aimed at reducing risk of CSF overdrainage in the vertical body position that is available on the market. It can be compared to an adjustable valve which is working in the vertical body position. In the horizontal position, it behaves as a normal fixed-pressure valve with low resistance. Therefore it cannot prevent overdrainage associated with vasocycling in the horizontal position. Historically, such an overdrainage is seen particularly frequently in paediatric cases.

The question arises whether such a sophisticated system is well targeted to work in combination with a fixed-pressure valve. A combination of a ProGAV (programmable valve) and the ProSA (replacing the fixed Shunt Assistant) is probably more comprehensive. It is true that it increases the total cost of the implant, but adjustability in both the horizontal and vertical position is unique and desirable in our opinion. Dr. Salomon Hakim used to say that an adjustable valve is a valve with a steering wheel. The ProGAV and ProSA will be a valve with two steering wheels: ProGAV useful for major setting of overall valve performance and ProSA for fine-tuning of specific aspects related to overdrainage in the vertical position (<10% of all complications in shunted patients are related to posture related overdrainage according to the UK Shunt Registry). It is not a valve

Fig. 3 (a) Pressure flow characteristics for different operating settings; (b) Operating pressure levels: mean values and 95% confidence intervals for different settings of the ProSA

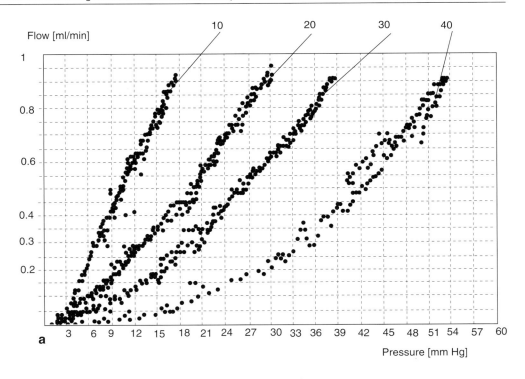
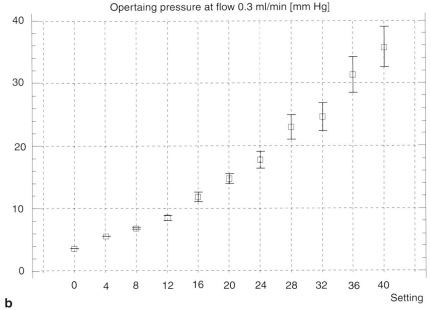

for fools; however, in experienced hands it may be useful to manage particularly difficult cases of hydrocephalus.

Conclusion

The ProSA does not change settings in the presence of an external magnetic field (up to 3 T in an MRI magnet). Because of image distortion, implantation of the valve on the chest rather than on the skull may be considered, if MRI scanning of the patient is likely in follow-up.

The valve is comfortable in programming. Verification of programmed setting can be done without the necessity of an X-ray.

Conflicts of interest statement This evaluation study was commissioned by B. Brown Ltd UK, in agreement with the University of Cambridge, which partly contributes to Z.C.'s salary. The study was conducted independently, and the manufacturer's comments were provided unabridged.

References

1. Aschoff A, Kremer P, Benesch C, Fruh K, Klank A (1995) Kunze S Overdrainage and shunt technology. A critical comparison of programmable, hydrostatic and variable-resistance valves and flow-reducing devices. Childs Nerv Syst 11(4):193–202
2. Czosnyka Z, Czosnyka M, Richards HK, Pickard JD (2002) Laboratory testing of hydrocephalus shunts – conclusion of the U.K. Shunt evaluation programme. Acta Neurochir (Wien) 144(6):525–38
3. Momjian S, Owler BK, Czosnyka Z, Czosnyka M, Pena A, Pickard JD (2004) Pattern of white matter regional cerebral blood flow and autoregulation in normal pressure hydrocephalus. Brain 127(Pt 5):965–72
4. Petrella G, Czosnyka M, Smielewski P, Allin D, Guazzo EP, Pickard JD, Czosnyka ZH (2009) In vivo assessment of hydrocephalus shunt. Acta Neurol Scand 120(5):317–23

Simulation of Existing and Future Electromechanical Shunt Valves in Combination with a Model for Brain Fluid Dynamics

Inga Margrit Elixmann, M. Walter, M. Kiefer, and S. Leonhardt

Abstract Several models are available to simulate raised intracranial pressure (ICP) in hydrocephalus. However, the hydrodynamic effect of an implanted shunt has seldom been examined. In this study, the simple model of Ursino and Lodi [14] is extended to include (1) the effect of a typical ball-in-cone valve, (2) the effect of the size of the diameter of the connecting tube from valve to abdomen, and (3) the concept of a controlled electromechanical shunt valve in overall cerebrospinal fluid dynamics.

By means of simulation, it is shown how a shunt can lower ICP. Simulation results indicate that P and B waves still exist but at a lower ICP level and that, due to the exponential pressure-volume curve, their amplitude is also considerably lowered. A waves only develop if the valve is partially blocked. The resulting ICP is above the opening pressure of the valve, depending on the drain and resistance of the shunt.

The concept of a new electromechanical shunt was more successful than the traditional mechanical valves in keeping ICP at a desired level. The influence of the patient's movements or coughing on ICP as well as the body position affecting the reference ICP, which can be measured, has not yet been modeled and should be addressed in future using suitable algorithms.

Keywords Hydrocephalus • Shunt • Mechatronic/electromechanical valve • Model • A waves • B waves

I.M. Elixmann (✉), M. Walter, and S. Leonhardt
Helmholtz-Institute for Biomedical Engineering,
RWTH Aachen University, Aachen, Germany
e-mail: krause@hia.rwth-aachen.de

M. Kiefer
Department of Neurosurgery, Saarland University,
Homburg-Saar, Germany

Introduction

Accumulation of fluid in the cerebrospinal region and peaks in intracranial pressure (ICP) in patients with hydrocephalus are caused by reduced intracranial storage capacity (compliance = dV/dP) and an increased resistance to outflow. According to the classic bulk cerebrospinal fluid (CSF) flow theory, CSF produced in the plexus choroidei passes through the ventricles (which are enlarged in hydrocephalus patients) and is absorbed in the granulationes arachnoideales. CSF is mostly absorbed in the capillary bed. According to Greitz [6], in communicating hydrocephalus, the enlarged ventricles can be explained by transmantle pulsatile stress. Much research has aimed at providing an explanation for the pathomechanisms observed in hydrocephalic patients. According to the Monroe-Kellie doctrine, the overall craniospinal volume can be expressed as the sum of tissue, blood, and CSF volume at any point in time

$$V_{total}(t) = V_{CSF}(t) + V_{blood}(t) + V_{tissue} \quad (1)$$

According to Marmarou et al. [10] and Avezaat et al. [2], a monoexponential pressure-volume (P-V) relationship exists with

$$ICP(t) = p_0 + k_0 e^{k_{elast} V(t)} \quad (2)$$

Thus, changes in blood volume will alter ICP. ICP oscillations may occur as a function of pulsating blood flow to the brain caused by heartbeats (P waves) or, even stronger, due to vasogenic volume alterations which induce the B waves and the dangerous A waves. Table 1 shows the period of time and amplitudes of these waves.

Ursino et al. [14, 15] developed a hemodynamic model which can simulate these waves. A waves are self-sustained ICP oscillations due to an unstable configuration with a decreased elastic coefficient and an increased outflow resistance due to venous congestion. B waves are induced by changes in the arterial vasotonus due to a change of oxygen

Table 1 Data on the dynamics of intracranial pressure

Wave type	Period of time	Amplitude (mmHg)
Pulse, P	0.25–1.5 s	1–20
B	20 s–2 min	>3
A	5–20 min	36–110

and carbon dioxide in the blood. Walter et al. [17] extended the model of Ursino et al. with a physiological model which describes the gas exchange between blood and cells.

In the present study, the model has been extended further by considering the effect of different shunt types on ICP, including a new electromechanical valve concept.

Implanting a shunt is common therapy for patients with hydrocephalus to drain CSF into another body compartment to reduce pressure peaks. Electronic sensors have been developed to measure ICP [5, 9, 11, 13], one of which has been approved for 28 days of use [9]. Flow sensors are also under development [7], although more research is needed before they can be applied in hydrocephalus therapy. However, no in vivo measurements are available for ICP and CSF flow, measured at the same time, through a shunt in another body compartment.

Current passive shunts have the disadvantage that they cannot automatically adapt to alterations in shunt resistance over time due to particles that adhere in the tube, or because the need for drainage may change over time due to variation in CSF production. However, these problems can be addressed by an electromechanical shunt which automatically changes its resistance, to maintain a certain ICP related to atmospheric pressure. Use of an electromechanical shunt can also enable a desired ICP course to be maintained over several days (as assessed by the physician). The effectiveness of the control mechanism for the electromechanical shunt can initially be explored by simulation using the hydrocephalus model.

Using the simulation model, Mnomani et al. [12] investigated the behavior of an electromechanical scheduled valve. However, a "scheduled" valve is a blind valve and does not change its opening behavior if the condition of the patient changes within a short time and might, therefore, be dangerous.

The present study shows (1) how a shunt influences ICP, (2) the extent to which a shunt has to be occluded by particles before it no longer prevents A waves, (3) how simulations reveal the change in ICP curves when changing the diameter of the tube connecting a typical ball-in-cone valve to the abdomen, and (4) a new electromechanical valve concept which automatically changes a tube's diameter to obtain a desired ICP.

Materials and Methods

The Model

The simulation model was implemented in the computer-aided engineering platform Matlab-Simulink (The MathWorks, Inc.). In our model, ICP results from the change in volume in the craniospinal space according to

$$C_{ic} \cdot \frac{dICP}{dt} = \frac{dV_a}{dt} + \frac{P_c - ICP}{R_f} - \frac{ICP - CVP}{R_0} - Q_s, \quad (3)$$

where C_{ic} is the intracranial compliance, V_a the blood volume in the arterial-arteriolar cerebrovascular bed, and P_c and CVP the capillary and venous pressures, respectively. R_f denotes the resistance to CSF formation, R_0 the resistance to CSF outflow, and Q_s is the volume flow through the shunt. Note that the compliance can also be expressed by the elastic coefficient k_{el} and the current ICP [10],

$$C_{ic} = \frac{1}{k_{el} \cdot ICP} \quad (4)$$

The parameters were the same as used by Walter [16], which means that a healthy resorption coefficient was considered to be 13.89 µl/(s kPa) and those for P and B waves were reduced by 67%, and for A waves by as much as 92%. An unhealthy elastic coefficient was considered to have an assigned value of 0.26 ml^{-1}.

In the simulation, the influence of shunts on A, B, and P waves with frequencies of 0.03 min^{-1}, 0.03 Hz, and 1.5 Hz, respectively, was tested (Table 1).

Shunts

The P-V flow characteristic of a shunt is determined by the opening pressure p_0 of the valve and the resistance of the valve with the connected tube and catheter. Note that a silicone tube of 90 cm length with an inner diameter of 0.7–1.3 mm can account for 80–90% of the overall resistance of the shunt – a fact that is often overlooked.

Aschoff [1] examined the hydrodynamic properties of a large number of valves in a test rig. His measurements reveal that different silicone slit valve models start drainage at ICP above zero, but differ in their flow-to-pressure characteristics. Some models have an exponential behavior whereas

Simulation of Existing and Future Electromechanical Shunt Valves in Combination with a Model for Brain Fluid Dynamics

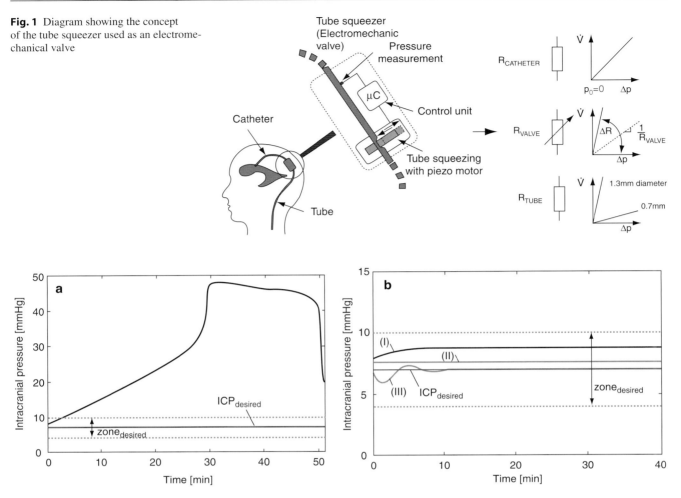

Fig. 1 Diagram showing the concept of the tube squeezer used as an electromechanical valve

Fig. 2 Simulation of (**a**) A wave, and (**b**) with additional ball-in-cone valve connected to a tube with inner diameters of 0.7 mm (*I*), 1.3 mm (*II*), and the tube squeezer (*III*). *ICP* intracranial pressure

others have a logarithmic relationship between flow and pressure. Ball-in-cone and membrane valves have a clear switching behavior at p_0. They do not drain for ICP below p_0 and can be approximated by a proportional pressure-flow characteristic for an ICP higher than p_0.

From previous measurements on a test rig, pressure-flow characteristics of current valves with a 90-cm long tube were determined [8]. Several ball-in-cone valves with a tube had a conductance of about 12.5 (ml/h)/mmHg. This value was taken as being representative for a current shunt. The opening pressure was set to 7 mmHg which equals the desired ICP for an adult in supine position for a ventriculo-peritoneal shunt.

As a new electromechanical valve concept, a "tube squeezer" has been simulated (Fig. 1). A control unit measures ICP and can change the diameter of a silicone tube over a length of 3 mm, using a piezo motor, to obtain the desired ICP of 7 mmHg. A simple control algorithm forcing the ICP to stay within a desired pressure zone has been implemented to adjust the tube diameter and hence the conductance. The overall conductance of the shunt (catheter, tube squeezer, and tube) can change between 0, when the tube is completely closed, to 22 (ml/h)/mmHg, when the tube is fully open with an inner diameter of 1.3 mm. A ball-in-cone valve drains CSF only if ICP is higher than p_0, whereas the tube squeezer drains at any positive ICP because p_0 equals zero.

Results and Discussion

Fig. 2a shows the simulated A wave. Fig. 2b illustrates that this wave can be prevented by a shunt. The ball-in-cone valve with the larger tube diameter of 1.3 mm achieves a final ICP

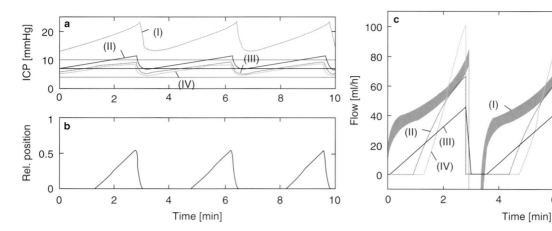

Fig. 3 Simulation of (**a**) B waves (*I*) with additional ball-in-cone valve connected to a tube with inner diameter = 0.7 mm (*II*), 1.3 mm (*III*, *dotted line*), and the tube squeezer (*IV*); and (**b**) the relative position of the tube squeezer (closed = 0); and (**c**) the appropriate flow through the valves (*II–IV*) and the change in blood volume (*I*)

which is closer to the desired ICP than the valve with a diameter of 0.7 mm. The tube squeezer needs some time for the desired ICP to be reached, but is eventually closest to the desired ICP compared with the ball-in-cone valve. Simulations have shown that a particle of minimum 1 mm in length, which blocks 50% of the cross-section of a tube with 0.7 mm diameter, can no longer prevent A waves.

The positive effect of the tube squeezer is less obvious for B waves, as shown in Fig. 3a, b. All shunts reduce average ICP up to 12 mmHg, and the tube squeezer reduces oscillations by up to 60%; however, unlike in the control of A waves, small oscillations still occur. The shunt reduces the average ICP and thus the amplitude in ICP by shifting the operating point down the monoexponential P-V relationship as determined by Marmarou et al. [10] and Avezaat et al. [2]. Hence the reduction amplitude was also observed for P waves. In the simulation with B waves using the shunt with the smaller tube diameter (0.7 mm) ICP increases beyond the desired ICP zone. This is because CSF is not drained sufficiently with the slow ramp up to 46 ml/h. Figure 3c indicates that the motor does not need to change the tube's diameter all of the time. It drains CSF up to 100 ml/h and then closes the valve. A decrease in blood volume (Fig. 3c(I)) is followed by a stop of drainage.

Conclusion and Outlook

The present simulation study provides some insight into how a shunt influences the typical patterns seen in hydrocephalic patients and how an electromechanical valve could improve therapy. It is shown that tube diameter plays a major role in the development of the ICP. The smaller the chosen diameter of the tube, the greater the difference in ICP with regard to the chosen opening pressure. If the diameter decreases too much (as in the case of a partial block of the tube), A waves can no longer be prevented. For A waves, the electromechanical shunt was the only one to achieve the desired ICP. Changes in ICP – e.g., due to B waves – could not be eliminated, but they could at least be reduced.

Although the simple algorithm used to control the tube squeezer can be modified, changes in ICP due to changes in cranial blood volume cannot be prevented entirely. A shunt can only reduce ICP due to drainage of CSF. If ICP decreases for a short period of time due to a reduction of intracranial blood volume (as it does in B waves due to a change in vasotonus), the shunt can only stop drainage but cannot inject additional CSF. Therefore, ICP drops below the target pressure of 7 mmHg.

These simulations are limited to the typical hydrocephalic patterns and, in the future, should address other situations – e.g., ICP fluctuations due to movement. In this case, an intelligent filter will be needed to obtain a reasonable ICP value as a control variable. Signal interpretation will also be needed for the patient coughing. A sudden steep increase in ICP should make the valve close in order to prevent overdrainage.

To obtain an objective measure of which shunt is most effective, particularly for the development of control algorithms for electromechanical valves, evaluation criteria should be applied. Mnomani et al. [12] introduced three different evaluation criteria, the so-called figures of merit (FOM): The first FOM indicates whether the mean ICP is within the physiologically desired zone, the second FOM is the fraction of time ICP stayed within the limits, and the third FOM is the fraction of time the valve was closed. Although this is a good approach it remains questionable which FOMs are really needed; for this reason, they were not used for the present simulation. We agree with the first FOM which indicates whether overdrainage or underdrainage has occurred. We also consider three other, new FOMs to be useful. One new FOM could measure the deviation of ICP from the desired zone, but only if ICP is out of that zone for longer than a specified period of time; this is because for short periods (such as during coughing) the ICP can be higher without having any effect. Another useful FOM could be the measure of control energy needed. It is not so important that the valve closes all the time but rather that the actuator position, and hence the resistance for a tube squeezer, changes as little as possible but has good control performance to achieve the first FOMs successfully. Energy-saving piezoelectric actuators only require energy when altering their position. Finally, another useful FOM could measure the amount of oscillation, since it is suggested that increased pulsation could be the cause of dilated ventricles in hydrocephalic patients [3, 4]. For all these evaluations, criteria-specific values are needed. For example, how long can the ICP surpass the desired zone? At which amplitude are oscillations tolerable? These are questions that still need to be addressed in order to design an optimally performing electromechanical shunt.

Acknowledgements The authors thank the German Federal Ministry of Science and Education (BMBF) for financial support of the BMBF project "iShunt".

Conflicts of interest statement Dr. M. Kiefer has received financial support in the past for activities other than this research, from Raumedic AG, Helmbrecht, Germany. All other authors declare that they have no conflict of interest.

References

1. Aschoff A (1994) In-vitro-Testung von Hydrocephalus-Ventilen. Professorial dissertation, Heidelberg University, Heidelberg, pp 86–179
2. Avezaat CJJ, Van Eijndhoven JHM (1979) Cerebrospinal fluid pulse pressure and intracranial volume-pressure relationships. J Neurol Neurosurg Psychiatry 42:687–700
3. Di Rocco C, Pettorossi VE, Caldarelli M, Mancinelli R, Velardi F (1978) Communicating hydrocephalus induced by mechanically increased amplitude of the intraventricular cerebrospinal fluid pressure: experimental studies. Exp Neurol 59:40–52
4. Egnor M, Zheng L, Rosiello A, Gutman F, Davis R (2002) A model of pulsations in communicating hydrocephalus. Pediatr Neurosurg 36:281–303
5. Ginggen A, Tardy Y, Crivelli R, Bork T, Renaud P (2008) A telemetric pressure sensor system for biomedical applications. IEEE Trans Biomed Eng 55:1374–1381
6. Greitz D (2004) Radiological assessment of hydrocephalus: new theories and implications for therapy. Neurosurg Rev 27:145–165
7. Hara M, Kadowaki C, Konishi Y, Ogashiwa M, Numoto M, Takeuchi K (1983) A new method for measuring cerebrospinal fluid flow in shunts. J Neurosurg 58:557–561
8. Krause I, Jetzki S, Rehbaum H, Linke S, Kiefer M, Walter M, Leonhardt S (2009) Dynamic bench testing of shunt valves. In: Hydrocephalus. Baltimore, p 98
9. Kunze G, Göhler KG, Reichenberger R. (2009) Entwicklung des Raumedic TD1 readP, ein erster Schritt auf dem Weg zum idealen, telemetrischen Hirndruckmesssystem. Sektionstagung, Congress Proceedings, Homburg, Germany, p 56
10. Marmarou A, Shulman K, Rosende RM (1978) A nonlinear analysis of the cerebrospinal fluid system and intracranial pressure dynamics. J Neurosurg 48:332–344
11. Miyake H, Ohta T, Kajimoto Y, Matsukawa M (1997) A new ventriculoperitoneal shunt with a telemetric intracranial pressure sensor: clinical experience in 94 patients with hydrocephalus. J Neurosurg 40:931–935
12. Mnomani L, Alkharabsceh AR, Al-Zu'bi N, Al-Nuaimy W (2009) Instantiating a mechatronic valve schedule for a hydrocephalus shunt. Conf Proc IEEE Eng Med Biol Soc 31:749–752
13. Richard KE, Block FR, Weiser RR (1999) First clinical results with a telemetric shunt-integrated ICP-sensor. Neurol Res 1:117–120
14. Ursino M, Lodi CA (1997) A simple mathematical model of the interaction between intracranial pressure and cerebral hemodynamics. J Appl Physiol 82:1256–1269
15. Ursino M, Ter Minassian A, Lodi CA, Bydon L (2000) Cerebral hemodynamics during arterial and CO_2 pressure changes: in vivo prediction by a mathematical model. Am J Physiol Heart Circ Physiol 279:H2439–H2455
16. Walter M (2002) Mechatronische Systeme für die Hydrozephalustherapie. Shaker, Aachen, pp 29–58
17. Walter M, Jetzki S, Leonhardt S (2005) A model for intracranial hydrodynamics. In: IEEE annual engineering in medicine and biology conference, Shanghai, Congress Proceedings, pp 5603–5606

Examination of Deposits in Cerebrospinal Fluid Shunt Valves Using Scanning Electron Microscopy

Constantinos Charalambides and Spyros Sgouros

Abstract Obstruction remains the most common complication of cerebrospinal fluid shunts. The valve constitutes an important site of potential malfunction. The aim of this pilot study was to investigate the extent and composition of debris depositions along the structural components of the shunt valve.

We examined three explanted Medos programmable valves. The valves were stored and examined wet. They were cut open and disassembled. All specimens were studied under a scanning electron microscope (SEM; Quanta 200; FEI, Hillsboro, OR, USA) operating at different levels of accelerating voltage and 110 µA beam current. Valve areas analyzed included the ruby ball and collar, the flat spring with its pillar, and the staircase cam. The elemental composition, in areas with abnormal deposits, was subsequently determined by energy-dispersive X-ray microanalysis (EDS) using a Si (Li) detector (Sapphire; EDAX, Mahwah, NJ, USA) with a super ultrathin Be window.

All explanted valves had varying degrees of deposits in all surveyed areas. The extent of the deposits was not related to the time since implantation. The effect of these deposits on proper functioning of the valve as well as their pathogenesis is difficult to establish.

Keywords Hydrocephalus • Cerebrospinal fluid shunt • Shunt valve • Scanning electron microscopy

Introduction

Mechanical failure remains a major complication of shunting for the treatment of hydrocephalus. Although, most commonly, this is due to ventricular catheter occlusion by choroid plexus or ependymal tissue, valve obstruction is the cause of the malfunction in a significant proportion of shunts. Recent studies have shown that even when ventricular catheter occlusion is the main cause of the obstruction, valves are underperforming [2]. Proper mechanical performance of the valve mechanism is largely dependent on its components remaining free of contaminants after implantation.

Previous studies utilizing electron microscopy confirmed the presence of deposits in explanted valves [5, 8, 9]. It seems that the metal components of the valves, as well as surface irregularities, are particularly prone to the adherence of blood cells, fibroblasts, and infectious organisms eventually leading to valve dysfunction [1]. It has to be kept in mind though that these studies were performed on dry specimens, which may not be an accurate representation of the situation as it exists when the valve is functioning in vivo.

The aim of the study was to investigate the extent and composition of debris depositions along the structural components of explanted shunt valves. Valves were kept wet after removal in an attempt to chart reality as closely as possible. Hydrodynamic function was not tested before disassembly because this could alter the physical state of any deposits within the valve.

Materials and Methods

Three Medos programmable valves were explanted from children who presented with shunt malfunction, all under the care of the senior author (S.S.). No clinical or laboratory findings were suggestive of infection preoperatively. Valves were stored wet in a sterile water bath straight after removal to exclude any postexplantation crystallization of material. No attempt was made to flush any material through the valves before they were examined in order to avoid alterations in the physical state of any deposits. All specimens, after disassembling, were studied under a scanning electron microscope (SEM; Quanta 200; FEI, Hillsboro, OR, USA) operating at various levels of accelerating voltage and a 110 µA beam current at the Materials Analysis Laboratory of the University of Athens School of Dentistry. No gold plating was required. Valve areas analyzed included the ruby ball and collar, the

C. Charalambides and S. Sgouros (✉)
Department of Neurosurgery,
'Attikon' University Hospital,
Athens, Greece
e-mail: sgouros@med.uoa.gr

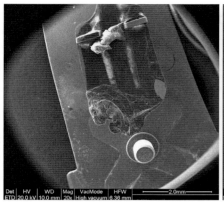 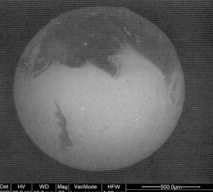 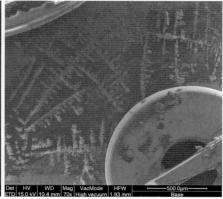

Fig. 1 *Left*: Scanning electron microscopy images obtained during the examination of the flat spring of a valve which had been implanted 12 months before its removal for a central catheter obstruction. The surface is covered with extensive deposits, especially in the area in contact with the staircase cam. Original magnification × 20; *Middle*: Scanning electron microscopy showing the synthetic ruby ball that was removed from a patient 6 months after implantation due to shunt malfunction. Interestingly, depositions are noted only on the part of the ball in contact with the CSF. Original magnification × 67; *Right*: Higher magnification, in a different patient, shows areas with heavy depositions simulating colonies of bacteria in a valve not formally declared infected

flat spring with its pillar, and the staircase cam; all of these parts are critical in the cerebrospinal fluid (CSF) flow path. The materials that constitute the valves are also important to the analysis. The Medos programmable valve rotating staircase has a titanium base, the flat spring is made of stainless steel, whereas the ball is made of synthetic ruby. The elemental composition in areas with abnormal deposits was determined by energy-dispersive X-ray microanalysis (EDS) using a Si (Li) detector (Sapphire; EDAX, Mahwah, NJ, USA) with a super ultrathin Be window.

Results

A total of three explanted Medos programmable valves were analyzed with implantation periods of 2, 6, and 12 months. During the revision operations, ventricular catheter obstruction was documented in all patients. Routine microbiological testing of intraoperative CSF samples was not supportive for the presence of infection in any of the patients.

All explanted valves had extensive, though of variable degree, deposits in all surveyed areas, critical to the performance of the valve, independent of the time from implantation (Fig. 1; left). An exception to this was the synthetic ruby ball: It had very few deposits in its lower half lying in the seat in contrast to the upper half which is in closer contact with the CSF and demonstrated heavy depositions (Fig. 1; middle). In one of the valves the sedimented material on the staircase cam had acquired the appearance of bacterial colonies developing in a culture medium (Fig. 1; right).

EDS in areas with abnormal deposits disclosed considerable peaks of sodium (Na), chloride (Cl), carbon (C), oxygen (O), and calcium (Ca) (Fig. 2). This spectrum was typical for

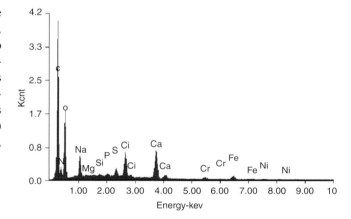

Fig. 2 An energy-dispersive X-ray microanalysis (EDS) spectrum from the flat spring of the valve shown in Fig. 1, specifically from the area corresponding to the maximum density of depositions. There are considerable peaks of C, Ca, Na, O, and Cl

all the areas analyzed with small deviations between specimens. This indicates that the deposits are mainly due to ions normally found in the CSF even in small concentrations (Ca) whereas the C peak illustrates the presence of organic precipitations despite the absence of infection.

Discussion

The in vivo interaction of the external surface of shunts with the surrounding tissues of the host is responsible for many of the problems encountered in shunted patients. It is well documented that the materials that constitute the shunt components gradually degrade over time due to the continuous action of surrounding cellular components such as macrophages [3, 4].

As a consequence, fractures and heavy calcification of the distal tubing causing shunt malfunction are seen in clinical practice [6]. In addition to the destruction of the external surface of shunt components, the internal environment is also disrupted over time because of material deposition. The lumina of the proximal and distal catheters as well as the intervening shunt valve comprise potential sites of debris depositions. It has already been shown that considerable ingrowth of extraneous tissue (choroid plexus or ependyma) occurs in the lumen of the central catheter [3, 7]. Protein derived from the CSF may also gradually accumulate and block the ventricular catheter. Furthermore, the inner surface of the shunt is isolated from the immune system and provides an environment for bacterial colonization [10]. Surface irregularities caused by material deposition aid bacterial adhesion [3].

A previous study by the senior author (S.S.) performed on 19 dry specimens (16 explanted valves and 3 new unused valves of various types) used SEM and EDS to investigate the degradation of shunt valve structure over time due to the deposition of debris, and compare them with the findings in unused valves [9]. At the time of the study, it was not possible to perform SEM on wet specimens, so all the specimens had to be dry and coated with gold (Au). They demonstrated that shunt valves suffer extensive material deposition over time, a finding that was not surprising bearing in mind earlier reported findings in catheter studies. These deposits were mainly formed from inorganic crystals originating from ions normally found in the CSF. Moreover, it was interesting to note the lack of a carbon (C) peak in some noninfected valves, indicating that the deposits did not contain protein. On the contrary, all the clinically infected valves were found to have a substantial C peak. What was surprising to notice was the extent and timing of the depositions: Extensive deposits were observed as early as 2 weeks after implantation. One would expect that it would take several months before such a development took place.

Conclusion

As mentioned earlier, in the present study all three valves utilized were examined as wet specimens to approach as close as possible the in vivo conditions and avoid any crystallization of material after removal. Our findings are coherent with the results of previous studies performed on dry specimens as mentioned above. Extensive material depositions in performance-critical areas of the valve were seen, originating from ions found in the CSF. The extent and consistency of the depositions were independent of the time since implantation; all three valves displayed similar SEM images despite the fact that the time of implantation before removal ranged from 2 to 12 months. This implies that several factors may be involved in the pathogenesis of the deposits, at varying degrees, including the implantation process itself, the narrow aperture of the resistance elements of the shunt system, and the material that the shunt is made of which may promote a slow filtration process. The effect of these deposits on proper functioning of the valve is difficult to establish, but it is reasonable to assume that valve function is impaired due to the deposits, based on their recorded extent and location.

These findings suggest that there is possibly a scope for improvement of the material that valves are made of and their design in order to produce valves less susceptible to debris deposition. Furthermore, from a clinical point of view, when a patient presents with a blocked shunt, it may be a good idea to change all of the shunt system, even if only a catheter obstruction is found, as an old valve may be functioning suboptimally due to debris material deposition.

Acknowledgements We would like to thank Prof. G. Iliadis and Dr. S. Zinelis of the Materials Analysis Laboratory of the School of Dentistry of the University of Athens for the substantial help with the technical aspect of this project.

Conflicts of interest statement We declare that we have no conflict of interest.

References

1. Browd SR, Gottfield ON, Ragel BT, Kestle JR (2006) Failure of CSF shunts: part I: obstruction and mechanical failure. Pediatr Neurol 34:83–92
2. Brydon HL, Bayston R, Hayward R, Harkness W (1996) Removed shunt valves: reasons for failure and implications for valve design. Br J Neurosurg 10:245–251
3. Del Bigio MR (1998) Biological reactions to cerebrospinal fluid shunt devices: a review of the cellular pathology. Neurosurgery 42(2):319–325
4. Echizenya K, Satoh M, Murai H et al (1987) Mineralization and biodegradation of CSF shunting systems. J Neurosurg 67: 584–591
5. Gower DJ, Lewis KC, Kelly DL Jr (1984) Sterile shunt malfunction. A scanning electron microscopic perspective. J Neurosurg 61:1079–1084
6. Griebel RW, Hoffmann HJ, Becker L (1987) Calcium deposits on CSF shunts. Clinical observations and ultrastructural analysis. Childs Nerv Syst 3:180–182
7. Guevara JA, Zuccaro G, Trevisan A et al (1981) Microscopic studies in shunts for hydrocephalus. Childs Brain 8:284–293
8. Schoener WF, Reparon C, Verheggen R, Markakis E (1991) Evaluation of shunt failures by compliance analysis and inspection of shunt valves and shunt materials using microscopic or scanning electron microscopic techniques. In: Matsumoto S, Tamaki N (eds) Hydrocephalus: pathogenesis and treatment. Springer, Tokyo, pp 452–472
9. Sgouros S, Dipple SJ (2004) An investigation of structural degradation of cerebrospinal fluid shunt valves performed using scanning electron microscopy and energy-dispersive x-ray microanalysis. J Neurosurg 100:534–540
10. Zhong Y, Bellamkonda RV (2008) Biomaterials for the central nervous system. J R Soc Interface 5:957–975

Microstructural Alterations of Silicone Catheters in an Animal Experiment: Histopathology and SEM Findings

Regina Eymann, Yoo-Jin Kim, Rainer Maria Bohle, Sebastian Antes, Melanie Schmitt, Michael Dieter Menger, and Michael Kiefer

Abstract *Introduction*: Biocompatibility of implants in humans has been classified as "inert," "tolerated," and "bioactive." In shunt-treated patients, catheter-induced complications account for up to 70% of all hardware failures. Our objective was to study whether foreign body reactions to silicone shunt catheters in subcutaneous tissue and at their distal, intraperitoneal ends leading to occlusion can be reproduced in an animal model.

Materials and Methods: Twelve different silicone catheters were implanted in 6-week-old Wistar rats: (a) purely in the subcutaneous tissue and (b) through the subcutaneous tissue into the peritoneal cavity. One of the catheters was of our own design with a silicated surface. After 1 year, all catheters were explanted and were examined by histopathology and scanning electron microscopy (SEM).

Results: Histopathological analysis revealed the development of collagenous membranes and chronic immune reactions around the catheters. Completely organized intraluminal obliteration was seen in six intraperitoneally inserted catheters. SEM demonstrated calcifications and signs of biodegradation. Silicated catheters showed the most extensive calcifications.

Discussion: Hydrocephalus shunt catheters cannot be termed "inert" or "biotolerated." Rather, they must be regarded as "bio-active" implants. The extensive reaction on silicated catheters can act as reference to estimate the biocompatibility of surface modifications. The model proved appropriate for further studies.

R. Eymann (✉), S. Antes, M. Schmitt, and M. Kiefer
Department of Neurosurgery, Saarland University Hospital and Saarland University Faculty of Medicine,
Homburg-Saar (Saarland), Germany
e-mail: regina.eymann@uks.eu

Y.-J. Kim and R.M. Bohle
Institute of Pathology, Saarland University Hospital and Saarland University Faculty of Medicine,
Homburg-Saar (Saarland), Germany

M.D. Menger
Institute of Clinical Experimental Surgery,
Saarland University Hospital and Saarland University Faculty of Medicine,
Homburg-Saar (Saarland), Germany

Keywords Hydrocephalus • Cerebrospinal fluid shunt • Catheters failure • Foreign body reaction • Silicone

Introduction

Silicone is the exclusive material used for shunt catheter production. According to several authors' reports of foreign body reaction on silicone shunt catheters [1, 2, 9, 10, 11], they cannot be classified as "biological inert" considering the standard classification of biocompatibility [15]. The classification separates between "inert," "tolerated," and "bioactive" according to tissue reactions on foreign material implants:

Definitions

Biologically inert: materials which do not initiate any reaction or interact with surrounding tissue after implantation. Further characteristics are:

- Corrosion resistant
- Thermally resistant
- Refractory
- Coatable

Biotolerant: minor reaction of surrounding tissue. Over the long term, the material is neither biologically inert nor bioactive. Long-term follow-up is characterized by

- No material degradation
- No cellular transformation of surrounding tissue
- No toxic injury during residence time.

Bioactive: Reaction of surrounding tissue on the implant with interplay adhesion. The connection is joined by material engagement with bone or other tissue, which affects tensile strength.

In hydrocephalic, shunted patients, catheter-induced complications are responsible for up to 70% of all complications. Catheter occlusions account for up to 50% of all shunt failures surveyed over a 12-year follow-up [14]. Such shunt obstructions can occur at any time after implantation and at any position within the shunt. The distal, intraperitoneal tube end can occasionally be obstructed by adhesions and abdominal viscera. The surgical procedure of implantation, using a trocar or open (on sight) technique for intraperitoneal catheter insertion, has no influence on the occurrence of shunt failure [2]. The aim of the present study was (1) to prove the validity and reliability of our new model to study catheter biodegradation in animals, (2) to compare our previous results [8] using now-modified surfaces and adding additionally tensile stress on catheters as in daily practice and as occurring with children's growth, (3) to prove the feasibility of extending the model for studies on intraperitoneal foreign body reaction after shunt catheter implantation.

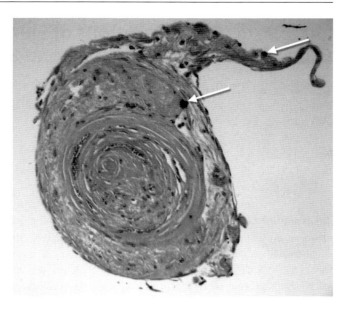

Fig. 1 The catheter lumen is occluded by loosely arranged repair tissue, and focally, regressive calcifications (*arrows*) are detectable. Von Kossa stain (as a standard to demonstrate calcium in mineralized tissue), ×5 objective

Materials and Methods

In 12 six-week-old Wistar rats, various silicone catheters commercially available silicone catheters were implanted. Additionally, a catheter with a modified silicated surface and an antibiotic-impregnated catheter (AIS) were explored. The silicated catheter was designed to provoke extensive foreign body reaction. Silicium oxide is the base for mesoporous ceramic implants designed to be bioactive [12].

All animals were operated on using latex-free gloves and in a latex-free environment to prevent foreign body reaction or allergy resulting from latex [13]. Anesthesia was initiated with CO_2 inhalation for rats' short-term sedation, followed by full anesthesia with intraperitoneally administered 1 mL 0.1% (RS)-(±)-2-(2-Chlorphenyl)-2-8methylamino)-cyclohexane (Ketavet®) (dosage: 1 mL/kg body weight) and 0.24 mL 2-(2,6-Dimethylphenylamino)-5,6-dihydro-4H-thiazin (Rompun®; 2%) (dosage: 2 mg/kg body weight), providing sufficient and long-lasting anesthesia without the need for artificial ventilation. Before operation, all animals were shaven, and the skin was disinfected with Polyvidon-Jod (10 mg Jod/1 mL solution) (Braunol®) for 10 min. A 60-mm-long catheter was inserted subcutaneously via a small skin incision over the right shoulder and hip region. Catheter ends were sutured and fixed on the muscles around the hip and the shoulder using nonabsorbable suture material. To mimic the typical implantation technique used during shunt insertion in humans, catheters were slightly stretched before implantation. The catheters' fixation served to simulate conditions comparable to those in growing children. Another catheter of the same type was fixed on the shoulder with a similar technique and intraperitoneally inserted with an intraperitoneal length of 100 mm via a third skin and small peritoneal incision. With a purse-string suture the opening of the abdominal wall was closed around the catheter to avoid undesired dislocation. All wounds were closed using absorbable subcutaneous suturing and octylcyanoacrylate tissue adhesive for superficial skin closure.

This model aimed at simulating the angular tensile strength and the shear forces for both catheters in the subcutaneous flexible tissue as in children during growth. In addition the intraperitoneal insertion should clarify differences between subcutaneous and intraperitoneal foreign body reactions. All implants remained inserted for 1 year. The adult animals were euthanized with intraperitoneally applied pentobarbital.

Thereafter, all catheters were explanted, including the surrounding tissue, for histopathological and scanning electron microscope (SEM) examination. Histopathological evaluation was conducted independently by two pathologists (R.M.B. and Y.J.K.) on formalin-fixed (buffered formalin 4%) and paraffin-embedded, 3-μm thick, hematoxylin-eosin and von Kossa stained slides.

Results

We could confirm the previous findings of our preceding pilot study [8]:
- All subcutaneous catheters showed:
  - Adherent surrounding tissue during explanation,
  - Fractures and grooves extending deep into the silicone material,
  - Calcifications on the surface area (Figs. 1 and 2).
- All intraperitoneally inserted catheters showed:
  - Calcification on the surface of its subcutaneous part,

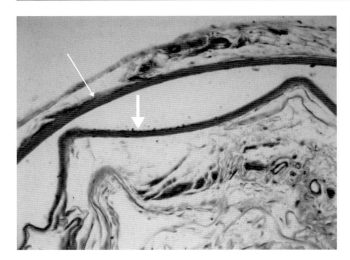

Fig. 2 Collagen fiber–rich capsule surrounding an antibiotic-impregnated catheter (*small arrow*). Interestingly, there is even evidence for calcification of the occlusive granulation tissue within the catheter lumen (*large arrow*). The occluding tissue consists of loosely arranged granulation tissue with a fiber-rich inner capsule pointing to the catheter. Von Kossa stain, ×5 objective

- Calcification of the intraperitoneal part, but more dispersed than on the subcutaneous parts,
- Occlusion of the distal, intraperitoneal lumen with various shapes.

The degree of distal intraperitoneal catheter occlusion varied in its extension. In one catheter type, intraluminal occluding tissue (as foreign body reaction) with an overall length of 140 mm could be measured, while others were just occluded by fibrous membranes at their tips. The occlusive tissue was mainly composed of granulation tissue showing some chronic inflammation and occasionally foreign body giant cells. The catheters were surrounded by a collagen fiber–rich capsule, especially the silicated catheter tips. In antibiotic-impregnated shunt catheters, we could additionally detect intraluminal calcifications.

Discussion

Obviously, our principal objective to ameliorate our recently described animal model for studying foreign body reactions on shunt catheters in a way to mimic the tensile stress and shear forces acting on the catheter in growing children could be achieved. The animal movements and growth added, furthermore, catheter deflexions and stretching, simulating excellently the naturally given conditions of growing shunted children during their daily activity. In the rat model presented here, histopathological findings similar to those found in humans could be reproduced, but in a much shorter time. This holds true also for the intraperitoneal findings. Hence the model can also serve to study details of immunological and pathophysiological processes provoked by silicone catheters in soft tissues and the

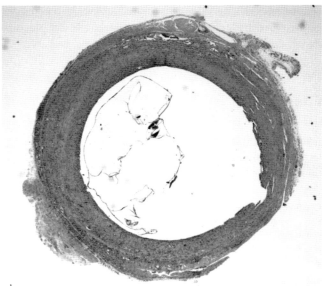

Fig. 3 Image from light-optical microscope showing a tissue-encapsulated Silk-coated catheter. The connective tissue capsule consists of a young granulation tissue with a mild chronic, aseptic inflammatory reaction, and with foreign body giant cells. Hematoxylin and eosin stain (H&E), ×2.5 objective

peritoneal cavity. As previously seen in patients [2, 5], we also found distal intraperitoneal shunt catheter occlusions due to foreign body reaction in our model. It can be argued that lacking flow within the tubes might facilitate intraluminal tissue growth. On the other hand, our proposed methodology provides the best proof that distal shunt occlusion does not necessarily result from cerebrospinal fluid (CSF) contents (proteins, cells, etc.). Some have argued, based on findings of astroglial cells' ingrowth through ventricular catheters' holes into its lumen despite CSF all around all of the catheters' holes, that such cells might play some role in distal shunt obstruction as well. In contrast, our findings underline the suggestion that such distal obstruction can be an autonomous process, emanating from the intraperitoneal cavity itself. Similar findings regarding foreign body reactions on silicone catheters used for continuous ambulatory peritoneal dialysis support this hypothesis [4, 10]. Further, episodes of lacking CSF flow also occur in shunted patients with more proximally occluded catheters [3, 6]. Our model without flow simulates a comparable condition and can now easily explain findings from our daily practice with shunt occlusion at two different positions, of which one is the distal obstruction.

Surprisingly, we found calcifications inside the intraperitoneal catheters' lumen too (Fig. 1). This intraluminal calcification argues for an autonomous process of biodegradation on the inner catheter surface occurring autonomously as a matter of silicone "aging"/degradation [7]. The influence of CSF itself and fluid flow within the tubes has yet to be studied.

As intended, the reaction on the silicated catheters was the greatest (Fig. 3). Accordingly, it can serve as a reference for serious reactions on silicone to study alternative materials or surface-modified silicone catheters with improved biocompatibility over those that have recently become available.

Conclusion

As intended, the reaction to…available. Silicone as a long-term implant, especially under the implant stressing conditions, can not be defined as biocompatible or biological inert.

Conflicts of interest statement This scientific work has been sponsored in part by a grant from the German Federal Ministry of Education and Research (BMBF). R.E. and M.K. have received some financial support in the past for other research work from Raumedic AG (Helmbrechts, Germany). Further, they have received honoraria and financial support for scientific congress attendance from Codman & Shurtleff Inc. (Raynham, MA, USA), a division of Ethicon (Somerville, NJ, USA) and Johnson & Johnson (New Brunswick, NJ, USA), and Aesculap AG (Tuttlingen, Germany) a division of B. Braun Melsungen AG (Melsungen, Germany).

M.S. and S.A. have received financial support for educational purposes from Codman & Shurtleff Inc. (Raynham, MA, USA), a division of Ethicon (Somerville, NJ, USA) and Johnson & Johnson (New Brunswick, NJ, USA) and Aesculap AG (Tuttlingen, Germany) a division of B. Braun Melsungen AG (Melsungen, Germany). R.M.B., M.D.M., and Y.-J.K. have nothing to declare.

References

1. Boch AL, Hermelin E, Sainte-Rose C, Sgouros S (1998) Mechanical dysfunction of ventriculoperitoneal shunts caused by calcification of the silicone rubber catheter. J Neurosurg 88:957–982
2. Browd SR, Ragel BT, Gottfried ON, Kestle JRW (2006) Failure of cerebrospinal fluid shunts: part I: obstruction and mechanical failure. Pediatr Neurol 34:83–92
3. Bruni JE, DelBigio MR (1986) Reaction of periventricular tissue in the rat fourth ventricle to chronically placed shunt tubing implants. Neurosurgery 19:337–345
4. Burkart JM (2002) Peritoneal dialysis. In: Brenner BM, Rectors FC Jr (eds) The kidney, vol 2, 5th edn. Saunders, Philadelphia, pp 2517–2545
5. Del Bigio MR (1998) Biological reactions to cerebrospinal fluid shunt devices: a review of the cellular pathology. Neurosurgery 42:319–325
6. Del Bigio MR, Bruni JE (1986) Reaction of rabbit lateral periventricular tissue to shunt tubing implants. J Neurosurg 64:932–940
7. Echizenya K, Satoh M, Murai H, Ueno H, Abe H, Komai T (1987) Mineralization and biodegradation of CSF shunting systems. J Neurosurg 67:584–591
8. Eymann R, Meier U, Kiefer M (2010) Animal experiments to evaluate complications of foreign materials on silicone with shunt catheters: preliminary results. Acta Neurochir Suppl 106:91–93
9. Hashimoto M, Yokota A, Urasaki E, Tsujigami S, Shimono M (2004) A case of abdominal CSF pseudocyst associated with silicone allergy. Childs Nerv Syst 20:761–764
10. Jörres A, Ludat K, Sander K, Dunkel K, Lorenz F, Keck H, Frei U, Gahl GM (1996) The peritoneal fibroblast and the control of peritoneal inflammation. Kidney Int Suppl 56:S22–S27
11. Kazan S, Açikba C, Rahat O, Tuncer R (2000) Proof of the patent subcutaneous fibrous tract in children with V-P shunt malfunction. Childs Nerv Syst 16:351–356
12. Kinnari TJ, Esteban J, Gomez-Barrena E, Zamora N, Fernandez-Roblas R, Nieto A, Doadrio JC, Lopez-Noriega A, Ruiz-Hernandes E, Arcos D, Vallet-Regi M (2009) Bacterial adherence to SiO2-based multifunctional bioceramics. J Biomed Mater Res A 89:215–223
13. Pires G, Morais-Almeida M, Gaspar A, Godinho N, Calado E, Abreu-Nogueira J, Rosado-Pinto J (2002) Risk factors for latex sensitization in children with spina bifida. Allergol Immunopathol (Madr) 30:5–13
14. Saint-Rose C, Piatt JH, Renier D, Pierre-Kahn A, Hirsch JF, Hoffman HJ, Humphreys RB, Hendrick EB (1991–1992) Mechanical complications in shunts. Pediatr Neurosurg 17:2–9
15. Wintermantel E, Shah-Derler B, Bruinink A, Petitmermet M, Blum J, Ha S-W (2008) Biokompatibilität. In: Wintermantel E, Ha SW (eds) Medizintechnik life science engineering, 4th edn. Springer, Berlin, pp 59–91

Expression Analysis of High Mobility Group Box-1 Protein (HMGB-1) in the Cerebral Cortex, Hippocampus, and Cerebellum of the Congenital Hydrocephalus (H-Tx) Rat

Mitsuya Watanabe, Masakazu Miyajima, Madoka Nakajima, Hajime Arai, Ikuko Ogino, Sinji Nakamura, and Miyuki Kunichika

Abstract High mobility group box-1 protein (HMGB-1), a protein expressed highly in developing neurons, is involved in the development and differentiation of neurons. At the same time, it functions as a transcriptional regulator of particular genes and as a cytokine: HMGB-1 released from a defective cell has been reported to induce damage to the adjacent cells.

With a view to examine the relationship between neuronal damage caused by hydrocephalus and HMGB-1, we analyzed the expression of HMGB-1 in the cerebellum, cerebrum, and hippocampus of 1-day-old congenitally hydrocephalic H-Tx rats.

As opposed to nonhydrocephalic H-Tx rats, the hydrocephalic H-Tx rats were observed to show stronger expression of HMGB-1 in the cerebellum, cerebrum, and hippocampus. Consequently, the protein was presumed to influence the development of neurons from an early postnatal stage not only in the cerebral cortex and hippocampus but also in the cerebellum, which is less susceptible to the direct effects of hydrocephalus. We expect that, in the future, regulating the expression or functions of HMGB-1 will lead to the possibility of impeding the progress of neuronal damage caused by hydrocephalus.

Keywords Congenital hydrocephalus • High mobility group box-1 protein (HMGB-1) • H-Tx rat

Introduction

Ventriculomegaly associated with hydrocephalus affects the cellular composition and structure of the cerebrum. In contrast, the cerebellum is not directly affected by ventriculomegaly and should thus be more appropriate as the subject of comparative investigation. We thus attempted to identify proteins involved in the development of hydrocephalus in the cerebellum by proteome analysis and reported a specifically higher expression of high mobility group box-1 (HMGB-1) in 1-day-old hydrocephalic rats than in normal rats [1].

HMGB-1 is a DNA-binding nuclear protein that comprises the chromatin and plays an important role in the maintenance of DNA conformation. It is also involved in the development and differentiation of neurons and thus is highly expressed in developing neurons [5].

The present study focused on HMGB-1 and analyzed the expression of the protein in the cerebellum, cerebral cortex, and hippocampus.

Materials and Methods

Five 1-day-old hydrocephalic H-Tx rats (H-Tx rats) and five nonhydrocephalic H-Tx control rats (non-H-Tx rats) were used.

Reverse Transcriptase Polymerase Chain Reaction

Brains were removed from H-Tx and non-H-Tx rats. The cerebral cortex, hippocampus, and cerebellum were dissected from the brains, fixed in liquid nitrogen, and stored at −80°C until analysis. RNAs were extracted from each sample using the guanidine hydrochloride method, and cDNAs were synthesized from the RNAs using reverse transcriptase (RT). Polymerase chain reaction (PCR) was performed with HMGB-1 primers (F: ccggatgcttctgtcaactt, R: ttgatttttgggcggtactc) and GAPDH

M. Watanabe (✉), M. Miyajima, M. Nakajima, H. Arai, I. Ogino, S. Nakamura, and M. Kunichika
Department of Neurosurgery, Juntendo University,
Bunkyoku, Tokyo, Japan
e-mail: mitsuya.med-juntendo@tamanan-hp.com

primers (F: accacagtccatgccatcac, R: tccaccaccctgttgctgta), using 20 cycles at 95°C for 30 s, 64°C for 1 min, and 72°C for 1 min.

Western Blot

Nuclear protein was extracted from the frozen samples of each brain region and subjected to electrophoresis using 10% gel. The separated protein was transferred to a PDVF membrane using the iBlot Dry Blotting System (Invitrogen), and protein bands were detected using the WesternBreeze Chemiluminescent Western Blot Immunodetection Kit (Invitrogen). The primary antibodies used were rabbit polyclonal HMGB-1 antibody (Abcam) diluted to 1:1,000 and mouse monoclonal GAPDH antibody (Abcam) diluted to 1:3,000.

Immunostaining

Paraffin-embedded sections were reacted with rabbit polyclonal-HMGB-1 antibody (Abcam) diluted to 1:200 as the primary antibody, then with DAKO ENVISION System Labeled Polymer (DAKO) as the secondary antibody, and then stained with DBA. The sections were further subjected to nuclear staining with hematoxylin.

Results

HMGB-1 mRNA expression was identified in the cerebral cortex, hippocampus, and cerebellum in both the H-Tx and non-H-Tx groups, but the expression in the hippocampus and cerebellum were higher in the H-Tx group than in the non-H-Tx group (Fig. 1). In the cerebral cortex, no significant difference in HMGB-1 mRNA expression was found between the two groups. Similarly, HMGB-1 protein expression was also identified in all of the brain regions tested in both groups, and the expression of the protein in the hippocampus and cerebellum was higher in the H-Tx group than in the non-H-Tx group (Fig. 2). Immunohistochemistry revealed a higher expression of HMGB-1 in the nuclei of neurons in the cerebral cortex, hippocampus, and cerebellum of the H-Tx group than in those of the non-H-Tx group (Fig. 3a–c).

Discussion

The observed higher expression of HMGB-1 in the hippocampus and cerebellum than in the cerebral cortex in 1-day-old rats may be related to the fact that both the hippocampus, especially the dentate gyrus, and the cerebellum are composed

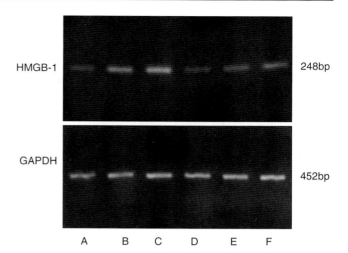

Fig. 1 Results of reverse transcriptase polymerase chain reaction (RT-PCR). Hydrocephalus(+): *A* cerebral cortex, *B* hippocampus, *C* cerebellum. Hydrocephalus (−): *D* cerebral cortex, *E* hippocampus, *F* cerebellum.

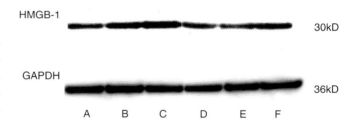

Fig. 2 Result of Western blot. Hydrocephalus (+): *A* cerebral cortex, *B* hippocampus, *C* cerebellum. Hydrocephalus (−): *D* cerebral cortex, *E* hippocampus, *F* cerebellum

of granule cells formed during almost the same period. The higher expression of HMGB-1 in the H-Tx group than in the non-H-Tx group is likely to be due to the retarded development of neurons associated with hydrocephalus, suggesting that the disturbance of neuronal development and differentiation in the early postnatal period may occur not only in the cerebral cortex and hippocampus, which are directly affected by ventriculomegaly, but also in the cerebellum, which is not affected by ventriculomegaly.

Recent studies suggest that HMGB-1 serves as a precipitating/inflammatory factor (cytokine) during cerebral infarction [3]. The proposed secretory mechanisms of HMGB-1 include passive secretion from the nucleus and cytoplasm in response to cell damage, such as apoptosis and necrosis, and active secretion from lysosomes following acetylation in the nucleus in response to inflammatory stimuli, such as cytokines. The secreted HMGB-1 acts on adjacent target cells via the receptor for advanced glycation end products (RAGE) and Toll-like receptor 2/4 (TLR 2/4). Eventually, nuclear factor kappa B (NF-κB) arising in the cytoplasm acts on the nucleus to again induce acetylation of HMGB-1, which is secreted from lysosomes. This chain reaction appears to be involved in the expansion of a cerebral ischemic lesion; the inhibition of

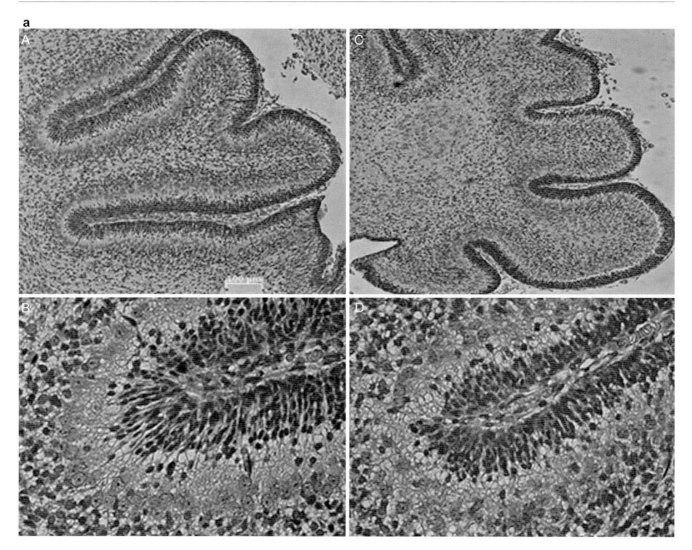

Fig. 3 (**a**) Photomicrographs of the immunostaining for HMGB-1 in the cerebellum. (A) H-Tx, original magnification×100; (B) H-Tx, original magnification×400; (C) non H-Tx, original magnification×100; (D) non H-Tx, original magnification×400. (**b**) Photomicrographs of the immunostaining for HMGB-1 in the hippocampus. (A) H-Tx, original magnification×100; (B) H-Tx, original magnification×400; (C) non H-Tx, original magnification×100; (D) non H-Tx, original magnification×400. (**c**) Photomicrographs of the immunostaining for HMGB-1 in the cerebral cortex. (A) H-Tx, original magnification×100; (B) H-Tx, original magnification×400; (C) non H-Tx, original magnification×100; (D) non H-Tx, original magnification×400

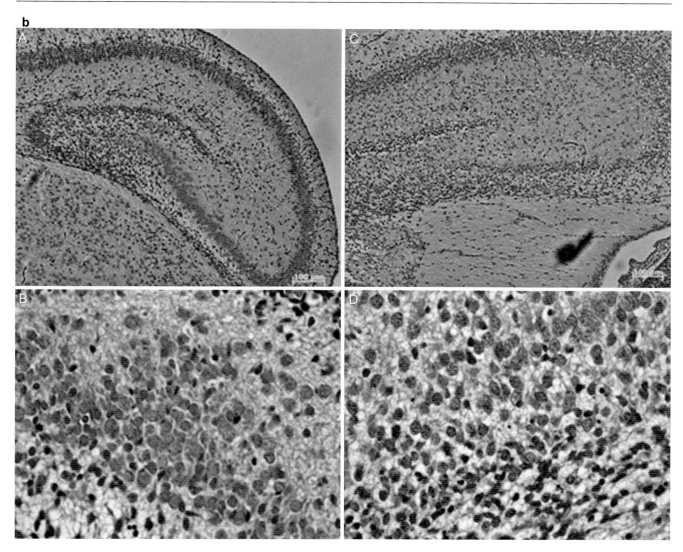

Fig. 3 (continued)

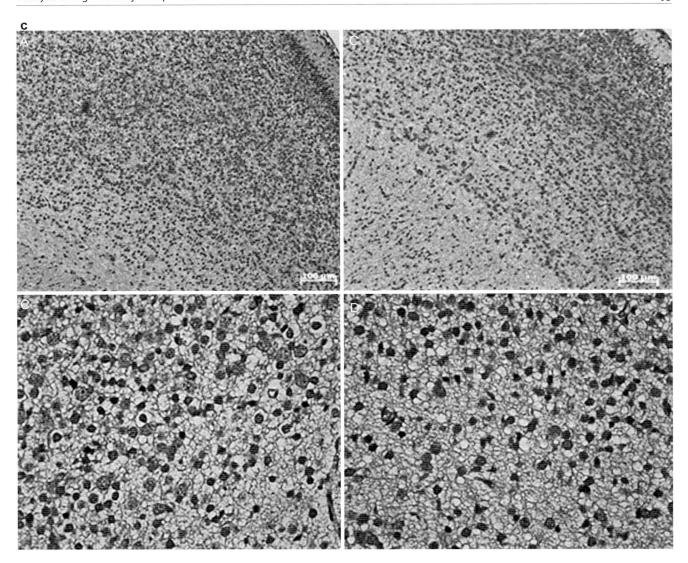

Fig. 3 (continued)

HMGB-1 with agents such as anti-HMGB-1 antibody, A-box peptide, soluble RAGE, and anti-RAGE antibody has been shown to delay the progression of cerebral ischemia [6].

We previously demonstrated that the hippocampus and cerebral cortex of 4-week-old H-Tx rats express IL-1β and IL-6 [2] and that neuronal cell death is observed even in the cerebral cortex of 8-week-old H-Tx rats that were considered to have developed compensatory hydrocephalus [4]. It is speculated that the HMGB-1 secretion chain is to some extent involved in neuronal cell damage caused by hydrocephalus. Thus, future studies may develop new treatment strategies for hydrocephalus based on the control of this secretion chain.

Conclusion

We observed developmental impairment of cerebellum at an early point after birth, where we had not expected so much influence of hydrocephalus.

Conflicts of interest statement We declare that we have no conflict of interest.

References

1. Li X, Miyajima M, Mineki R, Taka H, Murayama K, Arai H (2005) Analysis of cerebellum proteomics in the hydrocephalic H-Tx rat. Neuroreport 16(6):571–574
2. Miyajima M, Sato K, Arai H (1996) Choline acetyltransferase, nerve growth factor and cytokine levels are changed in congenitally hydrocephalic HTx rats. Pediatr Neurosurg 24(1):1–4
3. Mori S, Liu K, Takahashi HK, Nishibori M (2009) Therapeutic effect of anti-nucleokine monoclonal antibody on ischemic brain infarction. Yakugaku Zasshi 129(1):25–31
4. Nonaka Y, Miyajima M, Ogino I, Nakajima M, Arai H (2008) Analysis of neuronal cell death in the cerebral cortex of H-Tx rats with compensated hydrocephalus. J Neurosurg Pediatr 1(1):68–74
5. Parkkinen J, Raulo E, Merenmies J, Nolo R, Kajander EO, Baumann M et al (1993) Amphoterin, the 30-kDa protein in a family of HMG1-type polypeptides. Enhanced expression in transformed cells, leading edge localization, and interactions with plasminogen activation. J Biol Chem 268:19726–19738
6. Yang QW, Wang JZ, Li JC, Zhou Y, Zhong Q, Lu FL, Xiang J (2010) High-mobility group protein box-1 and its relevance to cerebral ischemia. J Cereb Blood Flow Metab 30(2):243–254

Brain Localization of Leucine-Rich α2-Glycoprotein and Its Role

Madoka Nakajima, M. Miyajima, I. Ogino, M. Watanabe, Y. Hagiwara, T. Segawa, K. Kobayashi, and H. Arai

Abstract *Objectives*: We have previously reported that the level of leucine-rich alpha-2-glycoprotein (LRG) expression is specifically increased in cerebrospinal fluid (CSF) of idiopathic normal pressure hydrocephalus (INPH). The objective of this study is to examine the localization of LRG – the cerebral areas where it is expressed.

Method: The histological sections of autopsied brain specimens from ten subjects, five adult cases (mean age 43.6 years; range 34–50 years) and five senile cases (mean age 76.0 years; range 67–88 years) were prepared, multi-stained with antibodies against human LRG, glial fibrillary acidic protein (GFAP), CD31, and aquaporin-4 (AQP4), and reviewed for the expression sites of LRG.

Results: Immunostains of GFAP and LRG were compared in standard brain specimens from elderly patients. The results indicated that LRG is distributed throughout the entire brain, with especially high expression in the deep cerebral cortex. In addition, the cells that express LRG showed similar morphology to astrocytes. Double staining of CD31 and LRG revealed a significant expression of LRG in the pericapillary regions. The expression was observed in resident astrocytes, as well as in the capillary vessel to which astrocytic processes grow and adhere. When age-related comparisons were made between senile and adult specimens, LRG expression increased with age.

Conclusion: LRG expression in resident astrocytes increased with age.

Keywords Leucine-rich alpha-2-glycoprotein • Astrocyte • Aquaporin-4

Introduction

Previously, we reported that leucine-rich α2-glycoprotein (LRG) is specifically elevated in idiopathic normal pressure hydrocephalus (INPH) patients, based on proteome analysis of CSF obtained by lumbar puncture [2, 4]. LRG in the brain is thought to be closely related to the pathophysiology of INPH, but its function and localization in the brain remain unknown. In the present study, immunostaining with various markers to clarify the localization of LRG was conducted on brain sections collected at autopsy.

Materials and Methods

Investigation of LRG Localization in Autopsied Human Brain (Section Staining)

We used anti-human LRG (329) rabbit IgG (Affinity Purify) custom antibodies produced by Immuno-Biological Laboratories Co. (IBL; Takasaki, Japan) for immunostaining of LRG within the brain.

LRG expression was localized within the cerebral parenchyma using autopsied brain specimens from ten subjects, five adult cases (mean age 43.6 years; range 34–50 years) and five senile cases (mean age 76.0 years; range 67–88 years) from the Juntendo University Department of Pathology (Table 1). Paraffin sections from each area of the autopsied human brain were immunostained with each of the following primary antibodies: anti-human LRG (329) rabbit IgG (IBL; 1:20), anti-myelin basic protein (MBP), goat IgG (sc-13914; Santa Cruz Biotechnology Inc.; 1:100), anti-GFAP rabbit

M. Nakajima (✉), M. Miyajima, I. Ogino, M. Watanabe, and H. Arai
Department of Neurosurgery, Juntendo University School of Medicine, Tokyo, Japan
e-mail: madoka66@juntendo.ac.jp

Y. Hagiwara
Department of Pathology and Oncology,
Juntendo University School of Medicine,
Tokyo, Japan and
Immuno-Biological Laboratories,
Gunma, Japan

T. Segawa and K. Kobayashi
Immuno-Biological Laboratories,
Gunma, Japan

Table 1 The differences in the expression patterns of LRG with age in the deep cerebral cortex

Adult cases (n=5)				Senile cases (n=5)			
Age	Sex	Disease	Count (mean)	Age	Sex	Disease	Count (mean)
43 years old	Male	Renal amyloidosis	8.2	88 years old	Male	Amyloid angiopathy	43
42 yeras old	Female	Systemic mycotic disease	13	69 years old	Male	Parkinson's disease	51.4
50 years old	Male	Amyotrophic lateral sclerosis	6.6	74 years old	Male	Pemphigoid	48.2
49 years old	Female	Malignant lymphoma	4.8	67 years old	Male	Cerebral infarction	43.8
34 years old	Male	Acute lymphocytic leukemia	8.2	82 years old	Male	Normal pressure hydrocephalus	52
mean ± SD; 8.68 ± 3.05				mean ± SD; 47.68 ± 4.18			

Brain sections were immunostained, and the number of positive cells in five visual fields at ×20 magnification was counted. t-Test: $p<0.01$
LRG leucine-rich α2-glycoprotein

IgG (AB1980; Chemicon International Inc.; 1:500), anti-human GLUT-5 rabbit IgG (GLUT5; IBL18905; 1:50), anti-human Olig2 rabbit IgG (Olig2; IBL18953; 1:100), anti-CD31 mouse IgG (ab9498; Abcam; 1:25), anti-neurofilament-L goat IgG (sc-12980; Santa Cruz Biotechnology Inc.; 1:200), and anti-AQP4 goat IgG (sc-9888; Santa Cruz Biotechnology Inc.; 1:1000).

For preprocessing, sections were autoclaved at 121 °C for 10 min with Glut-5, Olig2, and CD31 antibodies and blocked with 5× SEA BLOCK blocking buffer (Pierce) and 1% donkey serum phosphate-buffered saline (PBS). Staining was performed with DAB, following treatment with Dako Envision System-Labeled Polymer, HRP (Dako; Code: K1491), and Histofine Simple Stain MAX PO(G) (Nichirei Biosciences 414161) as secondary antibodies.

Sections were viewed under a Nikon E800 microscope, and images were captured with an AxioCam HRc CCD camera using AxioVison Rel 4.7 imaging processing software.

Specimens of cultured human astrocytes (1800; Science Cell), human glioblastoma, astrocytoma grade III, epithelial-like cell line (U373 MG), nuclear lysate (ab14902), and astrocytoma (grade 2) were immunostained with GFAP and LRG, and differences in LRG expression between resident astrocytes and reactive astrocytes were investigated.

Human LRG Reverse Transcriptase Polymerase Chain Reaction (RT-PCR) and Direct Sequence Analysis

Total RNA was extracted from cultured human astrocytes using Isogen (311–02501; Nippon Gene), and cDNA was amplified with the AccuScript High Fidelity 1st Strand cDNA Synthesis kit (Agilent Technologies – Stratagene Products) with 5 U/μL Taq DNA polymerase (11-146-173-001; Roche Applied Science) and the following primer sets: primer 1F (cgaccaaaaagcccaggggg) and primer 1R (ggttggctggcaggtgggtc) (32–270; 239 bp); primer 2F (cgtgcacctggccgtggaat) and primer 2R (accctggccagcttgttgcc) (221–763; 543 bp); and primer 3F (gccagacgctcctggcagtg) and primer 3R (tggccagggctcagctggaa) (1021–1648; 628 bp). PCR was carried out with 35 cycles of 72 °C for 30 s, 64 °C for 1 min, and 72 °C for 1 min.

Each target band was labeled with a Terminator Cycle Sequencing kit v3.1 (433690; Applied Biosystems) and then analyzed with ABI3100 capillaries (Applied Biosystems) and deposited in GenBank as Accession number NM_052972.2.

Results

Localization of LRG in the Brain

Comparison of MBP and LRG staining in a brain from an elderly subject (age 88 years, amyloid angiopathy) showed that LRG expression was localized mostly in the cerebral cortex, particularly the deep cortex (Fig. 1). LRG, GFAP, Olig2, and GLUT5 immunostaining of the brain of a 50-year-old with amyotrophic lateral sclerosis showed that cells expressing LRG were unlike oligodendroglia or microglia and had the same morphology as astrocytes with endfeet processes that extend toward the vessels and appear to wrap around the capillaries (Fig. 2).

LRG antibody staining of cultured human astrocytes showed LRG immunoreactivity, and RT-PCR and

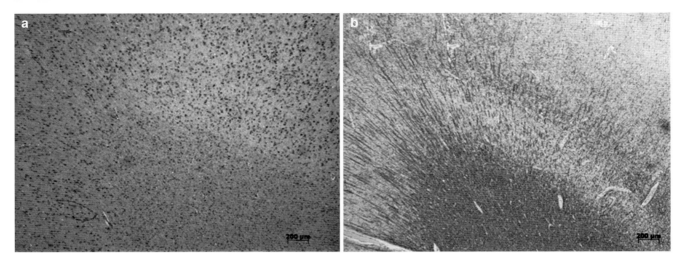

Fig. 1 Leucine-rich α2-glycoprotein (LRG) (**a**) and anti-myelin basic protein (MBP) (**b**) staining of autopsied brain sections from an 88-year-old subject with amyloid angiopathy. LRG expression localizes mostly in the cerebral cortex, particularly the deep cortex

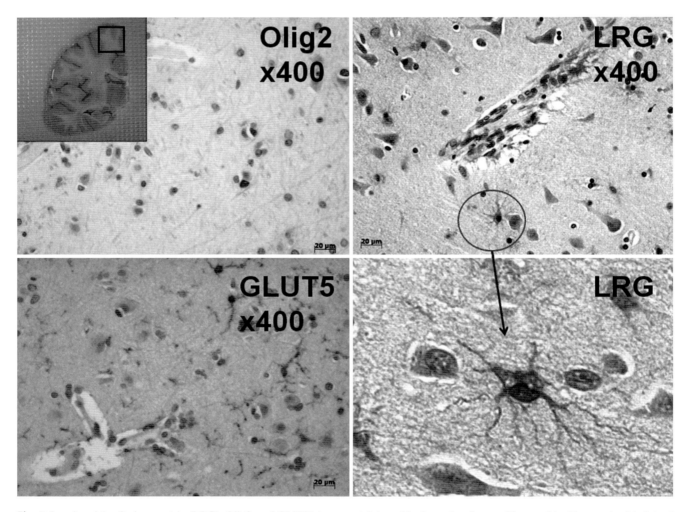

Fig. 2 Leucine-rich α2-glycoprotein (LRG), Olig2, and GLUT5 immunostaining of brain section from a 50-year-old with amyotrophic lateral sclerosis. LRG-positive cells appear to be astrocytes with endfeet processes extending to the capillaries, rather than oligodendroglia or microglia

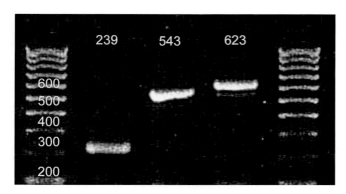

Fig. 3 Leucine-rich α2-glycoprotein (LRG) reverse transcriptase polymerase chain reaction (RT-PCR) Total RNA was extracted from cultured human astrocytes

sequencing confirmed LRG gene expression in astrocytes (Fig. 3). LRG expression appears to occur in a portion of the astrocytes. Double-staining with CD31 and LRG showed greater LRG expression in the astrocytes with processes that extend near the vessels. After LRG antibody immunostaining of astrocytoma (grade 2), no immunoreactivity to LRG could be observed, suggesting limited LRG expression in reactive astrocytes, but greater expression in some resident astrocytes.

Changes in LRG Expression in the Brain with Age

LRG immunostaining was followed by confocal microscopy of brain sections from the parietal cortex of five adult cases and five senile cases. To investigate the differences in the expression patterns of LRG with age in the deep cerebral cortex, brain sections were immunostained and the number of positive cells in five visual fields at a ×20 magnification was counted (Table 1). The number of positive cells in adult cases and in senile cases were 8.68±3.05 (mean±SD) and 47.68±4.18, respectively (t-test: $p<0.01$). LRG immunostaining showed a tendency for increased immunoreactivity with age.

Discussion

LRG was isolated in 1977 from human serum by Haupt and Baundner [1], and in 1985, its amino acid sequence was determined. LRG is a 38 kDa protein and consists of 312 amino acid residues, 66 of which are leucine. This protein contains periodic eight-unit repeats of a three-member amino acid sequence: leucine, proline, and asparagine. This consensus sequence, termed the leucine-rich repeat, has been found in over 55,000 sequences in the Pfam database of protein alignments [5, 6].

The human LRG gene is localized to chromosome subband 19p13.3, and its protein is known to exist in the extracellular space. LRG is coexpressed with transforming growth factor βI type II receptor (TGF βR-II) [3], and its amino acid sequence contains a putative membrane binding region, suggesting potential binding with TGF βR-II on the cell surface. LRG is thought to bind to collagen and fibronectin, as well as to TGF-β through collagen [3].

The results of the present study show that the high expression of LRG in a portion of astrocytes in the deep cortex causes these astrocytes to extend processes around the capillaries. Thus, LRG may bind to collagen and fibronectin and deposit on the capillaries, thereby contributing to arteriosclerotic changes. In the present study, LRG expression was observed in astrocytes of the deep cerebral cortex. Although the number of astrocytes tends to decrease with age, LRG expression tends to increase. The role of the increase of LRG expression with age is unclear and remains an issue for further study. The relationship of LRG with specific diseases in the elderly also requires further investigation.

Conclusion

The expression of LRG in the brain was found to be localized in the cerebral cortex. This included expression in astrocytes and processes, with significant expression in the processes around blood vessels. LRG expression in the brain increased with age.

Conflicts of interest statement We declare that we have no conflict of interest.

References

1. Haupt H, Baudner S (1977) Isolation and characterization of an unknown, leucine-rich 3.1-S-alpha2-glycoprotein from human serum (author's transl). Hoppe Seylers Z Physiol Chem 358:639–646
2. Li X, Miyajima M, Mineki R, Taka H, Murayama K, Arai H (2006) Analysis of potential diagnostic biomarkers in cerebrospinal fluid of idiopathic normal pressure hydrocephalus by proteomics. Acta Neurochir (Wien) 148:859–864; discussion 864
3. Meier U, Miethke C (2003) Predictors of outcome in patients with normal-pressure hydrocephalus. J Clin Neurosci 10:453–459
4. Nakajima M, Miyajima M, Ogino I, Watanabe M, Miyata H, Karagiozov KL, Arai H, Hagiwara Y, Segawa T, Kobayashi K Hashimoto Y (2011) Leucine-rich alpha-2-glycoprotein is a marker for idiopathic normal pressure hydrocephalus. Acta Neurochir (Wien) 153:1339–1346; discussion 1346

5. Okumura K, Ohkura N, Inoue S, Ikeda K, Hayashi K (1998) A novel phospholipase A2 inhibitor with leucine-rich repeats from the blood plasma of Agkistrodon blomhoffii siniticus. Sequence homologies with human leucine-rich alpha2-glycoprotein. J Biol Chem 273:19469–19475

6. Shirai R, Gotou R, Hirano F, Ikeda K, Inoue S (2010) Autologous extracellular cytochrome c is an endogenous ligand for leucine-rich alpha2-glycoprotein and beta-type phospholipase A2 inhibitor. J Biol Chem 285:21607–21614

Role of Artificial Cerebrospinal Fluid as Perfusate in Neuroendoscopic Surgery: A Basic Investigation

Masakazu Miyajima, Kazuaki Shimoji, Misuya Watanabe, Madoka Nakajima, Ikuko Ogino, and Hajime Arai

Abstract Neuroendoscopic surgery is distinct from usual craniotomy as it is performed in water. We have previously reported that the use of artificial cerebrospinal fluid (CSF) as perfusate in third ventriculostomy is more efficacious in minimizing severe host reaction than normal saline or lactated Ringer's solution. In this study, we investigated the effects of different perfusion solutions in human cultured astrocytes. We cultured human astrocytes in growth medium. Then each of them was further cultured for 6 h in artificial CSF, lactated Ringer's solution, or normal saline. Using DNA microarray, RNAs were extracted from each of the cells and were comprehensively analyzed to identify differences in patterns of gene manifestation. Compared to the use of artificial CSF, in cases where lactated Ringer's solution or normal saline was used, there was little difference in the pattern of gene manifestation, but there was an increase in gene manifestation related to apoptosis and inflammatory reaction. For neuroendoscopic surgery, the use of artificial CSF as a perfusate is considered effective in maintaining brain homeostasis compared to the use of normal saline or lactated Ringer's solution.

Keywords Neuroendoscope • Artificial cerebrospinal fluid • DNA microarray • Lactated Ringer's solution • Saline

Introduction

The use of artificial cerebrospinal fluid as a perfusate for neuroendoscopic surgery was first reported by Griffith et al. in 1990 [3]. They reported on the treatment of infantile hydrocephalus, during which they induced coagulation of the choroid plexus and then perfused it with artificial cerebrospinal fluid. The first to report on the significance of the use of artificial cerebrospinal fluid in neuroendoscopic surgery were Oka et al. [6]. According to that report by Oka et al., a comparison was conducted between two groups that used either normal saline solution or an artificial cerebrospinal fluid. In the normal saline solution group, clinical symptoms, including headache, high fever, and neck stiffness resulting from meningeal irritation, were present in all cases. In contrast, in the artificial cerebrospinal fluid group, while headache and high fever were present in one of the five cases, there were no apparent cases of neck stiffness. Furthermore, compared to the artificial cerebrospinal fluid group, an increased number of cells were apparent in the cerebrospinal fluid of the normal saline solution group. In addition, body temperature transitions tended to be higher for the normal saline solution group than the artificial cerebrospinal fluid group. These results suggested the possibility that the use of artificial cerebrospinal fluid as a perfusate during neuroendoscopic surgery could minimize the effects caused by the use of normal saline.

From the report by Oka et al., it is clear that the use of normal saline solution as a perfusate is not preferable for neuroendoscopic surgery. As such, among commercially available infusion solutions, we have continued to use lactated Ringer's solution, which has a composition that is relatively similar to cerebrospinal fluid. However, in comparing cerebrospinal fluid, artificial cerebrospinal fluid, and lactated Ringer's solution, we observed that the ion concentrations of K, Mg, Ca, etc. and pH vary dramatically. In 40 cases of endoscopic third ventriculostomy procedures that we conducted, we compared and evaluated the biological effects of lactated Ringer's solution and artificial cerebrospinal fluid, employing a reverse analytical approach. For postoperative changes in body temperature, we found that compared to lactated Ringer's solution, artificial cerebrospinal fluid presented fewer instances of abnormal

---

M. Miyajima (✉), K. Shimoji, M. Watanabe, M. Nakajima, I. Ogino, and H. Arai
Department of Neurosurgery, Juntendo University,
Tokyo, Japan
e-mail: mmasaka@juntendo.ac.jp

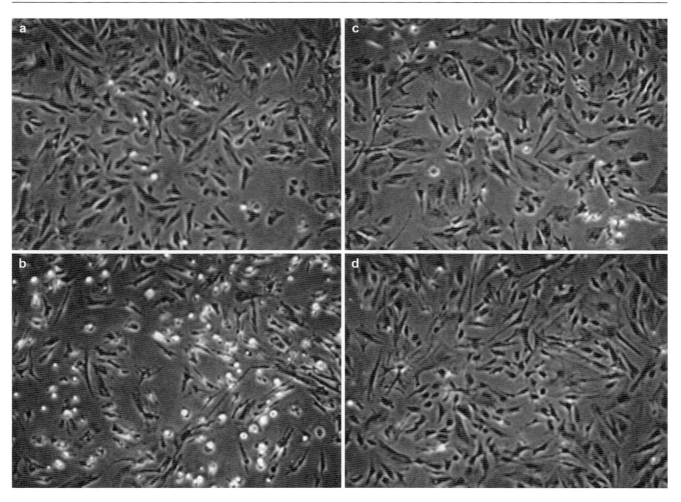

Fig. 1 Morphological characterization of astrocytes after exposure to various perfusates: (**a**) growth medium, (**b**) saline, (**c**) lactated Ringer's solution, and (**d**) artificial cerebrospinal fluid

increases in body temperature. Furthermore, while we saw no significant difference in postoperative headaches when comparing lactated Ringer's solution and artificial cerebrospinal fluid, nausea and vomiting tended to be more prevalent in cases where lactated Ringer's solution was used. On the basis of these results, we concluded that compared to artificial cerebrospinal fluid, lactated Ringer's solution might cause more significant damage to the brain. As such, we performed in vitro experiments.

Materials and Methods

Normal human astrocytes and astrocyte growth medium (AGM) BulletKit were obtained from Clonetics, BioWhittaker Inc. (Walkersville, MD, USA). Saline solution, lactated Ringer's solution, and artificial cerebrospinal fluid were supplied by Otsuka Pharmaceutical Factory Inc. (Tokushima, Japan).

We cultured human astrocytes in growth medium. Then each of them was further cultured for 6 h in artificial cerebrospinal fluid, lactate Ringer's solution, or normal saline. We isolated the total RNA from each of the cells using the single-step guanidium thiocyanate extraction method. The total RNA (20 µg) from the three independent experiments was then converted into double-stranded cDNA using the Ambion WT Expression Kit (Ambion) and transcribed in vitro into biotinylated cRNA according to the manufacturer's instructions (Affymetrix). The 20 µg of fragmented cRNA was hybridized for 16 h under constant rotation at 45°C in Human Gene 1.0 ST array (Affymetrix). After washing and staining the samples, fluorescence was determined using a GeneChip Scanner 3000 (Affymetrix). Data files were evaluated using the GeneChip Suite 5.0 software (Affymetrix). The data were generated using Ingenuity Pathway Analysis (Agilent Technologies).

Results

(1) From a morphological perspective, we observed significant cell death among astrocytes cultured in normal saline solution. In contrast, we detected no morphological changes with lactated Ringer's solution or artificial cerebrospinal fluid (Fig. 1).

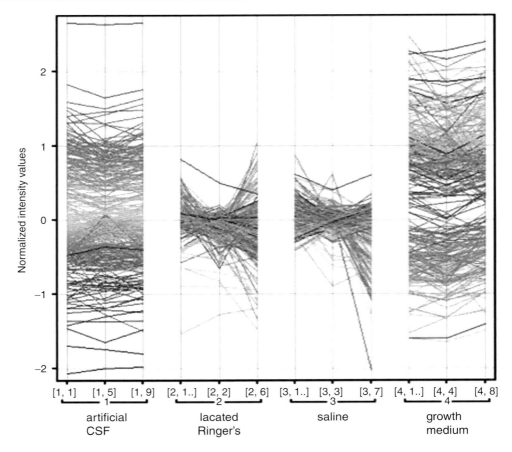

Fig. 2 DNA array gene expression analysis: Genes displayed high and low expression levels with artificial cerebrospinal fluid and cell culture medium, and a similar gene expression pattern was observed. However, with normal saline and lactated Ringer's solution, a comparatively average expression pattern was observed

(2) When comparing gene expression states using DNA array gene expression analysis, we found that with artificial cerebrospinal fluid and cell culture medium, genes displayed high and low expression levels and a similar gene expression pattern was observed. However, with normal saline and the lactated Ringer's solution, a comparatively average expression pattern was observed. From this, we found that compared to normal saline or lactated Ringer's solutions, artificial cerebrospinal fluid and cell culture medium resulted in more active RNA transcription, and from that we can assume that the cells functioned more actively (Fig. 2).

(3) In a volcano plot analysis, compared to artificial cerebrospinal fluid, 47 genes had altered expression in lactated Ringer's solution, and the expression of 42 genes was altered in normal saline solution. Furthermore, of these genes, 30 were common to both solutions (Fig. 3). Of these 30 genes, we looked at the genes for which expression increased; compared with the genes from the artificial cerebrospinal fluid, we found that there were 18 genes from the lactated Ringer's solution and 15 from normal saline. Of those genes, 12 were identical between the two groups (Table 1). Among these genes were the tumor necrosis factor (TNF) and nuclear factor kappa-B (NF-kB) genes, which are vital to apoptosis. The gene that showed the greatest increase, cation transport regulator homolog 1 (CHAC1), has recently been reported as being associated with apoptosis [5]. Similar to the normal saline solution, no changes in cell morphology were detected 6 h after exposure to lactated Ringer's solution; however, it is clear that there was an amplification of genes related to cell death.

Discussion

Although the area of the brain that absorbs cerebrospinal fluid is still unknown, there is no doubt that the choroid plexus is where most of the cerebrospinal fluid is produced. The interstitial blood vessels of the choroid plexus are fenestrated capillaries, which allow plasma to pass freely. However, tight junctions mutually integrate the epithelial cells of the choroid plexus. As such, ventricular communication is not possible, and a blood–cerebrospinal fluid barrier is formed. When comparing plasma and cerebrospinal fluids, there are significant variations in K, Mg, and Ca concentrations, and slight variations are also seen in other ion concentrations. Therefore, cerebrospinal fluid is not simply a filtered plasma solution but a fluid that is formed and excreted by choroid plexus epithelial cells. Furthermore, because cerebrospinal fluid communicates freely with the ventricular interstitial fluid, cerebrospinal fluid is thought to have a vital impact on the development and maintenance of the cerebrum [4].

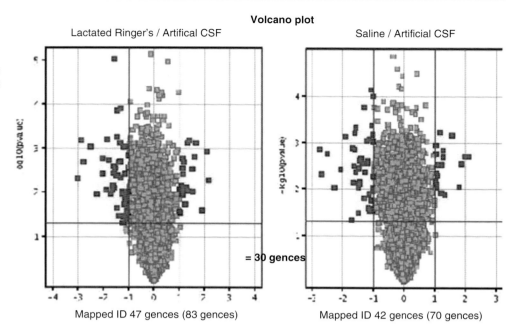

Fig. 3 In a volcano plot analysis, compared with artificial cerebrospinal fluid, the expression of 47 genes increased or decreased in the lactated Ringer's solution, and the expression of 42 genes increased or decreased in the normal saline solution. Of these genes, 30 were common to both solutions

Table 1 Genes for which expression increased, compared with those from artificial cerebrospinal fluid (ACSF)

Saline/ACSF	Fold change	Lactated Ringer's/ ACSF/ ACSF	Fold change
CHAC1	4	CHAC1	4
DUSP1	3	DUSP1	4
TNFAIP3	3	TNFAIP3	3
BHLHE40	2	BHLHE40	2
CD274	2	CD274	2
ERRF11	2	ERRF11	2
ID1	2	ID1	2
ID3	2	ID3	2
LIF	2	LIF	2
MYC	2	MYC	2
NFKBIA	2	NFKBIA	2
TUFT1	2	TUFT1	2
BDNF	2	RFC1	2
HBEGF	2	TOB2	2
HMGCS1	2	UIMC1	2
IFFO2	2	–	–
JUNB	2	–	–
RND3	2	–	–

Eighteen genes in the lactated Ringer's solution changed, as did 15 genes in normal saline. Of those genes, 12 were identical between the two solutions

The main condition requiring neuroendoscopic surgery is noncommunicating hydrocephalus, which often manifests as prominent ventricular dilation. Further, in cases of prominent ventricular dilation, the ventricular ependymal cells are damaged and the glial limiting membrane comes into direct contact with the cerebrospinal fluid. Even if the ependyma is intact, the cerebrospinal and interstitial fluids are able to communicate freely, acting as a vital cerebral regulator. This suggests that the perfusate used in neuroendoscopic surgery will have a direct impact on cerebral function.

In primary research comparing normal saline solution and artificial cerebrospinal fluid, human astrocytes were used, and cells were cultured using a culture medium, artificial cerebrospinal fluid, and normal saline. With normal saline solution, the ratio of surviving cells was low, and these solutions were reported to be associated with apoptosis [2]. Through in vitro research and clinical trials, it has been demonstrated that normal saline solutions have a poisonous effect on neurons. Furthermore, Doi et al. reported that in ventriculocisternal perfusion experiments using rats, both in vitro and in vivo, normal saline solution caused neural cell death in the cerebral cortex and hippocampus [1]. In observing ventriculocisternal perfusion for 24 h, it was determined that only normal saline solution resulted in apoptosis, while no morphological changes were observed with artificial cerebrospinal fluid or lactated Ringer's solution. Through these experiments, it is clear that, similar to normal saline, no morphological changes were apparent when using lactated Ringer's solution; however, there was an amplification of genes associated with cell death.

Conclusion

For neuroendoscopic surgery, the use of artificial cerebrospinal fluid as a perfusate is considered effective in maintaining brain homeostasis compared to the use of normal saline or lactate Ringer's solution.

Conflicts of interest statement We declare that we have no conflict of interest.

References

1. Doi K, Morioka Y, Nishimura M, Kawano T, Harada D, Naito S, Yamauchi A (2009) Perfusion fluids used in neurosurgery affect cerebrospinal fluid and surrounding brain parenchyma in the rat ventriculocisternal perfusion model. J Toxicol Sci 34(5):511–518
2. Enomoto R, Tatsuoka H, Komai T, Sugahara C, Takemura K, Yamauchi A, Nishimura M, Naito S, Matsuda T, Lee E (2004) Involvement of histone phosphorylation in apoptosis of human astrocytes after exposure to saline solution. Neurochem Int 44(6):459–467
3. Griffith HB, Jamjoom AB (1990) The treatment of childhood hydrocephalus by choroids plexus coagulation and artificial cerebrospinal fluid perfusion. Br J Neurosurg 4(2):95–100
4. Johanson CE, Duncan JA III, Klinge PM, Brinker T, Stopa EG, Silverberg GD (2008) Multiplicity of cerebrospinal fluid functions: new challenges in health and disease. Cerbrospinal Fluid Res 5:10
5. Mungrue IN, Pagnon J, Kohannim O, Gargalovic PS, Lusis AJ (2009) CHAC1/MGC4504 is a novel proapoptotic component of the unfolded protein response, downstream of the ATF4-ATF3-CHOP cascade. J Immunol 182(1):466–476
6. Oka K, Yamamoto M, Nonaka T, Tomonaga M (1996) The significance of artificial cerebrospinal fluid as perfusate and endoneurosurgery. Neurosurgery 38(4):733–736

Subdural or Intraparenchymal Placement of Long-Term Telemetric Intracranial Pressure Measurement Devices?

Melanie Schmitt, Regina Eymann, Sebastian Antes, and Michael Kiefer

Abstract We established a CE-certified telemetric device to measure intracranial pressure (ICP) noninvasively. To evaluate whether subdural or intraparenchymal insertion of such devices should be preferred, we implanted these telemetric ICP measurement devices (Raumedic, Rautel) in both locations. The study was performed in nine minipigs. The telemetric data were validated every 3 months using conventional intraparenchymal ICP measurement probes.

The intraparenchymal telemetric device failed in one animal 12 months after insertion. Computed tomography (CT) revealed first hints for failure: Despite the implantation in adult animals, the skull dimensions seemingly increased after implantation, and the sensor tip was dislocated on the tabula interna level. This finding could also be verified by histopathological examination which would explain the reason for mismeasurement. The subdural catheter failed after 9 months. CT and histopathological examination revealed a bony encapsulation of a large catheter part, which had been located correctly initially. We propose that chronic pulsatile stress on the device was the underlying reason for this phenomenon, comparable to that in meningeal arteries.

In some of the other animals, failure of subdural catheters could be detected. Histopathological examinations in these cases are still pending. Nevertheless, we assume similar underlying reasons for failure in these subdural probes.

In conclusion, we favour intraparenchymal placement of telemetric ICP measurement devices.

Keywords • Intracranial pressure • ICP • Telemetric • CSF shunts • ICP measurement

Introduction

The pathological conditions of the cerebrovascular system such as traumatic brain injury (TBI), stroke, hydrocephalus, or intraventricular haemorrhages are predisposing risk factors for elevated intracranial pressure (ICP). As a consequence, these conditions demand a continuous measurement of ICP, which is indispensable for appropriate ICP therapy management [8].

The conventional method for ICP measurement is the implantation of an external ventricular drain (EVD) with a pressure transducer, but intraparenchymal probes are also used . However, this type of ICP measurement should be removed according to several authors after about 10 days of implantation, because of an exponentially rising risk of infections after that period of time due to the external drainage [7]. Furthermore, a device which noninvasively measures the performance of CSF shunts and the ICP after ETV procedure is needed.

During the last three decades, attempts have been made to develop such a device to control intracranial pressure telemetrically [1, 3]. We have now succeeded in developing a CE-certified telemetric ICP measurement device. This probe allows the reading of the ICP through closed skin. For this reason, the insertion of this so-called Rautel (Raumedic®) is an elegant way to observe ICP without the risk of catheter-related infections and without frequent subsequent surgical interventions. Furthermore, the Rautel can remain in situ over the acute phase of TBI, whereas conventional EVD or external intraparenchymal probes to monitor ICP may require a revision due to infection (see above).

In general, there are two types of Rautel available: There is the possibility of either a subdural and an intraparenchymal insertion. The question is whether subdural or intraparenchymal placement of the telemetric ICP probes should be preferred. A possible argument for subdural implantation would be minor risks such as haemorrhages. The intraparenchymal insertion on the contrary is supposed to be more reliable.

M. Schmitt (✉), R. Eymann, S. Antes, and M. Kiefer
Department of Neurosurgery, Medical School, Saarland University, Homburg-Saar, Germany
e-mail: m.schmitt@uniklinikum-saarland.de

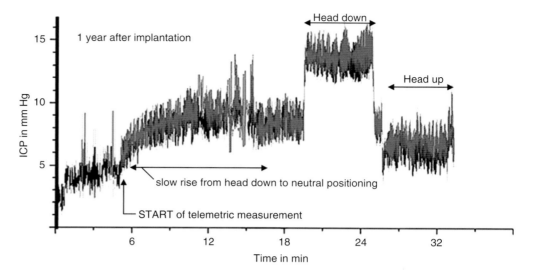

Fig. 1 Long-term overview of 30 min, comparing telemetric (*light grey*) and conventional (*black*) intracranial pressure (*ICP*) monitoring during different positioning

For this reason we conducted an animal experiment with the aid of minipigs, to determine whether preference should be given to subdural or intraparenchymal insertion of a Rautel.

Materials and Methods

We examined nine adult minipigs (at least 12 months old) in this experiment. Both subdural and intraparenchymal ICP measurement devices were implanted in each minipig. For this purpose, the animals were given a general anaesthetic (1.5% isoflurane, vaporised in an air–N_2O mixture, 0.15 mg/h fentanyl), intubated, and ventilated, by a veterinarian.

Due to the specific anatomical conditions of these animals, the craniotomy through the frontal sinus could not be avoided. Therefore, single-shot antibiotic treatment was given.

The subdural and the intraparenchymal ICP probes were inserted on the left and right sides, respectively. To validate the telemetric data, conventional ICP monitoring using intraparenchymal probes was performed. Such probes were inserted via a more frontally located access during the initial implantation and during quarterly routine follow-up. Correct positioning of both telemetric and conventional probes was verified routinely by X-ray.

To gather data in a wide pressure range, positioning of the animals was changed between 15° head-down, normal prone position, and 15° head-up. Total monitoring time of each device lasted at least 30 min. Before final wound closure, the conventional ICP measurement catheter was removed. To close the wound, subcutaneous stitches and gluing of the skin surface were performed to reduce infection risk [2]. Since neither subdural nor intraparenchymal probes provided reliable data after 12 months in one animal, computed tomography (CT) scans and histopathological tissue examinations were performed according to our study protocol.

Results

Our results indicated that the telemetric devices delivered reliable data in comparison with conventional ICP measurement probes, for at least 9 months. The quarterly comparison revealed that the telemetric system provides reliable measurements during the change of positioning of the animals as well, as shown in Fig. 1.

After the above-mentioned period of 9 months, the intraparenchymal telemetric probe failed in one animal. The reason underlying this failure was revealed by CT; even though the measurement probe was initially implanted correctly, the sensor tip had become dislocated on the level of the tabula interna of the skull, due to an increase in the size of the animal's skull (see Fig. 2), despite the fact that it was an adult animal that was chosen to avoid bone growth. This finding could also be verified by histopathological examinations, which were performed according to the study protocol in cases of device failure.

Regarding the subdural catheter, macroscopic inspection also revealed a reasonable cause for failure; the probe which was properly implanted was partially covered by a bony layer during the course of the study, as can be seen in Fig. 3.

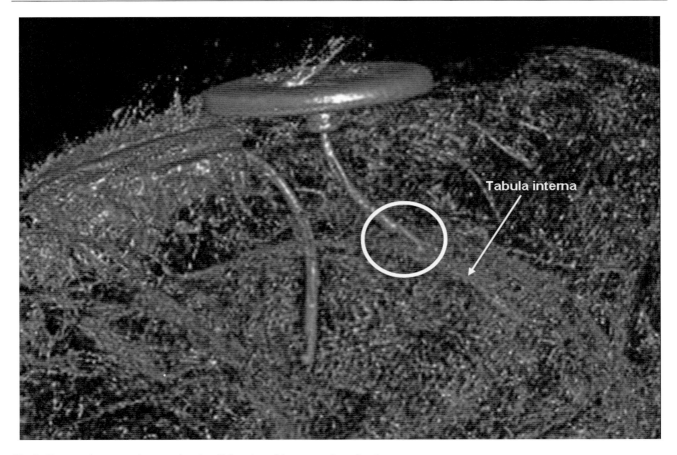

Fig. 2 Computed tomography scan showing dislocation of intraparenchymal catheter

The sensor tip was also included in this process of bony overgrowth, which can easily explain the probe's dysfunction.

Discussion

Our findings show that telemetric ICP measurement devices deliver reliable data for at least 9 months. For this period of time, subdural implantation of the telemetric probes seems feasible. Longer-term observations revealed the development of a bony chamfer around these implants, surrounding the catheter with its sensor tip as measuring part. This finding seems to be comparable with the skull chamfer of meningeal arteries. Consequently we also believe that the bony cover of the inserted catheters may be due to the chronic pulsatile stress of the brain.

Regarding the dislocation followed by the dysfunction of the intraparenchymally inserted probe, several underlying phenomena can be discussed.

1. As a part of the natural behaviour pattern of these animals, the telemetric devices are exposed to direct external forces, which might provoke subdural displacement and dislocation of the probes. Such forces can end up even with fractures. Ossification around and over the implant might also indicate a healing process.
2. For several reasons, the housing was developed using ceramics as a well-established material for long-term implants. Detailed analysis of the microstructure and chemistry of these ceramics revealed a broad range of foreign body reactions, even in terms of ossification [4–6, 9, 10]. For example, the pore size had a significant influence. To date, this point, which might be another reason for the ossification around the housing, has not been extensively analysed in our device.
3. Although we studied adult animals to avoid bone growth, some further minor growing of the animals occurring at the given age cannot be ruled out.

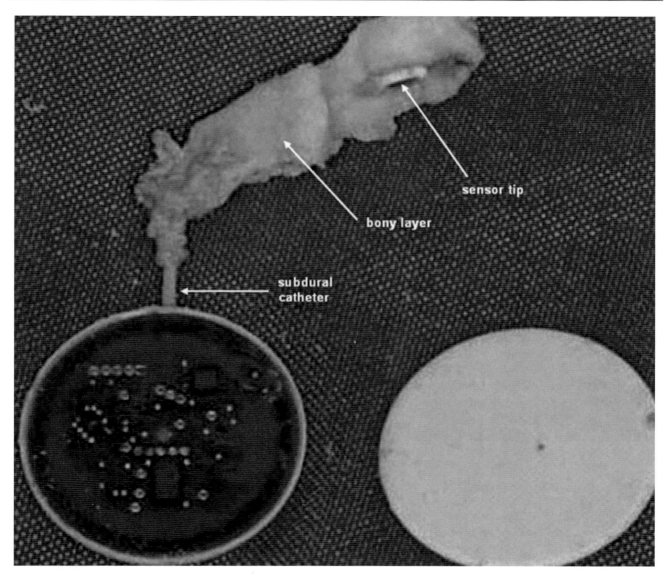

Fig. 3 Macroscopic finding of bony layer around subdural catheter

Conclusion

Reliable data could be gathered by intraparenchymal ICP measurement probes during long-term application (more than 9 months). Subdural catheters seem to have higher failure rates after 9–12 months, which can be attributed to several of the discussed reasons. From the current point of view, we favour an intraparenchymal placement of telemetric ICP measurement probes for long-term application, whereas for short-term usage both insertion sites seem feasible.

Conflicts of interest statement This scientific work has been sponsored in part by a grant from the Federal Ministry of Education and Research (BMBF), Germany.

R.E. and M.K. have received some financial support during the past for other research work from Raumedic AG, Helmbrecht, Germany.

M.S. and S.A. have received financial support for purposes of education from Codman (Johnsson and Johnsson Company), Raynham, MA, USA, and Aesculap (Miethke), Tuttlingen, Germany.

References

1. De Jong DA, Maas AI, den Ouden AH, de Lange SA (1983–1984) Long-term intracranial pressure monitoring. Med Prog Technol 10:89–96
2. Eymann R, Kiefer M (2010) Glue instead of stitches: a minor change of the operative technique with a serious impact on the shunt infection rate. Acta Neurochir Suppl 106:87–89
3. Frischholz M, Sarmento L, Wenzel M, Aquilina K, Edwards R, Coakham HB (2007) Telemetric implantable pressure sensor for short- and long-term monitoring of intracranial pressure. Conf Proc IEEE Eng Med Biol Soc 2007:514
4. Landor I, Vavrík P, Jahoda D, Pokorný D, Ballay R, Sosna A (2009) Long-term experience with the combined ARBOND hydroxyapatite

coating in implant osteointegration. Acta Chir Orthop Traumatol Cech 76:172–178
5. Nelson JF, Stanford HG, Cutright DE (1977) Evaluation and comparisons of biodegradable substances as osteogenic agents. Oral Surg Oral Med Oral Pathol 43:836–843
6. Park JB, Kelly BJ, Kenner GH, von Recum AF, Grether MF, Coffeen WW (1981) Piezoelectric ceramic implants: in vivo results. J Biomed Mater Res 15:103–110
7. Scheithauer S, Bürgel U, Ryang YM, Haase G, Schiefer J, Koch S, Häfner H, Lemmen S (2009) Prospective surveillance of drain associated meningitis/ventriculitis in a neurosurgery and neurological intensive care unit. J Neurol Neurosurg Psychiatry 80:1381–1385
8. The Brain Trauma Foundation, The American Association of Neurological Surgeons, The Joint Section on Neurotrauma and Critical Care (2000) Recommendations for intracranial pressure monitoring technology. J Neurotrauma 17:497–506
9. Tran N, Webster TJ (2009) Nanotechnology for bone materials. Wiley Interdiscip Rev Nanomed Nanobiotechnol 1:336–351
10. Zywicka B, Czarny A, Zaczy ska E, Kara J (2006) Activation of nuclear factor kappaB (NF-kappaB), induction of proinflammatory cytokines in vitro and evaluation of biocompatibility of the carbonate ceramic in vivo. Polim Med 36:23–35

Twelve-Year Hospital Outcomes in Patients with Idiopathic Hydrocephalus

George Stranjalis, T. Kalamatianos, C. Koutsarnakis, M. Loufardaki, L. Stavrinou, and D.E. Sakas

Abstract *Objective*: The aim of this study was to examine patients who were admitted for the first-ever shunting for idiopathic normal pressure hydrocephalus (INPH) during a 12-year period, in terms of variation rate, patient demographic characteristics, shunt procedures, postoperative complications, and hospital outcome.

Methods: An electronic database which included all shunted patients (1998 to 2009) was used to retrieve demographic, clinical, and hospital outcome data. INPH patient identification was based on clinical and imaging diagnostic criteria.

Results: INPH patients ($n=238$) who had undergone shunting were identified. The mean age and male to female ratio of INPH patients were 73.3 ($\pm$ 7) years and 1.28:1, respectively.

The number of surgically managed INPH cases and proportion of INPH-related shunting procedures rose consecutively during the second and last third of the study period. Ventriculoperitoneal shunts ($n=129$; 54.2%) were the most commonly used configurations, followed by ventriculoatrial ($n=108$; 45.4%) and lumboperitoneal ($n=1$; 0.4%). Intrahospital shunt-related complications were hematomas (0.84%), meningitis (0.42%), and status epilepticus (0.42%). A favorable outcome was reported for 66.8% of patients; 31.5% showed no change. Overall inpatient mortality was 1.7%.

Conclusion: The quantitative findings indicate a progressive rise in the number of surgically managed INPH patients that parallels a rise in the proportion of INPH-related shunting procedures. Contributing factors are likely to include improved diagnosis and an increase in awareness of the INPH syndrome by referring physicians.

Keywords Idiopathic normal pressure hydrocephalus • Hospital outcome • Complications • Audit • Retrospective

G. Stranjalis (✉), T. Kalamatianos, C. Koutsarnakis, M. Loufardaki, L. Stavrinou, and D.E. Sakas
Department of Neurosurgery, University of Athens, Athens, Greece
e-mail: ekne@neurosurgery.org.gr

Hellenic Centre for Neurosurgical Research (HCNR), "Professor Petros S. Kokkalis", Athens, Greece

Introduction

Idiopathic normal pressure hydrocephalus (INPH), the clinical syndrome characterized by gait disturbance, cognitive impairment, and urinary incontinence [3], typically manifests in the elderly [2]. While the pathophysiological mechanisms that give rise to INPH remain imperfectly understood [4], cerebrospinal fluid (CSF) shunting remains the most widely practised treatment option.

The University of Athens, Department of Neurosurgery, at Evangelismos Hospital is the largest of its kind in Greece, in recent years caring for over 1,500 patients annually [7]. Our department is committed to the generation and maintenance of electronic neurological disorder/disease databases for the evaluation of health care provision, the analysis of health trends, and formulation of future programmes/preventative strategies for various clinical entities.

The present clinical audit focused on surgically managed patients for INPH who had undergone a first-ever shunt operation in our department, and aimed at determining the (a) 12-year variation rate, (b) age and sex of patient, (c) shunt type, (d) postoperative shunt-related complications, and (e) hospital outcomes.

Methods

Identification of all patients who had undergone shunting for hydrocephalus from 1998 to 2009 was based on our departmental electronic database and took place following a data-mining strategy incorporating the search tags: *cerebrospinal fluid disorder*, *hydrocephalus*, and *shunt surgery*. Retrospective demographic, clinical, and hospital outcome data for all patients were collected. INPH patients were subsequently identified when the following clinical and imaging diagnostic criteria were met: (1) presence of at least two Hakim's symptoms, (2) ventriculomegaly on computed tomography (CT) or magnetic resonance imaging (MRI) scans, and (3) lack of secondary causes. Patient records typically included measures of gait performance

Table 1 Cumulative data (1998–2009) on INPH patients: demographic characteristics, type of shunt, postoperative complications, and hospitalization time

	No. (%) or mean (SD)
INPH patients	238 (32.4%)
Sex	
Male (%)	134 (56.3%)
Age (years)	73.3 (±7)
Shunt type	
VP, no. (%)	129 (54.2%)
VA, no. (%)	108 (45.4%)
LP, no. (%)	1 (0.4%)
Postoperative complications	
Shunt-related	
Meningitis	1 (0.42%)
Hematoma	2 (0.84%)
Status epilepticus	1 (0.42%)
Other	
Pneumonia	1 (0.42%)
Hospitalization (days)	11.5 (±10)

INPH idiopathic normal pressure hydrocephalus, *LP* lumboperitoneal, *VA* ventriculoatrial, *VP* ventriculoperitoneal

(incorporating time and steps needed to walk 10 m and steps needed to make a turning) assessed by the responsible neurosurgeons.

Results

From a total of 734 patients who underwent 955 shunt operations/reoperations during the 12-year study period, 238 patients (32.4%) were identified with INPH. Table 1 shows cumulative data on INPH patients with respect to age/sex, shunt-types, shunt-related complications, and hospitalization time. The number of patients surgically managed for INPH as well as the percentage of INPH-related shunts rose consistently during the second and last third of the study period (Fig. 1a, b). The mean age and male to female ratio of INPH patients were 73.3 (± 7) years and 1.28:1, respectively. Average length of hospitalization for those patients was 11.5 (± 10) days. Intrahospital postoperative shunt-related complications were hematomas ($n=2$; 0.84%), meningitis ($n=1$; 0.42%), and status epilepticus ($n=1$; 0.42%). No more than a single postoperative shunt-related complication was recorded per year. Ventriculoperitoneal (VP) shunts were the most commonly used shunt configurations ($n=129$; 54.2% of patients), closely followed by ventriculoatrial (VA) shunts

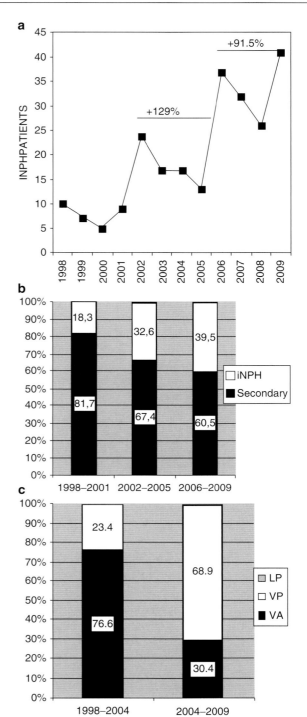

Fig. 1 (a) Annual number of idiopathic normal pressure hydrocephalus (INPH) patients who underwent shunting during the 12-year study period (1998–2009). Note the consecutive rise in the number of INPH patients during the second (+129%) and last (+91.5%) third of the study period. (b) A rise in the percentage of shunts for the treatment of INPH is apparent during the second and the last third of the study period. (c) Percentage of ventriculoperitoneal (*VP*), ventriculoatrial (*VA*), and lumboperitoneal (*LP*) shunts placed in INPH patients during the first (1998–2003) and second (2004–2009) half of the study period

($n=108$; 45.4% of patients). A single patient underwent lumboperitoneal (LP) shunting ($n=1$; 0.4%) due to a serious hematological disorder. A marked increase in the proportion of VP shunts was apparent during the second half of the study period (Fig. 1c). An improvement in gait (assessed at discharge by the responsible clinician) was reported in 66.8% of all shunted patients. Thus, a reported 77% of patients with VP shunts ($n=129$), 54.6% of patients with VA shunts ($n=108$), and the single patient with an LP shunt showed improved gait performance. Of all patients, 31.5% were reported to show no overt change in gait performance following shunting (22% of patients with VP shunts, $n=28$; 43% of patients with VA shunts, $n=47$). Overall hospital mortality for the entire study period was 1.7% (three shunt-related deaths, one shunt-independent).

Discussion

Surgical management of the elusive INPH syndrome [3] remains a widely practised treatment option. Increasing evidence suggests that shunting for INPH presents acceptable risk-to-benefit ratios [1, 6].

The present clinical audit examined admissions (1998–2009) related to first-ever shunt placement for INPH. The present data on patient demographic characteristics and surgical procedures indicate (1) that the majority of INPH patients were male, (2) the mean age for the whole INPH sample was over 70 years, and (3) VP shunts were the most commonly used configurations. Factors contributing to the marked increase in the proportion of VP shunts during the second half of the study period remain to be established. While no prospective or retrospective studies have previously supported the use of a specific shunt configuration, it is worth noting that the present data indicate a trend toward increased rates of recorded gait improvement (77%) following VP shunting. An earlier prospective study by Raftopoulos et al. [5] reported a 55% improvement in gait, 9 days postoperatively, for a small cohort of INPH patients who underwent VA shunting. The overall rate of gait improvement following VA shunts reported here (54.6%) appears comparable.

Conclusion

The present findings indicate a progressive rise in the number of surgically managed INPH patients that parallels a rise in the proportion of INPH-related shunting. Factors contributing to the observed rise may include improved diagnosis, an increase in awareness of the INPH syndrome by referring neurologists and general practitioners, as well as increasing patient quality of life requirements. A significant limitation of the present retrospective analysis concerns variability in records of gait assessment methodology. Standardization of gait assessment is necessary in future studies.

Conflicts of interest statement The authors have no conflicts of interest to disclose.

References

1. Bergsneider M, Black PM, Klinge P, Marmarou A, Relkin N (2005) Surgical management of idiopathic normal-pressure hydrocephalus. Neurosurgery 57:S29–S39
2. Black PM, Ojemann RG, Tzouras A (1985) CSF shunts for dementia, incontinence, and gait disturbance. Clin Neurosurg 32: 632–651
3. Hakim S, Adams RD (1965) The special clinical problem of symptomatic hydrocephalus with normal cerebrospinal fluid pressure: observations on cerebrospinal fluid hydrodynamics. J Neurol Sci 2:307–327
4. Krauss JK, von Stuckrad-Barre S (2008) Clinical aspects and biology of normal pressure hydrocephalus. Handb Clin Neurol 89:887–902
5. Raftopoulos C, Deleval J, Chaskis C, Leonard A, Cantraine F, Desmyttere F, Clarysse S, Brotchi J (1994) Cognitive recovery in idiopathic normal pressure hydrocephalus: a prospective study. Neurosurgery 35:397–404
6. Stein SC, Burnett MG, Sonnad SS (2006) Shunts in normal-pressure hydrocephalus: do we place too many or too few? J Neurosurg 105:815–22
7. Stranjalis G, Sakas DE (2004) A history of the department of neurosurgery at the Evangelismos Hospital, Athens. Acta Neurochir (Wien) 146:1165–1169

What Is the Appropriate Shunt System for Normal Pressure Hydrocephalus?

Christos Chrissicopoulos, S. Mourgela, K. Kirgiannis, A. Sakellaropoulos, N. Ampertos, K. Petritsis, and A. Spanos

Abstract Normal pressure hydrocephalus (NPH) represents a common disorder among older people with mild elevation of cerebrospinal fluid pressure and certain clinical manifestations. We present a patient with such a disorder in whom a programmable valve was implanted. With the use of a lower opening pressure, the patient developed a subdural hematoma although the symptoms subsided. After evacuating the hematoma and by setting the valve pressure higher, the patient recovered without any symptomatology. We observed that only the higher pressure was the right one, although in two different pressure values the symptoms had subsided.

Keywords Normal pressure hydrocephalus (NPH) • Programmable shunt system • Subdural hematoma • Ventriculomegaly

Introduction

Normal pressure hydrocephalus (NPH) syndrome was first described by Hakim and Adams in 1965 as symptomatic occult hydrocephalus with "normal cerebrospinal fluid pressure" [3]. NPH is a chronic type of communicating hydrocephalus in adults, and therefore patients do not exhibit the classic signs of increased intracranial pressure, such as headache, nausea, vomiting, or altered consciousness. The etiology behind NPH is still unknown; it may be that NPH is due to an alteration in fluid reabsorption and brain tissue compliance. All these years an important question has been, what type of shunt system and shunting procedure are best for

C. Chrissicopoulos (✉), S. Mourgela, K. Kirgiannis, N. Ampertos, K. Petritsis, and A. Spanos
Neurosurgical Department, "Agios Savvas" Anticancer Institute, Athens, Greece
e-mail: md.christos@yahoo.it

A. Sakellaropoulos
Pulmonary and Critical Care Medicine, "Neon Athineon" Hospital, Athens, Greece

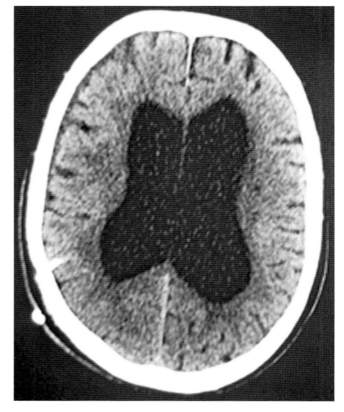

Fig. 1 Computed tomography scan showing ventricular enlargement in normal pressure hydrocephalus (NPH) patient

NPH patients? We report a case of an NPH patient to show that although there are programmable valve systems, there is still a need for more precise pressure determination.

Case Presentation

A 72-year-old man with a history of Parkinson's disease, diabetes mellitus type 2, and coronary artery disease was admitted to our clinic with symptoms of NPH (abnormal "magnetic" gait, "dementia," and urinary incontinence). Brain computed tomography (CT) revealed ventricular enlargement (Fig. 1). A

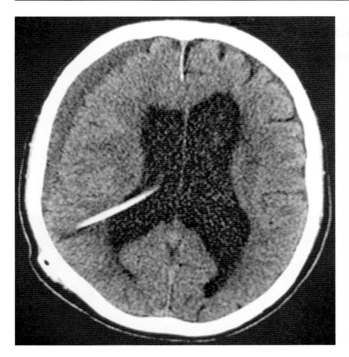

Fig. 2 Computed tomography scan showing shunt with subdural hematoma

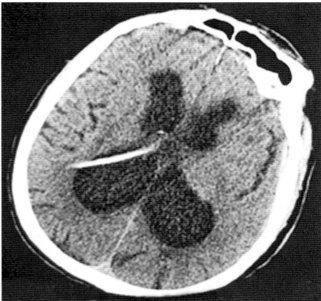

Fig. 3 Ventricular system with valve pressure at 110 mmH$_2$O

lumbar puncture (LP) for radionuclide cisternography (RC) was performed. We have been using RC in our clinic for the last 20 years, and by correlating the imaging patterns with the surgical outcomes, we can in certain cases deliver an indication of the most suitable shunt system. Cerebrospinal fluid was under normal pressure, and RC revealed communicating hydrocephalus. We decided to use a programmable valve (Delta type Strata, Medtronic) of 80 mmH$_2$O (1.5 indication position), and the implantation site was the occipital horn of the right ventricle. The patient recovered postoperatively, and symptoms such as abnormal gait and urinary incontinence subsided, although the patient still suffered from apathy. Three weeks later on a follow-up brain CT, a subdural hematoma was revealed on the right parietal lobe at the site of the valve implantation (Fig. 2). In our opinion, the hematoma was due to overdrainage, and we decided that the initial setting was incorrect. Although we readjusted the programmable valve and set the pressure to 110 mmH$_2$O (two indication position) the symptoms of the patient reappeared, and the hematoma increased slightly. After evacuation of the subdural hematoma by trepanation and lowering the valve pressure to the 80 mmH$_2$O, the patient gradually recovered 1 month later (Fig. 3).

Discussion

NPH is a type of hydrocephalus that occurs in older adults, with average age older than 60 years. NPH develops slowly over time. The slow enlargement of the ventricles means that the fluid pressure in the brain may not be as high as in other types of hydrocephalus.

There are two forms of NPH: the secondary form which is caused by subarachnoid hemorrhage, head injury, cranial surgery, or central nervous system infection, and the idiopathic form where the cause is at present unknown.

NPH is often misdiagnosed as Parkinson's disease, Alzheimer's disease, or senility, due to its chronic nature and its presenting symptoms. Although the exact mechanism is unknown, it is thought to be a form of communicating hydrocephalus with impaired cerebrospinal fluid (CSF) reabsorption at the arachnoid villi.

The most typical NPH cases with the clinical triad (dementia, magnetic gait, and urinary incontinence) have every possibility of responding to a shunting operation, and the patient may dramatically improve after CSF drainage [1]. In patients with symptomatic ventriculomegaly and features of NPH, one goal of therapy should be reduction of the ventricular size, although ventriculomegaly is not related to the positive clinical outcome[2].

Complications of CSF diversion include subdural hematoma formation, ventriculitis, catheter-related hemorrhage, or introduction of air into the ventricles. Subdural hematoma formation resulting from "overdrainage" of the ventricles and laceration (tearing) of bridging veins is an important clinical concern [4].

Most studies performed for evaluation of NPH patients, such as neuropsychological assessment, neuroimaging techniques, removal of CSF, RC, measurements of cerebral blood flow and metabolism, pressure monitoring, and hydrodynamic tests, do not always predict the outcome after the CSF diversion (shunting) [3, 5].

From our case study, we observed that only the higher valve pressure was the right one, although in the two different pressure value settings, the symptoms had subsided. When the valve pressure was regulated to the lower value, the patient had complications. This case study perhaps suggests that not only pressure but also CSF flow parameters must be taken into account at the same time in determining the right valve system. Another option for us could be to implant flow valves in NPH patients.

Conclusion

Since we do not have tests with predictive accuracy, the treatment for suspected NPH varies. Although there are many choices of shunt devices, there is still a need for more precise determination of valve opening pressure. It is very difficult to make the right choice for a shunt device in a patient with NPH. Even in NPH patients who are candidates for shunt surgery, we cannot obtain a good outcome without performing an ideal shunting operation using an appropriate shunt system.

Conflicts of interest statement We declare that we have no conflict of interest.

References

1. Bejjani GK, Hammer MD (2005) Normal-pressure hydrocephalus. Another treatable "dementia": part II contemporary. Neurosurgery 27(17):1–4
2. Bergsneider M, Warwick JP, Mazziotta JC, Becker DP (1999) Beneficial effect of siphoning in the treatment of adult hydrocephalus. Arch Neurol 56:1224–1229
3. Mori K, Mima T (1997) Can we predict the benefit of a shunting operation for suspected normal pressure hydrocephalus? Crit Rev Neurosurg 7:263–275
4. Pratt RW, Mayer SA (2005) Normal pressure "herniation". Neurocrit Care 2(2):172–175
5. Vanneste JA (1994) Three decades of normal pressure hydrocephalus: are we wiser now? J Neurol Neurosurg Psychiatry 57:1021–1025

Indications for Endoscopic Third Ventriculostomy in Normal Pressure Hydrocephalus

Nikolaos Paidakakos, S. Borgarello, and M. Naddeo

Abstract *Background*: Controversies remain regarding the proper diagnostic studies and prediction of outcome in patients with normal pressure hydrocephalus (NPH), and their management remains controversial. We propose a preoperative assessment routine the aim of which is to correctly select NPH patients, and to differentiate between them in terms of surgical treatment, identifying probable endoscopic third ventriculostomy (ETV) responders.

Materials and methods: We prospectively considered a group of 44 patients with suspected NPH on the basis of clinical symptoms and neuroradiological evidence, who have undergone supplemental diagnostic testing (tap test, external lumbar drainage, cerebrospinal fluid outflow resistance [Rout] determination through lumbar and ventricular infusion test). All 44 of these patients were treated with either shunt procedures or ETV.

Results: To choose the kind of treatment (shunt or ETV), we evaluated the individual response during infusion tests. The efficacy of both surgical techniques was approximately 70%, with a significantly lower complication rate for ETV.

Conclusions: We evaluated the correlation between the various tests and the postoperative outcomes both for shunting and for ETV. Rout proved useful for preoperative assessment and choice of treatment. In carefully selected patients, ETV had qualitative results similar to shunting, presenting significantly fewer complications.

Keywords Normal pressure hydrocephalus (NPH) • External lumbar drainage (ELD) • Infusion test • CSF outflow resistance (Rout) • Endoscopic third ventriculostomy (ETV) • Shunt

N. Paidakakos
Department of Neurosurgery, C.T.O. Hospital, Turin, Italy and Kriezi 38, Ilioupoli 16342, Athens, Greece
e-mail: n.paidakakos@gmail.com

S. Borgarello and M. Naddeo
Department of Neurosurgery, C.T.O. Hospital, Turin, Italy

Introduction

The term *normal pressure hydrocephalus* (NPH) was coined in 1964 by Salomon Hakim [8]. In 1965, Adams et al. introduced the term into the English-language literature [1], and then Hakim went on to describe the classic triad of gait disturbance, incontinence, and dementia, which improved after cerebrospinal fluid (CSF) removal [11].

Since then, considerable controversy has evolved on the appropriate diagnosis and treatment, due to the lack of universally accepted and evidence-based guidelines. Both our personal experience and a review of the literature confirm the difficulty in identifying diagnostic and prognostic tests with high predictive value and accuracy, which can help not only in predicting the postoperative outcome, but also in choosing the type of treatment. All tests we utilize are associated with both false-negative and false-positive results. Furthermore, the most commonly employed treatment (shunting) carries a very high rate of complications, often severe. The choice of endoscopic third ventriculostomy (ETV), a less invasive technique with a very low complication rate, has seldom been considered. In recent years, in the light of newer theories on CSF dynamics and pathophysiology, various studies have identified ETV as a valuable alternative [3, 4, 7, 12, 14].

In the present study, we propose a diagnostic and prognostic routine aiming to select the right NPH patients and to differentiate between them in terms of surgical treatment, identifying probable ETV responders.

Materials and Methods

From October 2002 through April 2008, 44 NPH patients were identified by our hydrocephalus outpatient clinic, on the basis of clinical history, physical examination, and neuroradiological findings, and studied prospectively. The patients included in the study satisfied all of the following parameters: insidious onset, progression over time, at least 6-month duration, age over 50 years, presence of one or more of the classic triad of symptoms, ventriculomegaly (Evans index >0.30) disproportionate to the grade of cerebral atrophy, and no macroscopic obstruction to CSF flow. Reported symptoms were corroborated by a source familiar with the patient's premorbid and current condition. The presence of any other major neurological, psychiatric, or general medical condition that would have been sufficient to explain the presenting symptoms was excluded.

As far as demographics were concerned, 21 patients were men and 23 women, and mean age was 72.2 years (range 54–85). Seventeen patients (38.6%) presented with the classical symptomatological triad, while the rest presented with one or two of the three symptoms at the time of diagnosis. The onset symptom was gait apraxia in 35 patients (79.5%), urinary urgency in seven (16%), and cognitive deficit in two (4.5%). The latency from onset to diagnosis ranged from 6 to 90 months (mean 29.8). Causative factors could be identified in eight patients (traumatic brain injury in five, subarachnoid hemorrhage in two, and meningitis in one). In the remaining 36 patients, no anamnestic feature possibly related to the hydrocephalic state was identified (idiopathic NPH). Follow-up ranged from 6 to 36 months (mean 21.9).

All patients underwent cerebral computed tomography (CT) scan, magnetic resonance (MR) and phase-contrast cine-MR imaging both preoperatively and postoperatively. To consolidate the diagnosis and to obtain prognostic elements, supplemental testing was undertaken. These consisted of subtractive tests, CSF outflow resistance (Rout) determination, and cognitive function assessment.

External lumbar drainage (ELD) was performed in all but four patients. The CSF evacuation rate was 10 mL/h for 3 days. Two of the latter four patients refused ELD, and in two, catheter placement was impossible: These patients underwent a tap test (50 mL of CSF evacuation). To evaluate improvement after CSF subtraction, the Hauser Ambulatory Index was used [9]; this test assesses the time and effort used by the patient to walk 25 ft (8 m). It was also reconsidered postoperatively.

Rout was measured in the lumbar and the ventricular compartment. The constant infusion test described by Katzman and Hussey was used [10]. Ringer lactate was used, at a 2 mL/min infusion rate until steady state was reached. Rout was calculated by the formula:

$$\left[\text{Rout} = (P_1 - P_0)/V_{\text{IN}} \right]$$

where P_1 represents the maximum pressure at steady state, P_0 the opening pressure, and V_{IN} the infusion rate. Values up to 15 mmHg/mL/min were considered normal. Rout scores were used as the main criterion for treatment choice (ventriculoperitoneal (vp) shunting vs. ETV). Patients with a high lumbar Rout (>15 mmHg/mL/min) were shunted (shunt system with programmable valve and antisiphon device). All of them presented lower ventricular values. Patients with normal or low lumbar Rout values, but high ventricular Rout values, underwent ETV. A high Rout in the intracranial compartment demonstrates, in our opinion, a gradient between the supraventricular and infraventricular compartments in favor of the former, thus justifying an indication for ETV (Fig. 1a, b).

The eventual cognitive impairment was assessed using the Mini-Mental State Examination (MMSE) [15]. The test assesses seven cognitive areas, using 30 items. Scores, adjusted for age and educational level, were calculated both preoperatively and postoperatively.

Finally, as far as outcome is concerned, Black's scale [2] slightly modified was the main measure utilized (Table 1). On that basis, outcome was classified as excellent, good, modest, temporary, or null. To more easily group patients, we considered excellent and good results to represent a favorable outcome, while modest, temporary, or null improvement defined an unfavorable outcome. The Hauser Ambulatory Index, MMSE, and clinical re-evaluation of the patient were also performed postoperatively.

Surgical Technique for ETV

ETV was performed using the standard procedure through a right precoronal burr hole. A rigid fiberscope was used in the free-hand manner. In all patients, fenestration on the third ventricle floor was performed between the mammillary bodies and the tuber cinereum. The opening was created by gently pushing the tip of the probe and then progressively enlarging it with a Fogarty balloon catheter. The arachnoid of the interpeduncular cistern was also opened. Soon after the fenestration, pulsations of the third ventricle floor were observed intraoperatively in most cases.

Results

Out of 44 operated patients, 30 presented a favorable outcome (68.2%). Specifically, 28 patients demonstrated increased lumbar Rout values and were shunted, in accordance with our algorithm, and of these, 19/28 (67.85%) showed a good or excellent result. The remaining 16 patients demonstrated increased ventricular Rout values, and thus underwent ETV. Of these, 11/16 had a favorable outcome (68.75%). It became evident that the two treatment modalities presented analogous qualitative results (Fig. 2).

The lumbar Rout values in the vp shunt group ranged from 16.3 to 29.3, with a mean 19.6 mmHg/mL/min, while in the ETV group, the values ranged from 5.3 to 14.1, with a mean value of 9.1. It is noteworthy that there was no overlapping

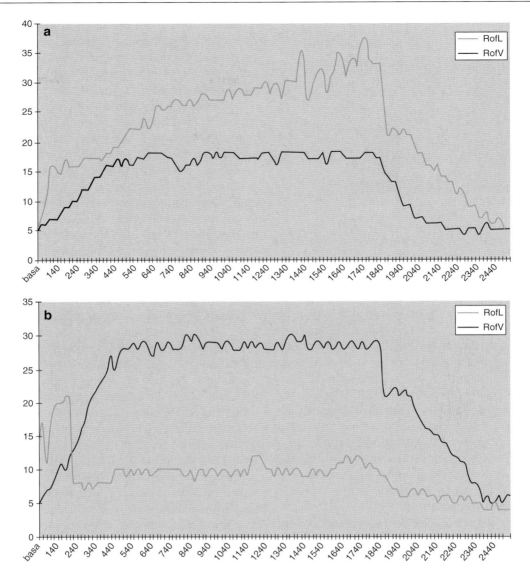

Fig. 1 Different results of lumbar (*gray curve*) and ventricular (*black curve*) infusion tests demonstrating gradient between supratentorial and infratentorial compartments. (**a**) Patient with higher lumbar values (indication for shunting); and (**b**) patient with higher ventricular values (indication for endoscopic third ventriculostomy [ETV])

between the two groups. Within the vp shunt group, we can identify two subgroups: the patients who had a favorable outcome had slightly higher mean lumbar Rout values than the ones with unfavorable outcome (20.15 vs. 18.7), even though the difference is not to be considered significant.

Table 1 Black's scale, modified

Outcome	Description
Excellent	Resumed pre-illness activity without deficit
Good	Resumed pre-illness activity with deficit; improvement of two or more symptoms
Modest	Improved but did not return to previous work; improvement of one symptom
Temporary	Temporary major improvement
Null	No change or worsening

The ventricular Rout values presented similar but inverted patterns, being higher in the ETV group than in the shunt group. In the former group, Rout ranged from 15.3 to 21.3, with a mean 19.1, while in the latter, the respective values were 7.3 to 15.2 (mean 10.8). We did not find any overlapping in this case, even if the ranges were closer. On the other hand, if we look within the ETV group, the mean values between patients with favorable and unfavorable outcome were identical (19.1 vs. 19).

The patients who had gait disturbance as the onset symptom presented a significantly higher rate of improvement. Of these, 22/35 had an excellent or good outcome (63%). Overall, if we consider the percentage that this subgroup represents within the total of 30 patients with favorable outcome, the rate grows even higher (22/30, 73%).

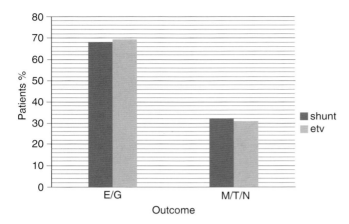

Fig. 2 Percentage of patients with favorable (*G/E* good/excellent) and unfavorable (*M/T/N* modest/temporary/null) outcomes, after shunting (*dark gray*) or endoscopic third ventriculostomy (*ETV*) (*light gray*). Success rates were similar, regardless of treatment modality

ELD was another parameter that proved to be very highly correlated to outcome. Out of seven patients with negative ELD response, only one had a good outcome, two had a modest result, and four did not improve at all. Out of the remaining 33 patients (ELD was administered in 40/44 patients) with a positive response to ELD, only four presented an unfavorable outcome (three modest, one temporary). In contrast, 29/33 patients (88%) had a good or excellent result. If we recalculate, considering the sum of patients with favorable outcomes ($n=30$), we can see how 97% (29/30) of good or excellent results were correctly predicted by ELD. The test's sensitivity was as high as 96.6%, with a positive predictive value of 87.8%.

The other parameters that were evaluated in terms of outcome did not show any significant correlation (latency from onset to diagnosis, Evans index, periventricular hyperintensity, cine MR [void], MMSE score, Hauser score, tap test, opening pressure – lumbar/ventricular).

Five of 16 patients treated with ETV had an unfavorable outcome. Of these patients, three had a negative ELD response preoperatively. After ETV failure, two of them were shunted with no benefit. The third refused further treatment. The other two had positive ELD results. One was shunted and showed a good outcome. Another one demonstrated occlusion of the stoma on postoperative cine MR imaging, was re-ETVed, and obtained a modest result (same as after first operation).

Discussion

Chronic communicating hydrocephalus does not represent an established indication for ETV; the hypothesis remains under intensive investigation. Nevertheless, many authors have lately reported their experience on the use of ETV for NPH cases, with more than acceptable results [3, 4, 7, 12, 14]. The rationale behind its use cannot be explained by means of the classic bulk flow theory. According to recent research into the dynamics of hydrocephalus, communicating hydrocephalus is a disorder of intracranial pulsations caused by decreased compliance [7], rather than a CSF absorption deficit.

The modern theory considers hydrocephalus as ventricular enlargement caused by an increased regional force directed from the ventricle toward the subarachnoid spaces (transmantle pressure gradient or transmantle pulsatile stress). Chronic transmantle pulsatile stress results in decreased compliance of the brain tissue and ventricular enlargement [4]. Conversely, CSF malabsorption and increased mean pressure are secondary to the more general vascular disturbances occurring in hydrocephalus [5]. ETV reduces the systolic pressure in the brain by simply venting ventricular CSF through the stoma [6], thus increasing intracranial compliance. In doing so, it produces similar results to shunting, in a more physiological modality [6], and with a considerably smaller complication rate.

Since CSF outflow resistance reflects the systems compliance, which can be altered by ETV, it is not arbitrary to hypothesize that Rout determination could provide essential information for selecting NPH patients in terms of treatment modality: in other words, patients who could benefit from ETV. The use of the infusion test to establish an indication for ETV in NPH patients has previously been reported. Meier et al. argued that patients whose Rout is increased in the ventricular system, while being normal in the lumbar region, should be considered for ETV [12, 13]. It has also been demonstrated that a subgroup of NPH patients is characterized by a functional dissociation of hydromechanical properties of the intracranial and spinal compartments [16].

It also became obvious from our study, considering the lumbar and ventricular Rout values obtained and correlated to the outcome, that this element can be exploited in terms of treatment choice. While ELD is an invaluable tool for selecting probable responders, regardless of type of treatment, Rout seems to have a major role in selecting the kind of treatment. Even if our numbers cannot support statistical significance, the correlation is pretty strong.

Furthermore, it is clear that patients selected through this algorithm demonstrated qualitative results similar to those either with shunting or with ETV (Fig. 2). The latter method is less invasive, presents fewer complications, and has a minor psychological impact on the patient; thus it should always be considered in carefully selected patients.

Conclusion

The authors believe that ETV should be part of the armamentarium of all neurosurgeons who treat NPH patients and that Rout determination could prove to be an important treatment selection element. Patients with low or normal lumbar Rout and high ventricular Rout should be strongly considered for ETV. However, our data must be confirmed in further studies. Multicenter randomized controlled studies are needed to address these issues.

Conflicts of interest statement   We declare that we have no conflict of interest.

References

1. Adams RD, Fisher CM, Hakim S, Ojemann RG, Sweet WH (1965) Symptomatic occult hydrocephalus with "normal" cerebrospinal-fluid pressure: a treatable syndrome. N Engl J Med 273:117–126
2. Black PM (1980) Idiopathic normal-pressure hydrocephalus: results of shunting in 62 patients. J Neurosurg 52:371–377
3. Gangemi M, Maiuri F, Buonamassa S, Colella G, de Divitiis E (2004) Endoscopic third ventriculostomy in idiopathic normal pressure hydrocephalus. Neurosurgery 55:129–134
4. Gangemi M, Maiuri F, Naddeo M, Godano U, Mascari C, Broggi G, Ferroli P (2008) Endoscopic third ventriculostomy in idiopathic normal pressure hydrocephalus: an Italian multicenter study. Neurosurgery 63(1):62–7; discussion 67–9
5. Greitz D (2004) Radiological assessment of hydrocephalus: new theories and implications for therapy. Neurosurg Rev 27:145–165
6. Greitz D (2007) Paradigm shift in hydrocephalus research in legacy of Dandy's pioneering work: rationale for third ventriculostomy in communicating hydrocephalus. Childs Nerv Syst 23(5):487–9
7. Hailong F, Guangfu H, Haibin T, Hong P, Yong C, Weidong L, Dongdong Z (2008) Endoscopic third ventriculostomy in the management of communicating hydrocephalus: a preliminary study. J Neurosurg 109(5):923–30
8. Hakim S (1964) Some observations on CSF pressure: hydrocephalic syndrome in adults with "normal" CSF pressure. Javeriana University School of Medicine, Bogata (Thesis no. 957)
9. Hauser SL, Dawson DM, Lehrich JR et al (1983) Intensive immunosuppression in progressive multiple sclerosis: a randomized, three-arm study of high-dose intravenous cyclophosphamide, plasma exchange, and ACTH. N Engl J Med 308:173–180
10. Katzman R, Hussey F (1970) A simple constant-infusion manometric test for measurement of CSF absorption: part I—rationale and method. Neurology 20:534–544
11. Marmarou A, Bergsneider M, Relkin N, Klinge P, Black PM (2005) Development of guidelines for idiopathic normal-pressure hydrocephalus: introduction. Neurosurgery 57(3 Suppl):S1–3; discussion ii-v
12. Meier U, Zeilinger FS, Schönher B (2000) Endoscopic ventriculostomy versus shunt operation in normal pressure hydrocephalus: diagnosis and indication. Acta Neurochir Suppl 76:563–566
13. Meier U, Zeilinger FS, Schönher B (2000) Endoscopic ventriculostomy versus shunt operation in normal pressure hydrocephalus: diagnosis and indication. Minim Invasive Neurosurg 43:87–90
14. Mitchell P, Mathew B (1999) Third ventriculostomy in normal pressure hydrocephalus. Br J Neurosurg 13:382–385
15. Rovner BW, Folstein MF (1987) Mini-mental state exam in clinical practice. Hosp Pract (Off Ed) 22(1A):99, 103, 106, 110
16. Trantakis C, Helm J, Keller M, Dietrich J. Meixensberger J (2004) Third ventriculostomy in communicating hydrocephalus in adult patients — the role of lumbar and cranial cerebrospinal fluid outflow measurement. Minim Invasive Neurosurg 47:140–144

Role of Endoscopic Third Ventriculostomy in Treatment of Selected Patients with Normal Pressure Hydrocephalus

Kostas N. Fountas, Eftychia Z. Kapsalaki, Konstantinos N. Paterakis, Gregory P. Lee, and Georgios M. Hadjigeorgiou

Abstract *Objective*: The purpose of our study was to evaluate the results of endoscopic third ventriculostomy (ETV) in the management of patients with idiopathic normal pressure hydrocephalus (INPH).

Methods: Our prospective study included seven patients (five men and two women; ages ranging between 68 and 78 years) with two or more typical NPH symptoms of short duration (<6 months), with no other morbidity factors, with a Mini-Mental State Examination (MMSE) score ≥18, aqueductal cerebrospinal fluid (CSF) stroke volume ≥42 μL, and positive lumbar drain test. The etiology of NPH was idiopathic in all of these cases. Their preoperative work-up included brain magnetic resonance imaging (MRI) and cine-MR, MMSE test, and CSF lumbar drain test, in all cases. The clinical status of all participants was graded using the Japanese intractable hydrocephalus system. An ETV was performed in all participants. Follow-up included periodic clinical evaluations, MMSE, and MRI with cine-MR studies. The follow-up time range was 12–72 months.

Results: The mean postoperative clinical grade was 3.1, while the preoperative was 6.1. Gait disturbance and urinary incontinence were the most responsive symptoms. The mean postoperative MMSE score was 23.6, while the preoperative score was 20.3. The mean postoperative aqueductal CSF stroke volume, 6 months after the procedure, was 31.6 μL, while the preoperative volume was 48.8 μL.

Conclusions: ETV may be a safe alternative surgical option for a limited number of carefully selected INPH patients.

Keywords Endoscopic • Complication • Hydrocephalus • Normal pressure • Outcome • Third ventriculostomy

Introduction

The term *normal pressure hydrocephalus* (NPH) was first described by Salomon Hakim, as a syndrome consisting of ventricular dilatation in the absence of elevated intracranial pressure, with gait disturbances, urinary incontinence, and dementia [7]. Since that original description, NPH has remained one of the most controversial topics in neurosurgery. When surgical intervention is decided upon, shunting of cerebrospinal fluid (CSF) is presently the only widely accepted method of treatment [1]. The relatively high incidence of complications associated with CSF shunt insertion, and the frequent necessity for revising these shunts, has spurred some clinical investigators to employ endoscopic third ventriculostomy (ETV) in the management of NPH patients [3, 6, 8–10].

Recently, however, ETV has also been employed in the management of meticulously selected patients with idiopathic NPH. Although the responsiveness to ETV varies significantly among the previously published series, there are certainly a limited number of patients, whose symptoms significantly improve after undergoing ETV [2, 4–6].

In our current communication, we present our results from a series of patients with idiopathic NPH undergoing ETV.

K.N. Fountas (✉) and K.N. Paterakis
Department of Neurosurgery, School of Medicine,
University Hospital of Larissa, University of Thessaly,
Larissa, Greece
e-mail: fountas@med.uth.gr

E.Z. Kapsalaki
Department of Diagnostic Radiology, School of Medicine,
University Hospital of Larissa, University of Thessaly,
Larissa, Greece

G.M. Hadjigeorgiou
Department of Neurology, School of Medicine,
University Hospital of Larissa, University of Thessaly,
Larissa, Greece

G.P. Lee
Department of Neurology,
Medical College of Georgia, Augusta, GA, USA

Table 1 Demographic data, symptomatology, and duration of symptoms in our cohort, as well as diagnostic tests and their results employed in our series

Patient	Sex	Symptoms	Symptom duration (m)	MMSE score	INPH grade	MRI/cine-MR (μL)	Lumbar drain test	Radionuclide cisternogram	ICP monitor	CT
S.F. 68 y.o.	♀	Gait disturbances, dementia, urinary incontinence	6	20	7 (3+1+3)	+ (48)	+	−	+	+
H.S. 70 y.o.	♂	Gait disturbances, dementia, urinary incontinence	4	19	8 (3+2+3)	+ (43)	+	+	+	+
J.D. 78 y.o.	♂	Gait disturbance, dementia	3	21	3 (2+1+0)	+ (42)	+	−	+	+
T.W. 72 y.o.	♂	Gait disturbance, dementia	4	20	4 (2+2+0)	+ (48)	+	+	+	+
S.M. 72 y.o.	♂	Gait disturbance, dementia	5	21	7 (4+3+0)	+ (50)	+	+	−	+
L.W. 72 y.o.	♀	Gait disturbances, dementia, urinary incontinence	4	19	8 (4+2+2)	+ (61)	+	−	−	+
L.S. 74 y.o.	♂	Gait disturbances, dementia, urinary incontinence	3	22	6 (3+2+1)	+ (50)	+	−	+	+

CT computed tomography, *ICP* intracranial pressure, *INPH* idiopathic normal pressure hydrocephalus, *MMSE* Mini-Mental State Examination, *MRI* magnetic resonance imaging, *y.o.* years old

Materials and Methods

Study Design

Our prospective clinical study covered a 6-year period (2002–2007). The study was approved by the institutional review boards of both participating institutions.

The inclusion criteria in our study were: (1) patient's age <80 years, (2) duration of symptoms <6 months, (3) absence of any other clinically evident comorbidity, (4) preoperative Mini-Mental State Examination (MMSE) score ≥18, (5) hyperdynamic CSF flow in the aqueduct demonstrated on the preoperative cine magnetic resonance (MR) study (aqueductal CSF stroke volume >42 μL), (6) symptom improvement after performing a lumbar CSF drain test, and (7) no previous shunt insertions.

Patient Population

A total of 133 patients were admitted to our facilities with the diagnosis of NPH. Only 15 patients (11.3%), however, met our inclusion criteria, and ultimately 7 patients (5.3%) consented to participate in our study. All participants had at least two symptoms of the classic triad of symptoms. No previous insults or any other pathologic conditions predisposing to NPH were identified in any of these patients, making the etiology idiopathic in all our study participants. The severity of their symptoms was evaluated using the grading system proposed by the Japanese Committee for Scientific Research on Intractable Hydrocephalus [11]. The analytical demographic data and the symptomatology of our patients are presented in Table 1.

Their preoperative evaluation included detailed neurologic examinations, MMSE, brain magnetic resonance imaging (MRI), and phase contrast cine MR studies, head computed

Table 2 Preoperative and postoperative INPH grades, MMSE scores, visual field, and MRI findings in our series

Patient	INPH grade		MMSE		Cine MR		Evans ratio	
	Pre-op	Post-op	Pre-op	Post-op	Pre-op (μL)	Post-op (μL)	Pre-op (%)	Post-op (%)
S.F.	7 (3+1+3)	4 (2+1+1)	20	22	48	31	45	45
H.S.	8 (3+2+3)	5 (1+2+2)	19	20	43	34	40	40
J.D.	3 (2+1+0)	1 (0+1+0)	21	23	42	28	50	45
T.W.	4 (2+2+0)	2 (0+2+0)	20	22	48	33	45	45
S.M.	7(4+3+0)	4(2+2+0)	21	25	50	34	50	45
L.W.	8(4+2+2)	3(0+2+1)	19	26	61	32	50	40
L.S.	6(3+2+1)	3(1+1+1)	22	27	50	29	50	40

INPH idiopathic normal pressure hydrocephalus, *MMSE* Mini-Mental State Examination, *MR* magnetic resonance

tomography (CT) scan, and lumbar CSF drain tests in all cases. The Evans ratio as well as the aqueductal CSF stroke volume was calculated in all patients preoperatively and postoperatively. The CSF drain test was performed by inserting a closed lumbar CSF drain system, draining 10 mL/h for a total of 72 h. In addition, radionuclide cisternogram (in 3/7) and intracranial pressure monitoring (in 5/7) were obtained in selected cases (Table 1).

Surgical Technique

All procedures were performed under general endotracheal anesthesia. A burr hole was placed just anterior to the coronal suture, approximately 3 cm from the midline. A rigid, 2.7 mm, 0° straight endoscope (Aesculap, AG & CO.KG, Tuttlingen, Germany) was utilized in all cases.

Follow-up

The follow-up of our patients included clinical evaluation in our outpatient clinic at 1, 4, and 12 weeks and at 6 and 12 months postoperatively, followed by standard annual examinations. Postoperative evaluation also included brain MRI and cine MR study; these were obtained at 4 weeks and then 6 months after discharge. The follow-up time ranged between 12 and 72 months (mean follow-up time: 36.7 months).

Results

The MRI study results obtained showed significant ventricular enlargement with Evans ratio >30% in all of our patients (Table 2). Characteristic flow void signal in the aqueduct area was present in all the preoperative MRI studies, indicating adequate CSF aqueductal circulation.

Significant improvement of their symptoms was observed in all patients after draining an adequate amount of CSF through a lumbar drain. The intracranial pressure measurements obtained in selected cases demonstrated normal variation of intracranial pressure with occasional recording of B waves in all monitored patients. The radionuclide cisternograms obtained in 3/7 (42.8%) patients demonstrated hyperdynamic CSF circulation.

In regard to the observed improvement of our patients postoperatively, gait disturbance responded better than any of the other symptoms (Table 2). With respect to the overall clinical outcome of our patients, there was significant improvement in their preoperative clinical hydrocephalus grades (Table 2). Improvement in the imaging findings of our patients was also observed. The calculated preoperative and postoperative MRI Evans ratios are summarized in Table 2. Interestingly, following ventriculostomy, the mean aqueductal CSF stroke volume decreased from 48.8 to 31.6 μL at the completion of 6 months after the procedure. No shunt insertion was required in any of our patients, and the observed initial improvement in their symptomatology has remained stable.

Although the number of participants in our current study was limited and therefore the drawing of any statistically powerful conclusions is impossible, we analyzed our results to detect any trends in our study population. Statistical analysis of our collected data demonstrated that there was no relationship between the patients' age, sex, and preoperative MMSE score, and the idiopathic normal pressure hydrocephalus (INPH) postoperative score improvement. Contrariwise, a relationship between surgical outcome and the preoperative INPH grade of our patients was demonstrated in our study (Spearman rank correlation test, $Rho=0.881$, $p=0.02$).

Analysis of our results in regard to the association of the clinical outcome (postoperative INPH score improvement) to the preoperative imaging findings showed that there was no relationship between the preoperative Evans ratio and the observed outcome. However, there was an association between clinical outcome and the preoperative aqueductal CSF flow velocity. Higher preoperative CSF flow velocity was associated with better clinical outcome in our study.

Discussion

NPH constitutes a common clinicopathologic entity. Despite the recent advances in understanding the pathologic changes associated with NPH, the exact pathophysiologic mechanisms implicated in the pathogenesis of NPH have remained unclear. A pathophysiologic mechanism proposed by Meier et al. postulates that in a subgroup of patients with NPH, there is a functional aqueduct stenosis [8, 9]. This acts as a valve-like mechanism compromising the CSF flow at pressure gradients ranging between 15 and 30 mmHg [8, 9]. In pressures higher than 30 mmHg, the flow resistance is overcome and the CSF circulation is restored. Patients whose NPH is the result of functional aqueduct stenosis may be ideal candidates for ETV.

The role of ETV in the treatment of NPH has remained controversial, and the selection criteria are ill-defined. In our current series, we considered ETV only for those patients who presented with symptoms of short duration. Short preoperative symptom duration most probably indicates well-preserved brain compliance and a minor, if any, permanent, irreversible damage of periventricular structures. Similarly, Gangemi et al. found that patients with short duration of symptoms responded better to ETV [2]. They concluded that short duration of symptoms was one of the strongest favorable prognostic factors for patients undergoing ETV for NPH [2].

We considered ETV only for patients younger than 80 years. We believe that relatively younger patients likely have more preserved brain parenchyma compliance, and less compromised cerebral blood flow. Similarly, we considered ETV only for NPH patients with CSF stroke volume higher than 42 µL on the preoperative cine MRI studies obtained. Meier et al. reported that the presence of suspected aqueductal stenosis on the preoperative MRI study of NPH patients was a strong indication for ETV [8, 9]. We believe that the larger the CSF stroke volume is, the more prominent the aqueduct obstruction becomes, in patients with NPH. It has to be emphasized that patients with functional aqueductal stenosis may represent a subgroup of patients diagnosed as idiopathic cases, who actually have an underlying pathology causing hydrocephalus. Routine employment of cine MR along with improvement and evolution of MRI software packages may accurately identify patients with functional aqueductal stenosis, in the near future.

Gait disturbances and urinary incontinence problems were improved postoperatively in 100% and 80% of our patients, respectively. Contrariwise, dementia showed some degree of improvement in only 32.5% in our series. Our findings are in agreement with those reported by Gangemi et al., who found postoperative improvement of gait difficulties in 73% of their patients, while their improvement rates for urinary incontinence and dementia were 31% and 16%, respectively [2].

The limitations of our current study have to be emphasized. The size of our series is limited, thus making the extraction of any statistically powerful conclusions impossible. Unfortunately, this is also a characteristic of the previously published ETV series in NPH patients [2, 6, 8–10]. A multi-institutional, prospective clinical study is necessary to evaluate the role of ETV in the treatment of patients with NPH.

Conclusions

ETV appears to be a valid surgical option for a very limited number of patients with NPH caused by a functional obstruction of the aqueduct. Although the indications for ETV remain to be defined, patients with evidence of hyperdynamic aqueductal CSF circulation, and/or increased CSF stroke volume (≥42 µL) seem to respond well to ETV. In addition, patients with symptoms of short duration responded well to ETV in our series. Gait disturbance and urinary incontinence were more responsive than dementia in our cohort. A prospective, multicenter clinical study is necessary for assessing the efficacy of ETV in the treatment of NPH.

Conflicts of interest statement We declare that we have no conflict of interest.

References

1. Bergsneider M, Black PM, Klinge P, Marmarou A, Relkin N (2005) Surgical management of idiopathic normal-pressure hydrocephalus. Neurosurgery 57(3 Suppl):S2, 29–39
2. Gangemi M, Maiuri F, Buonamassa S, Collela G, deDivitiis E (2004) Endoscopic third ventriculostomy in idiopathic normal pressure hydrocephalus. Neurosurgery 55:129–134
3. Gangemi M, Maiuri F, Collela G, Magro F, Seneca V, deDivitiis E (2007) Is endoscopic third ventriculostomy an internal shunt alone? Minim Invasive Neurosurg 50:47–50
4. Krauss JK, Droste DW, Vach W, Regel JP, Orszagh M, Borremans JJ et al (1996) Cerebrospinal fluid shunting in idiopathic normal-pressure hydrocephalus of the elderly: Effect of periventricular and deep white matter lesions. Neurosurgery 32:292–299
5. Larsson A, Wikkelso C, Bilting M, Stephensen H (1991) Clinical parameters in 74 consecutive patients shunt operated for normal pressure hydrocephalus. Acta Neurol Scand 84:475–482

6. Longatti PL, Fiorindi A, Martinuzzi A (2004) Failure of endoscopic third ventriculostomy in the treatment of idiopathic normal pressure hydrocephalus. Minim Invasive Neurosurg 47:342–345
7. Marmarou A, Bergsneider M, Relkin N, Klinge P, Black PM (2005) Development of guidelines for idiopathic normal-pressure hydrocephalus: introduction. Neurosurgery 57(3 Suppl):2, 1–3
8. Meier U, Zeilinger FS, Schonherr B (2000) Endoscopic ventriculostomy versus shunt operation in normal pressure hydrocephalus: diagnostics and indication. Acta Neurochir Suppl 76:563–566
9. Meier U, Zeilinger FS, Schonherr B (2000) Endoscopic ventriculostomy versus shunt operation in normal pressure hydrocephalus: diagnostics and indication. Minim Invasive Neurosurg 43:87–90
10. Mitchell P, Mathew B (1999) Third ventriculostomy in normal pressure hydrocephalus. Br J Neurosurg 13:382–385
11. Mori K (2001) Management of idiopathic normal-pressure hydrocephalus: a multiinstitutional study conducted in Japan. J Neurosurg 95:970–973

Endoscopic Third Ventriculostomy in Obstructive Hydrocephalus: Surgical Technique and Pitfalls

D. Bouramas, Nikolaos Paidakakos, F. Sotiriou, K. Kouzounias, M. Sklavounou, and N. Gekas

Abstract *Background*: Reviewing our experience in the variety of pathological entities causing obstructive hydrocephalous, we evaluate the effectiveness of endoscopic treatment, with particular attention to surgical technique, nuances, and pitfalls.

Materials and methods: We reviewed the cases of 57 consecutive patients with obstructive hydrocephalus of various origins in the last 9 years. They were treated by endoscopic third ventriculostomy (ETV). A septostomy was also performed in ten cases. Operative videos were reassessed, and surgical nuances reconsidered.

Results: ETV was accomplished in all but three cases. The overall rate of good results (shunt-independent patients with clinical remission or improvement) was 81.5% (44/54). From ten patients with ETV failure, five were re-ETVed successfully, and five were shunted. Patients with benign aqueductal stenosis and tumor compressing the aqueduct received the greatest benefit from the ETV. There were no permanent morbidities or any mortality. Fundamentals of preoperative planning, postoperative evaluation, and technical pitfalls have been considered.

Conclusion: ETV for obstructive hydrocephalus of various origins is safe and effective, and should be considered as a first-line treatment. Familiarity with the ventricular anatomy and its variations in hydrocephalus is key to success. Preoperative planning is mandatory. Awareness of potential pitfalls minimizes the risk.

Keywords Endoscopic third ventriculostomy (ETV) • Obstructive hydrocephalus • Aqueductal stenosis • Pitfalls • Cine MRI

D. Bouramas, N. Paidakakos (✉)
Department of Neurosurgery, Athens Naval Hospital, Athens, Greece

Department of Neurosurgery, Athens Bioclinic, Athens, Greece
e-mail: n.paidakakos@gmail.com

F. Sotiriou, K. Kouzounias, and N. Gekas
Department of Neurosurgery, Athens Naval Hospital, Athens, Greece

M. Sklavounou
Department of Neurosurgery, Athens Bioclinic, Athens, Greece

Introduction

The first ever endoscopic third ventriculostomy (ETV) was performed in 1923 by William Mixter, an urologist who used an urethroscope for the purpose [12]. Tracy J. Putnam then borrowed this urethroscope and modified it to optimize its use for the ventricular system. He specifically designed his ventriculoscope for cauterization of the choroid plexus in children with hydrocephalus [15]. Until the 1950s, various efforts were made to improve the technique, but technical limitations of the endoscope led to high mortality and morbidity rates [6]. At that point, valve-regulated shunt systems were introduced and gained great popularity. Since then they have been widely used to treat hydrocephalous. Nevertheless, high complication and failure rates have been reported, and an ideal shunt system still does not exist.

More recently, in the 1980s and first half of the 1990s, the concept of minimally invasive neurosurgery led to a renewed interest in neuroendoscopy [6]. Since then numerous indications for ETV have been established, and the procedure has become the treatment of choice for obstructive hydrocephalus [2, 5–7, 9, 10, 21].

In the present study, the authors report their experience in treating obstructive hydrocephalus of various origins by ETV. The effectiveness of endoscopic treatment has been evaluated within the various patient subgroups in terms of etiology. Particular attention has been paid to the technique's nuances and pitfalls, and for that purpose all operative videos have been reviewed.

Materials and Methods

We have retrospectively evaluated the cases of 57 consecutive patients with obstructive hydrocephalous treated by ETV in the last 9 years. Their age ranged from 43 to 89 years. Male to female ratio was 26:31. Follow-up period ranged from 4 to 36 months. The etiology of the hydrocephalic state (Table 1) was malformative (benign) aqueductal stenosis in 30 cases (53%), compression by tumors of the mesencephalic and

Table 1 Patient profiles and outcomes

Etiology of hydrocephalus	Number	Failed	Improvement	No improvement	Second ETV	Shunt
Sylvius stenosis	30	1	25	4	2	2
Postinfection	3	–	2	1	1	–
Cyst	5	–	4	1	1	–
Tumor	15	1	11	3	1	2
Hemorrhage	4	1	2	1	–	1
Total	57	3	44	10	5	5

ETV endoscopic third ventriculostomy

pineal regions and posterior fossa in 15 cases (26%), intraventricular cysts in 5 (9%), intraventricular or subarachnoid hemorrhage in 4 (7%), and postinfection aqueductal stenosis in 3 (5%). Patients with previous shunt insertion were excluded from this study, even though such patients are routinely considered for ETV in our practice. Patients with colloid cysts are also not being considered in this study.

All the patients were studied by magnetic resonance (MR) and phase-contrast cine MR imaging both preoperatively and postoperatively. The authors used a rigid endoscope to perform a blunt fenestration of the third ventricle floor. A septostomy was also performed in ten cases. The operative procedure videos of all cases have been reviewed and reassessed along with operative reports and preoperative neuroimaging.

Surgical Technique

We use the Aesculap neuroendoscopic system (B. Braun, Tuttlingen, Germany), comprising a rigid ventriculoscope, the long version with four channels (optical, working, irrigation, and outflow); the NeuroPilot IV steering system; and the UNITRAC holding arm. This system allows optimal fixation of the neuroendoscope, precise three-dimensional steering, safe maneuvering by defined movements in the sub-millimeter area, and optimal positioning of the neuroendoscope in situ, not to mention a much less fatiguing operation.

ETV is performed under general anesthesia, using the standard procedure through a right precoronal burr hole. In all patients, fenestration on the third ventricle floor is performed between the mammillary bodies and the tuber cinereum. The opening is created by gently pushing the tip of the probe and then progressively enlarging it with a Fogarty balloon catheter. Monopolar or bipolar cautery is used at times to help open a thick floor. Arachnoid remnants around the stoma are routinely cauterized to prevent reocclusion. Liliequist's membrane [11] is also opened whenever possible. Soon after the fenestration, pulsations of the third ventricle floor are observed intraoperatively in most cases.

Results

ETV was accomplished in all but three cases. Cerebrospinal fluid (CSF) flow through the stoma was demonstrated by postoperative cine magnetic resonance imaging (MRI). In the three cases, performing the stoma was not possible due to limited space on the third ventricle floor. These patients were later shunted, but were excluded from the study's statistics, so as not to bias the procedure success rate.

The overall rate of good results, defined as shunt-independent patients with clinical remission or improvement, was 81.5% (44/54). Ten of 54 patients with anatomically successful ETV, as shown by cine MRI, did not demonstrate a lasting clinical effect. A new cine MRI at 6 months demonstrated occlusion of the stoma in five patients; they underwent a second ETV operation and a new phase-contrast MR study to confirm patency of the stoma. The remaining five patients, without stoma occlusion, were shunted.

For more details see Table 1: out of 30 patients with benign Sylvius stenosis, we were able to perform ETV in 29, of whom 25 improved (86.2%). Of the four remaining patients, two were re-ETVed successfully, and two were shunted. If we consider the two successful reinterventions, the success rate in this patient subgroup rises to 93.1%. Fifteen patients presented with neoplastic pathology. In 14 patients, ETV was possible, and 11 showed a good outcome (78.6%). In seven of these patients, with a visible exophytic tumoral part within the ventricle, a biopsy was also obtained. Of the three patients with unfavorable outcome, two were shunted; the third patient underwent a second ETV procedure with success (including this patient, the success rate was 85.7%). ETV was accomplished in all three patients with postinfectious hydrocephalus. Two of three improved after the procedure (66.6%); the third underwent a reoperation but again with unfavorable outcome. He refused further treatment. Four of five patients with intraventricular cysts obtained a favorable result after ETV (75%). The fifth patient was re-ETVed, without clinical success. Finally, four patients presented with posthemorrhagic hydrocephalus. In three we were able to perform an ETV; two of them improved (75%); the third did not, despite anatomical patency of the stoma.

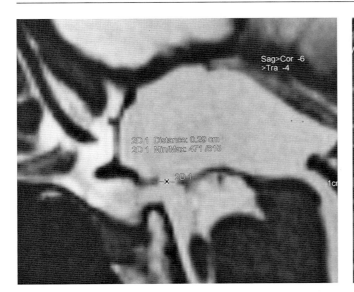

Fig. 1 Postoperative evaluation of the dimensions of the fenestration on magnetic resonance imaging (MRI). The measurement of anteroposterior diameter of the stoma was in this case 0.29 cm

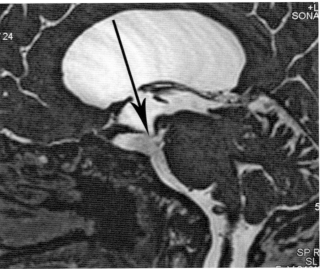

Fig. 2 Paramedian sagittal magnetic resonance (MR) scan. *Arrow* indicates correct trajectory through Monro foramen to the premammillary diaphragm

Apart from qualitatively controlling the patency of the stoma, with the use of cine MRI, quantitative measures have been obtained in the last seven patients. The maximum flow velocity at the stoma was calculated, thus providing us with a hydrodynamic evaluation of the fenestration. Results, of course, are not yet supportive of any evidence. Furthermore, postoperative MR scans were used to measure the anteroposterior diameter of the fenestration (Fig. 1). Out of the five patients with occlusion of the stoma after the first ETV, three demonstrated a smaller than average fenestration (<2.5 mm). In one patient we had not inspected the interpeduncular fossa. In the last patient, no apparent reason for reocclusion became evident. The vast majority of patients with anatomically successful ETVs demonstrated fenestration dimensions of 3 mm or more.

There were no permanent morbidities or any mortality. Complications were venous bleeding in three cases, which was controlled intraoperatively by abundant irrigation and compression applied by an inflated Fogarty balloon, and intracerebral bleeding in one case, which automatically resolved within the first 30 postoperative days with no major consequences. Three patients had transient memory loss; in two of them stretching of the fornix (contusion) was identified in reviewing the procedure video.

Discussion

The results of this study demonstrate that ETV for obstructive hydrocephalus of various origins is safe and effective. This has already been widely reported in the literature [1, 3–6, 8, 14].

Patients with benign aqueductal stenosis and tumor compressing the aqueduct receive the greatest benefit from ETV, both based on our results and other reports [3, 6].

Nevertheless, in obtaining a successful ETV, many parameters have to be considered. The given patient's anatomical characteristics must be thoroughly studied by meticulous preoperative neuroradiological evaluation; planning is crucial to tailor the trajectory to the individual anatomical relationship; postoperative stoma patency evaluation and follow-up are no less important. And last, but not least, common pitfalls must be kept in mind, both preoperatively and intraoperatively.

Familiarity with the ventricular anatomy [16, 18] and its variations [13, 19, 20] in hydrocephalus is fundamental. Long-standing hydrocephalus and postinflammatory states may result in unusual anatomical variants, resulting in disorientation during surgery or erroneous trajectory positioning. The structures that need to be carefully assessed on MRI preoperatively are the third ventricle and its dimensions, the aqueduct of Sylvius, the premammillary diaphragm, the pituitary diaphragm and its eventual downward displacement, the foramen of Monro and its specific anatomy, the prepontine cistern, the neurovascular structures beneath the floor of the third ventricle. The anatomic alignment of the endoscopic shaft with the Monro foramen and the premammillary space is crucial, both for the avoidance of stretching of the fornix or the brain parenchyma and for the feasibility of the ventriculostomy (Fig. 2). For this reason, preoperative approach planning, based on anatomical landmarks, is of the utmost importance.

MRI is an indispensable tool for both planning, as mentioned above, and follow-up [6]. The calculation of the stoma

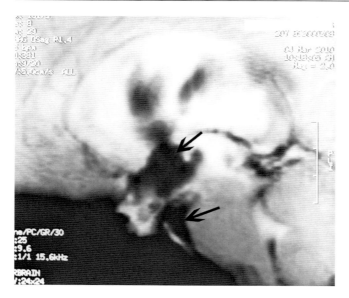

Fig. 3 The postoperative evaluation of cerebrospinal fluid (CSF) dynamics after endoscopic third ventriculostomy (ETV) in cine magnetic resonance imaging (MRI). Significant flow void in the anterior chamber of the third ventricle (*upper arrow*) and the prepontine cistern (*lower arrow*) demonstrating the diversion of CSF flow

dimensions, in our series, showed that an anteroposterior diameter of 3 mm or more, along with the cauterization of the remnants of arachnoid, may represent the most reliable factors for the long-term function of the ventriculostomy. Phase-contrast cine MR studies are useful before surgery, since they can demonstrate abnormal or limited or null aqueduct flow, but they are mostly valuable in the follow-up period. Flow void in the anterior chamber of the third ventricle and in the prepontine cistern are helpful indicators of CSF flow diversion and stoma patency (Fig. 3). Because postoperative failures occur early, radiological (and clinical) control studies must be performed particularly in the first years after the neuroendoscopic procedure [3].

On the basis of our experience and from a review of all operative videos and reports, we consider certain situations to be most critical for the success of ventriculostomy. To begin with, chronic, complicated hydrocephalic conditions, with distortion of the normal anatomy are the major obstacles in obtaining a successful ETV. In these cases, multiple septal fenestrations and choroid plexus atrophy are not rare, contributing to difficulty in orientation. Furthermore, the septal vein in these patients becomes more fragile and can rupture more easily during the operative maneuvers, due to the lack of tissular support by the septum.

A higher than normal position of the basilar artery tip, an aberrant posterior cerebral artery, or a short distance from clivus to mammillary bodies may result in no effective space for fenestration and failure to achieve ETV. On the other hand, a thickening of the premammillary arachnoid may render the floor of the third ventricle resistant and the perforation process more laborious and hence more dangerous. Thus it calls for special attention [6, 17].

Postinfectious states also represent technical challenges, because the presence of scarring tissue and adhesions, both in the ventricles and in the prepontine cistern, distorts anatomical landmarks and provokes ependymal thickening. Supracellar arachnoid cysts need special consideration too. Even if there is no consensus on their management [6], in our opinion the cyst must be removed/opened into the ventricles, and then an ETV with opening of the Liliequist's membrane must be performed (cystoventriculocysternostomy).

Finally, we stress the importance of navigating the prepontine cistern and dissecting the arachnoid trabeculae of Liliequist's membrane that may intervene with CSF flow, especially in chronic inflammatory states. Attention must be paid to this, keeping in mind that in this case the operator is working in front of the basilar artery and its perforators.

Conclusion

ETV for obstructive hydrocephalus of various origins is safe and effective, and should be considered as the first-line of treatment. Familiarity with the ventricular anatomy and its variations in hydrocephalus is key to success. Careful patient selection and effective fenestration are also key elements. Preoperative planning is mandatory. Awareness of potential pitfalls minimizes the risks.

Conflicts of interest statement We declare that we have no conflict of interest.

References

1. Bognar L, Markia B, Novak L (2005) Retrospective analysis of 400 neuroendoscopic interventions: the Hungarian experience. Neurosurg Focus 19(6):E10
2. Buxton N, Ho KJ, Macarthur D et al (2001) Neuroendoscopic third ventriculostomy for hydrocephalus in adults: report of a single unit's experience with 63 cases. Surg Neurol 55:74–78
3. Gangemi M, Mascari C, Maiuri F, Godano U, Donati P, Longatti PL (2007) Long-term outcome of endoscopic third ventriculostomy in obstructive hydrocephalus. Minim Invasive Neurosurg 50(5): 265–269
4. Grant JA, McLone DG (1997) Third ventriculostomy: a review. Surg Neurol 47:210–212
5. Hailong F, Guangfu H, Xiaoling L, Kai F, Haibin T, Hong P, Yong C, Weidong L, Dongdong Z (2004) Endoscopic third ventriculostomy in the management of obstructive hydrocephalus: an outcome analysis. J Neurosurg 100:626–633
6. Hellwig D, Grotenhuis JA, Tirakotai W, Riegel T, Schulte DM, Bauer BL, Bertalanffy H (2005) Endoscopic third ventriculostomy

for obstructive hydrocephalus. Neurosurg Rev 28(1):1–34; discussion 35–38
7. Hopf NJ, Grunert P, Fries G et al (1999) Endoscopic third ventriculostomy: outcome analysis of 100 consecutive procedures. Neurosurgery 44:795–806
8. Iantosca MR, Hader WJ, Drake JM (2004) Results of endoscopic third ventriculostomy. Neurosurg Clin N Am 15:67–75
9. Jones RFC, Kwok BCT, Stening WA et al (1994) The current status of endoscopic third ventriculostomy in the management of non communicating hydrocephalus. Minim Invasive Neurosurg 37:28–36
10. Kunz U, Goldmann A, Bader C et al (1994) Endoscopic fenestration of the 3rd ventricular floor in aqueductal stenosis. Minim Invasive Neurosurg 37:42–47
11. Liliequist B (1956) The anatomy of the subarachnoid cisterns. Acta Radiol 46:61–71
12. Mixter WJ (1923) Ventriculoscopy and puncture of the floor of the third ventricle. Boston Med Surg J 188:277–278
13. Morota N, Watabe T, Inukai T, Hongo K, Nakagawa H (2000) Anatomical variants in the floor of the third ventricle; implications for endoscopic third ventriculostomy. J Neurol Neurosurg Psychiatry 69:531–534
14. Murshid WR (2000) Endoscopic third ventriculostomy: towards more indications for the treatment of non-communicating hydrocephalus. Minim Invasive Neurosurg 43:75–82
15. Putnam TJ (1934) Treatment of hydrocephalus by endoscopic coagulation of the choroid plexus. N Engl J Med 210:1373–1376
16. Resch KDM, Perneczky A, Tschabitscher M, Kindel S (1994) Endoscopic anatomy of the ventricles. Acta Neurochir (Wien) 61:57–61
17. Riegel T, Alberti O, Hellwig D, Bertalanffy H (2001) Operative management of third ventriculostomy in cases of thickened, non-translucent third ventricular floor: technical note. Minim Invasive Neurosurg 44:65–69
18. Riegel T, Hellwig D, Bauer BL, Mennel HD (1994) Endoscopic anatomy of the third ventricle. Acta Neurochir (Wien) 61:54–56
19. Rohde V, Gilsbach JM (2000) Anomalies and variants of the endoscopic anatomy for third ventriculostomy. Minim Invasive Neurosurg 43:111–117
20. Rohde V, Krombach GA, Struffert T, Gilsbach JM (2001) Virtual MRI endoscopy: detection of anomalies of the ventricular anatomy and its possible role as a presurgical planning tool for endoscopic third ventriculostomy. Acta Neurochir (Wien) 143:1085–1091
21. Vandertop WP, van der Zwan A, Verdaasdonk RM (2001) Third ventriculostomy. J Neurosurg 95:919–921

Benign Cerebral Aqueductal Stenosis in an Adult

Christos Chrissicopoulos, S. Mourgela, N. Ampertos, A. Sakellaropoulos, K. Kirgiannis, K. Petritsis, and A. Spanos

Abstract We present a patient with partial stenosis of aqueduct of Sylvius which was an incidental finding without any clinical symptoms. That in our opinion means that the ventricular brain system has many reserves that are being activated before symptoms appear.

Keywords Aqueductal stenosis (AS) • Adult • Hydrocephalus • CSF circulation

Introduction

The cerebral aqueduct of Sylvius is a channel that connects the third and fourth ventricles and is located in the midbrain. It is a very narrow pathway for the cerebrospinal fluid (CSF) flow and hence may be a privileged site for the development of hydrocephalus [2]. There is surprising variation in the size and shape of normal aqueducts. In cross-section, the opening may be oval, round, diamond-shaped, T-shaped, or slit-like [6]. Normal CSF circulation requires an open aqueduct. If stenosis exists, symptoms of hydrocephalus may appear.

We report a case of benign aqueductal stenosis, which was an incidental finding.

Case Report

A 42-year-old male patient, suffering from dizziness of 1 month duration brought on when changing head position, was examined in our outpatient clinic. He had a history of mild

C. Chrissicopoulos (✉), S. Mourgela, N. Ampertos, K. Kirgiannis, K. Petritsis, and A. Spanos
Neurosurgical Department, "Agios Savvas" Anticancer Institute, Athens, Greece
e-mail: md.christos@yahoo.it

A. Sakellaropoulos
Pulmonary and Critical Care Medicine, "Neon Athineon"
MD Hospital, Athens, Greece

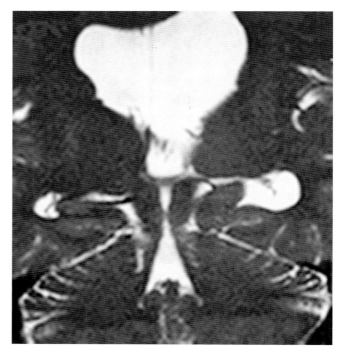

Fig. 1 Magnetic resonance imaging (MRI)-T2 scan: Coronal view showing a hourglass shape of the aqueduct and fourth ventricle

headache, without nausea or vomiting. Brain computed tomography (CT) and magnetic resonance imaging (MRI) showed a dilatation of the third ventricle with a normal appearing fourth ventricle (Fig. 1). The other anatomical formations were normal without signs of pathological distortions. Brain cine MRI revealed chronic dilatation of lateral and third ventricles, with mild stenosis of the aqueduct of Sylvius (Fig. 2). Meanwhile the headache subsided. The patient received no surgical treatment and is undergoing 1-year-interval follow-ups.

Discussion

Aqueductal stenosis (AS) is the most common form of non-communicating (obstructive) hydrocephalus in adults [5]. Primary AS is an isolated stenosis of the aqueduct (it can be

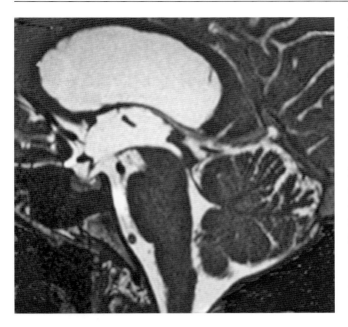

Fig. 2 Magnetic resonance imaging (MRI)-T2 scan: Sagittal view depicting a total black defect in the aqueduct of Sylvius without any cerebrospinal fluid (CSF) passing downwards in this static examination

congenital), while secondary AS is caused by compression of the aqueduct by space-occupying intracranial lesions [3]. Primary AS has been described by Russel and classified into four histological types: simple stenosis, forking or atresia, neuroglial septum formation, and periaqueductal gliosis [4]. Traumatic head injuries have been claimed to cause AS in a few cases, but the causal relationship is unclear.

In obstructive hydrocephalus due to benign AS in adults, the lack of communication between the ventricles across the tentorium creates a pressure differential between the supratentorial and infratentorial compartments. This creates a significant anatomical distortion of structures located at the level of the tentorial hiatus that is well tolerated because of the slow progression of the aqueductal obstruction [1]. Shunt placement resolves the situation by inverting the pressure differential and reestablishing a normal anatomy.

Conclusion

In benign AS, which may be of congenital origin, there is a critical point that must be reached so that in cases of previous compensation of the symptomatology, the compensatory mechanism does not work and symptoms appear. Benign AS remains a significant challenge.

Conflicts of interest statement We declare that we have no conflict of interest.

References

1. Cinalli G, Sainte-Rose C, Simon I, Lot G, Sgouros S (1999) Sylvian aqueduct syndrome and global rostral midbrain dysfunction associated with shunt malfunction. J Neurosurg 90(2):227–236
2. Fin L, Grebe R, Baledent O, Idy-Peretti I (2001) Numerical study of the cerebrospinal fluid (CSF) dynamics under quasistatic condition during a cardiac cycle engineering in medicine and biology society (2001). In: Proceedings of the 23rd annual international conference of the IEEE1. pp 274–276
3. Kao CD, Liao KK (2007) Adult aqueductal stenosis. Acta Neurol Taiwan 16(2):121–122
4. Nag TK, Falconer MA (1966) Non-tumoral stenosis of the aqueduct in adults. Br Med J 2(5523):1168–1170
5. Tisell M (2005) How should primary aqueductal stenosis in adults be treated? A review. Acta Neurol Scand 111:145–153
6. Turnbull IM, Drake CG (1966) Membranous occlusion of the aqueduct of Sylvius. J Neurosurg 24(1):24–33

Efficacy and Versatility of the 2-Micron Continuous Wave Laser in Neuroendoscopic Procedures

Florian H. Ebner, Christoph Nagel, Marcos Tatagiba, and Martin U. Schuhmann

Abstract Laser-assisted techniques offer a huge potential in neurosurgery, but have achieved little acceptance to date. One reason is the concern regarding heat production, uncontrollable and distant penetration, and tissue interaction.

We describe our experience with a 2-micron continuous wave laser (RevoLix jr.; LISA Laser Products OHG, Katlenburg-Lindau, Germany) for neuroendoscopic intraventricular procedures.

The laser beam is delivered through flexible fibers. In an aqueous medium, the effect is restricted to <2 mm in front of the tip with tissue penetration depth of 500 µm.

Forty-four patients (25 adults, 19 children) were operated on using the endoscopic, laser-assisted technique for treatment of obstructive hydrocephalus ($n=39$), pure cyst fenestration ($n=4$), or pure tumor biopsy ($n=1$). All 53 procedures were successfully performed in those 44 operations, with the laser being the main effective instrument used (except for biopsy). Besides one clinically silent small intracisternal hemorrhage and one worsening of a preexisting oculomotor palsy (following fenestration of multiple midbrain cysts), no procedure-related complications occurred.

The 2-micron continuous wave laser is a most valuable and useful tool, in our experience with safe applicability for endoscopic intracranial procedures in patients of all ages.

Keywords Laser • Neuroendoscopy • ETV • Obstructive hydrocephalus

Introduction

Technical advancements influence surgical techniques. This statement is of particular importance in neurosurgery. The field has been strongly influenced by the advent of the operating microscope, development of neuroendoscopic devices, introduction of the Cavitron ultrasonic aspirator, and establishment of intraoperative monitoring. The impressive improvement in postoperative outcomes achieved in the treatment of intracranial pathologies over the last 50 years would have been unimaginable without the support and integration of technological developments. The laser (light amplification by stimulated emission of radiation) as a surgical device was described by Maiman in 1966 [14]. With the introduction of continuous-wave lasers, the tool was applied to the field of neurosurgery [17]. In the meantime lasers with different wavelengths for different indications have been described and used [1, 3, 16, 18]. However, despite their huge potential, laser-based techniques have achieved little acceptance to date, and currently only a minority of neurosurgeons make use of them.

In the present article we describe our experience with a new laser device, the 2-micron continuous-wave laser, in neuroendoscopic intraventricular procedures and discuss the advantages and limitations of this particular type of laser.

Materials and Methods

Clinical Study

From February 2009 until June 2010, 44 consecutive patients were prospectively included in this study. All patients were scheduled for neuroendoscopic treatment of intracranial pathologies, mostly in conjunction with obstructive hydrocephalus. The endoscopic equipment consisted of rigid endoscopes with 30° optics and at least one working channel (Genitori, Karl Storz Company, Tuttlingen, Germany; MINOP, Aesculap, Tuttlingen, Germany) and the AIDA recording system (Karl Storz Company, Tuttlingen, Germany). The endoscopes were used free-hand with the steering left arm resting on an arm support. During laser surgery, safety eyewear has to be worn.

The neurological status before surgery, at discharge, and during the follow-up period was documented. Routinely performed postoperative imaging, computed tomography (CT) or magnetic resonance imaging (MRI) scans, were critically assessed.

F.H. Ebner, C. Nagel, M. Tatagiba, and M.U. Schuhmann (✉)
Department of Neurosurgery, Section of Pediatric Neurosurgery, Eberhard-Karls-University, Tübingen, Germany

Technical Description 2-Micron Laser

The RevoLix jr. is a 2-micron continuous-wave laser (LISA Laser Products OHG, Katlenburg-Lindau, Germany). Its technical specifications (Laser system: continuous-wave diode pumped solid state [DPSS] laser; wavelength: 2.0 micron; power to tissue: 1–15 W continuous wave; chopped mode: 50–1,000 ms; repetition rate 0.5–10 Hz) are designed for soft tissue surgery. The laser beam is delivered through flexible fibers. Water molecules selectively absorb the 2-micron wavelength. Thus, in an aqueous medium, the effect is restricted to <2 mm in front of the tip. More distant tissue is not affected. The tissue penetration is approximately 500 μm [12].

Surgical Technique

After endoscopic localization of the anatomic region of interest, the thin and flexible laser fiber is inserted through a working channel (Fig. 1a, b). For endoscopic third ventriculostomy (ETV) or other stoma creations, we started laser treatment with a power of 8 W continuous wave. When the tip of the fiber touches the target, the laser is briefly activated via a pedal switch. Stepwise perforations are blanched in a ring-like fashion marking the outer limits of the stoma, in case of ETV, in the floor of the third ventricle, between the infundibular recess anteriorly, hypothalamus laterally, and mammillary bodies posteriorly (Fig. 2a, b, d and e). The tissue within the marked stoma boundaries was evaporated with the laser, only rarely it had to be removed with a grasping forceps. The remaining adhesions were divided with mechanical shearing movements of the laser tip or by direct laser coagulation/cutting.

For cutting stronger arachnoid membranes, the laser power can be increased up to 15 W.

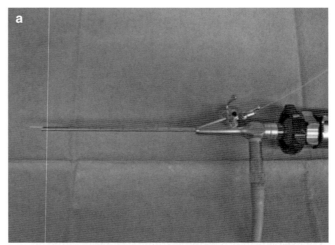
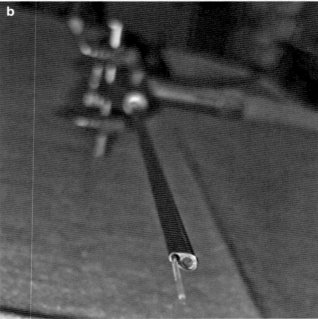

Fig. 1 The flexible laser fiber is introduced through the working channel. Frontal (**a**) and lateral (**b**) view

Results

Of the 44 patients included in the study, 25 were adults (18–72 years, mean 43.5 years) and 19 were in the pediatric age group (1 month–17 years, mean 5 years).

We performed the endoscopic, laser-assisted interventions for treatment of obstructive hydrocephalus ($n = 39$), pure cyst fenestration ($n = 4$), or pure tumor biopsy ($n = 1$). A total number of 53 laser-assisted procedures was performed in 44 operations. Thirty procedures were ETVs. In three patients, septostomy and tumor biopsy were combined. Twice we performed ETV and tumor biopsy, once ETV and cyst fenestration, and twice ETV and retroclival fenestration. During the same operation twice, the decision was made to implant in addition a ventriculoperitoneal shunt, once to revise a preexisting shunt, because of extensive membranous/arachnoidal retroclival adhesions.

Within the patient group with obstructive hydrocephalus, 16 patients suffered from aqueductal stenosis, combined in 3 cases with outflow obstruction of the fourth ventricle; in 11 cases, the obstruction was tumor related, in 7 cases it was due to obstruction of the fourth ventricle; 2 suprasellar arachnoid cysts and 2 colloid cysts caused an obstructive hydrocephalus; and one girl presented with connatal occlusion of the left foramen of Monro.

Four of the laser-assisted procedures were not related to obstructive hydrocephalus (frontal arachnoid cyst, temporal arachnoid cyst, cyst in the brainstem, and germinoma).

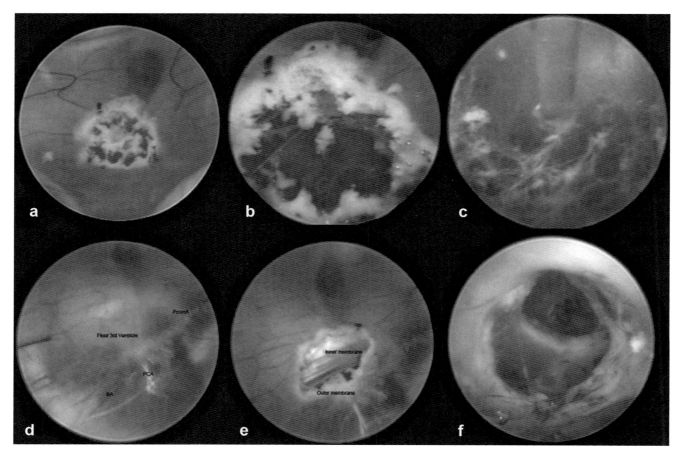

Fig. 2 Some illustrative examples of laser application. After placing an endoscopic third ventriculostomy (ETV) in a typical position (**a**), the basal cistern was encountered, filled with dense thin membranes and without any cerebrospinal fluid (CSF) flow (**b**). The laser was used to evaporize the intracisternal membranes (**c**), followed by opening of a second membrane. An overview is shown of the anatomical structures and local vessel topography at the floor of the third ventricle (**d**). The outer membrane of the floor of the third ventricle is opened with the laser (**e**). Multiple midbrain cysts treated by laser fenestration of three cystic compartment within the brainstem are shown (**f**). *BA* basilar artery, *ETV* endoscopic third ventriculostomy, *PcomA* posterior communicating artery, *PCA* posterior cerebral artery

All procedures were successfully performed mainly with the 2-micron continuous-wave laser as the only tool employed, except for biopsies, which were sampled with the biopsy forceps, with the laser used for hemostasis. The additional mechanical removal of floating membrane flaps after opening of the desired stoma was necessary only in a few cases.

One child suffered a clinical worsening of a preexisting oculomotor palsy after combined ETV and fenestration of several midbrain cysts; however, this was without functional relevance. The postoperative CT scan of one patient showed a bleeding in the basal interpeduncular cisterns despite an intraoperatively totally bloodless ETV. The patient was asymptomatic, however. Besides these two findings, no procedure-related complications occurred. Ten of the 30 patients with ETV required a ventriculoperitoneal shunting within 4 months after the endoscopic procedure. One patient needed a single lumbar puncture. No unintended or problematic vascular lesion occurred due to the use of laser. No clinical signs or symptoms occurred in any patients suggesting thermic damage to surrounding structures.

Discussion

Today ETV is the treatment of choice for obstructive hydrocephalus [4, 5]. The endoscopic procedure is performed either freehand or with a holding device, with or without frameless neuronavigation [6]. Different techniques are employed for opening the floor of the third ventricle [5]. The methods may be grossly divided into two categories: mechanical and energetic. The former includes use of the endoscope's tip, wires, (dilating) forceps, and balloon catheters [4, 8, 9]; the latter unipolar or bipolar electrodes [11] and lasers. Among laser devices, the neodymium:yttrium-aluminium-garnet (Nd:YAG) contact laser is the most widely used [2, 10, 20]. A matter of surgical concern regarding intraoperative use of the laser is the potential to cause serious lesions because of uncontrollable penetration and remote tissue interaction, causing, for example, vascular injury [4, 15].

Analyzing data in the literature, a relatively high rate of vessel injury with argon, KTP, and Nd:YAG lasers is found to be reported [13]. However, even with mechanical techniques, both arteries [7, 19] and veins may be injured [6].

The introduction of the 2-micron continuous-wave laser offers a new option in endoscopic laser-assisted neurosurgery [12, 13]. The laser energy is absorbed by water and thus has an extremely short range of action; since the laser beam penetrates only 500 μm deep in the tissue, it causes only a focal well-controllable lesion. The 2-micron continuous-wave laser combines the high tissue effectiveness of the CO_2 laser, but can be applied through a fiber as a contact laser working at submillimeter distances under water (Fig. 2a, b, c, f). At the same time it offers the hemostatic capacity of the Nd:YAG laser.

These characteristics – application through a flexible fiber, short penetration in cerebrospinal fluid (CSF), and good hemostatic capacity – render the laser useful for intraventricular neuroendoscopic procedures. In the reported series, no clinically relevant bleeding or structural damage such as memory impairment, hypothalamic dysfunction, or clinically relevant cranial nerve deficit occurred. The laser was applied with success both in children and adults. The ability to shrink tissue was used both in ETV and suprasellar arachnoid cysts. Touching consecutively the (tissue) borders with low laser power tightens floppy membranes and facilitates cutting a clean hole in the planished surface. A floating floor may hinder blunt perforation attempts [6] or promote reclosure of the stoma. A targeted laser cut allows a more controlled lesion in a membrane next to delicate surrounding structures than pushing with a blunt instrument.

From the ergonomic point of view, the use of the laser is time-saving and efficient. In most neuroendoscopic intraventricular procedure, a hole (a stoma) is created, which is often done with bipolar, forceps, and balloon dilatation. Therefore multiple instruments have to be exchanged. Using the laser fiber – most of the time – the whole procedure is done with a single instrument (the fiber) in a totally bloodless way. Another advantage of the laser is its ability to create holes in tissue surfaces approached at very flat angles, where other mechanical instruments slip and fail. Ergonomic disadvantages of the device are the necessary precautions and the obligation to wear safety eyewear. Additional instruments are required to take tissue samples or to mechanically remove membranes.

Regarding the time factor, no reasonable statistical analysis can be given, since the reported 44 patients include cases operated on by residents being introduced to the endoscopic laser technique. This fact, however, illustrates the sufficient safety level of the technique.

Conclusion

Summarizing our present experience, the 2-micron continuous-wave laser has turned out to be a most valuable, versatile, and "handy" tool with good usability and applicability for endoscopic intracranial procedures in patients of all ages.

Conflicts of interest statement We declare that we have no conflict of interest.

References

1. Bucholz RD, Pittman T (1991) Endoscopic coagulation of the choroid plexus using the Nd:YAG laser: initial experience and proposal for management. Neurosurgery 28(3):421–426; discussion 426–427
2. Buki A, Doczi T, Veto F, Horvath Z, Gallyas F (1999) Initial clinical experience with a combined pulsed holmium-neodymium-YAG laser in minimally invasive neurosurgery. Minim Invasive Neurosurg 42(1):35–40
3. Devaux BC, Joly LM, Page P, Nataf F, Turak B, Beuvon F et al (2004) Laser-assisted endoscopic third ventriculostomy for obstructive hydrocephalus: technique and results in a series of 40 consecutive cases. Lasers Surg Med 34(5):368–378
4. Ersahin Y, Arslan D (2008) Complications of endoscopic third ventriculostomy. Childs Nerv Syst 24(8):943–948
5. Hellwig D, Grotenhuis JA, Tirakotai W, Riegel T, Schulte DM, Bauer BL et al (2005) Endoscopic third ventriculostomy for obstructive hydrocephalus. Neurosurg Rev 28(1):1–34; discussion 35–38
6. Hopf NJ, Grunert P, Fries G, Resch KD, Perneczky A (1999) Endoscopic third ventriculostomy: outcome analysis of 100 consecutive procedures. Neurosurgery 44(4):795–804; discussion 804–806
7. Horowitz M, Albright AL, Jungreis C, Levy EI, Stevenson K (2001) Endovascular management of a basilar artery false aneurysm secondary to endoscopic third ventriculostomy: case report. Neurosurgery 49(6):1461–1464; discussion 1464–1465
8. Jones RF, Stening WA, Brydon M (1990) Endoscopic third ventriculostomy. Neurosurgery 26(1):86–91; discussion 91–92
9. Jones RF, Kwok BC, Stening WA, Vonau M (1994) Neuroendoscopic third ventriculostomy. A practical alternative to extracranial shunts in non-communicating hydrocephalus. Acta Neurochir Suppl 61:79–83
10. Krishnamurthy S, Powers SK (1994) Lasers in neurosurgery. Lasers Surg Med 15(2):126–167
11. Kunz U, Goldmann A, Bader C, Waldbaur H, Oldenkott P (1994) Endoscopic fenestration of the 3rd ventricular floor in aqueductal stenosis. Minim Invasive Neurosurg 37(2):42–47
12. Ludwig HC, Bauer C, Fuhrberg P, Teichmann HH, Birbilis T, Markakis E (1998) Optimized evaluation of a pulsed 2.09 microns holmium:YAG laser impact on the rat brain and 3 D-histomorphometry of the collateral damage. Minim Invasive Neurosurg 41(4):217–222
13. Ludwig HC, Kruschat T, Knobloch T, Teichmann HO, Rostasy K, Rohde V (2007) First experiences with a 2.0-micron near infrared laser system for neuroendoscopy. Neurosurg Rev 30(3):195–201; discussion 201
14. Maiman TH (1966) Biomedical lasers evolve toward clinical applications. Hosp Manage 101(4):39–41
15. McLaughlin MR, Wahlig JB, Kaufmann AM, Albright AL (1997) Traumatic basilar aneurysm after endoscopic third ventriculostomy: case report. Neurosurgery 41(6):1400–1403; discussion 1403–1404
16. Pinto FC, Chavantes MC, Fonoff ET, Teixeira MJ (2009) Treatment of colloid cysts of the third ventricle through neuroendoscopic Nd:YAG laser stereotaxis. Arq Neuropsiquiatr 67(4):1082–1087
17. Ryan RW, Spetzler RF, Preul MC (2009) Aura of technology and the cutting edge: a history of lasers in neurosurgery. Neurosurg Focus 27(3):E6

18. Schroeder HW, Gaab MR (1999) Endoscopic aqueductoplasty: technique and results. Neurosurgery 45(3):508–515; discussion 515–518
19. Schroeder HW, Warzok RW, Assaf JA, Gaab MR (1999) Fatal subarachnoid hemorrhage after endoscopic third ventriculostomy. Case report. J Neurosurg 90(1):153–155
20. Vandertop WP, Verdaasdonk RM, van Swol CF (1998) Laser-assisted neuroendoscopy using a neodymium-yttrium aluminum garnet or diode contact laser with pretreated fiber tips. J Neurosurg 88(1):82–92

Complications of Endoscopic Third Ventriculostomy: A Systematic Review

Triantafyllos Bouras and Spyros Sgouros

Abstract *Introduction*: Endoscopic third ventriculostomy (ETV) is an established treatment for hydrocephalus. Most studies focus on success rates, and complications are insufficiently charted. The aim of this study was to perform a systematic review of ETV complications.

Methods: A Medline search discovered 24 series of ETV (seven in children, five in adults, and 12 in a mixed-age group) with detailed complications reports.

Results: The analysis included 2,672 ETVs performed on 2,617 patients. The cause of hydrocephalus was aqueductal stenosis in 25.9%, tumor 37.0%, meningomyelocele–Chiari II 6.1%, posthemorrhagic 5.8%, postinfectious 1.4%, cysts 3.3%, Chiari I 0.4%, Dandy-Walker malformation 0.3%, cerebellar infarct 0.9%, normal pressure hydrocephalus 1.3%, and not recorded 16.8%. Overall complication rate was 8.8%. Permanent morbidity was 2.1%, neurologic in 1.2% (hemiparesis, gaze palsy, memory disorders, and/or altered consciousness), hypothalamic in 0.9% (diabetes insipidus, weight gain, or precocious puberty). Intraoperative hemorrhage was present in 3.9%, severe in 0.6% (including four cases [0.14%] of basilar rupture). Other surgical complications were 1.13% (three thalamic infarcts, six subdural, six intracerebral, and two epidural hematomas). Cerebrospinal fluid (CSF) infections occurred in 1.8%, CSF leak in 1.7%, anesthetic complications (bradycardia and hypotension) in 0.19% of cases. Postoperative mortality was 0.22% (six patients; sepsis two, hemorrhage three, and thalamic injury one). Another two children suffered delayed "sudden death" (after 25 and 60 months), caused by acute hydrocephalus due to stoma occlusion. There were no differences between pediatric and adult patients or short and long series (cutoff 100 patients). All deaths were reported in long series. Complication rates were insignificantly higher in short series.

Conclusions: Permanent morbidity after ETV is 2.1%, mortality is 0.22%. The incidence of delayed "sudden death" is 0.07%.

Keywords Endoscopic third ventriculostomy (ETV) • Hydrocephalus • Complications

Introduction

Endoscopic third ventriculostomy (ETV) is an established operation used to treat hydrocephalus of various etiologies in children and adults. Compared with the other main method used for the treatment of hydrocephalus – namely, the placement of ventriculoperitoneal shunt – it presents several advantages, among which the most important is the avoidance of lifetime shunt dependency. Nevertheless, the exact indications for ETV are still under discussion, as the success rate of the procedure is strongly influenced by the underlying pathology.

Several studies have been published aiming to elucidate this issue, and also to investigate other possible factors that influence the success rate and to record possible complications of ETV. The assessment of these factors is of major importance in considering the choice of treatment method in various cases of hydrocephalus, between ETV and shunt placement.

Despite the number of studies, there still exist unresolved issues concerning ETV complications; an exact overall complication rate of the procedure itself, regardless of the indication and the specific anatomic particularities in each case, is not clearly described. There is a wide variation in the reported complication rates, which is attributed to methodological issues, as some incidents are variably reported as complications (e.g., nonrelated to infection postoperative fever), but they are also attributed to true differences among various centers. This could imply that there is a relation between the center's experience and the complication rate; in some cases, the authors of a study state that their own complication rate was lower at later times, when their experience had grown [22].

Another important issue concerns the sporadic incidents of rapid and often lethal deterioration, even long after the

T. Bouras and S. Sgouros
Department of Neurosurgery, "Attikon" University Hospital,
Athens, Greece
e-mail: sgouros@med.uoa.gr

Table 1 The included series

n	Author	Center	Patients	Procedures	Age range
1	Garton et al. [11]	Vancouver, Canada	28	29	69 days–17 years
2	Er ahin et al. [9]	Izmir, Turkey	155	173	2 months–77 years
3	Hader et al. [15]	Calgary, Canada	131	131	1 months–89 years
4	Hopf et al. [18]	Mainz, Germany	95	100	3 weeks–77 years
5	Baldauf et al. [2]	Greifswald, Germany	10	10	25–85 years
6	Ray et al. [23]	Baltimore, USA	43	50	8 weeks–21 years
7	Amini et al. [1]	Salt Lake City, USA	36	36	18–72 years
8	Navarro et al. [22]	Chicago, USA	129	143	6 months–17 years
9	Gangemi et al. [10]	Naples, Italy	25	25	58–75 years
10	Ruggiero et al. [24]	Naples, Italy	63	24	6 months–17 years
11	van Beijnum et al. [28]	Utrecht, Netherlands	202	213	2–83 years
12	Kadrian et al. [20]	Sydney, Australia	203	203	2 days–78 years
13	Santamarta et al. [26]	Salamanca, Spain	66	66	27–67 years
14	Dusick et al. [8]	Los Angeles, USA	108	110	17–88 years
15	Baykan et al. [3]	Istanbul, Turkey	210	210	2 months–10 years
16	Hayhurst et al. [17]	Liverpool, UK	11	11	9–74 years
17	de Ribaupierre et al. [5]	Lausanne, Switzerland	24	24	0–18 years
18	Sacko et al. [25]	Toulouse, France	350	368	2 months–77 years
19	Jenkinson et al. [19]	Liverpool, UK	190	190	18–69 years
20	Schroeder et al. [27]	Greifswald, Germany	188	193	1 months–85 years
21	Hailong et al. [16]	Sichuan, China	58	58	5–67 years
22	Gorayeb et al. [12]	Sao Paulo, Brazil	36	36	3 days–11 months
23	Grunert et al. [13]	Mainz, Germany	159	171	10 days–77 years
24	Brockmeyer et al. [4]	Salt Lake City, USA	97	98	1 days–29.5 years

operation, which have been reported either in case reports or as short series of cases. The frequency of this phenomenon, albeit apparently very low, is not clearly outlined.

This study consists of a systematic review of 24 series of ETV regarding intraoperative, immediate postoperative, and delayed complications.

Methods

A thorough Medline search was performed, which recovered 24 series of ETV performed for various reasons in various populations, with valid reports of both short- and long-term morbidity and mortality rates, along with detailed lists of complications, which was the main inclusion criterion.

All complications reported were recorded and grouped as intraoperative, immediate postoperative, or delayed. Morbidity was categorized as neurologic and hormonal, and as temporal or permanent. Mortality was recorded as immediate postoperative, or delayed, with the last comprising cases of delayed "sudden death."

The possible influence of certain factors on the complication rate – namely, population age and number of patients treated in each series, has been investigated using the chi-square test, with the help of the Statistical Package for the Social Sciences (SPSS, version 17.0; SPSS Inc., Chicago, IL, USA).

Results

A total number of 2,672 ETVs performed on 2,617 patients were recorded; seven series were based on pediatric, five on adult populations, and 12 series on a mixed population. The mean follow-up was 26.7 months. The series characteristics are presented in Table 1.

Regarding the underlying pathologies, the cause of hydrocephalus was aqueductal stenosis in 25.9% of patients, posterior fossa or tectal tumor in 37%, meningomyelocele–Chiari II–related in 6.1%, posthemorrhagic in 5.8%, postinfectious in 1.4%, cyst in 3.3%, Chiari I–related in 0.4%, Dandy-Walker malformation in 0.3%, cerebellar infarct in 0.9%, normal pressure hydrocephalus in 1.3%, and either unknown or not mentioned in 16.8% of cases.

The overall complication rate was 8.8%. Permanent morbidity was recorded in 2.1% of patients, and it was either neurologic (1.2% in total: hemiparesis 0.4%, gaze palsy 0.3%, memory disorders 0.1%, permanent consciousness disorders 0.4%), or hormonal-hypothalamic (0.9% in total: diabetes insipidus 0.5%, weight gain 0.4%, precocious puberty 0.04%). A list of transient complications, including neurologic deficits (hemiparesis, gaze palsy, decreased consciousness, memory disorders, akinetic mutism, and seizures), systemic complications (bradycardia, hypotension, hyponatremia, urinary retention, deep vein thrombosis, and pulmonary embolism), and hormonal disorders (diabetes insipidus) was also recorded.

Important intraoperative technical issues were recorded as follows: 3.9% of ETVs were complicated by intraoperative hemorrhage. In 0.66%, the bleeding was severe and led to important intraventricular hemorrhage. Four cases (0.14%) of basilar rupture were recorded. Intraoperative neural trauma was cited to have occurred in 0.2% of procedures. It affected the fornix (0.08%), the thalamus (0.08%), or the midbrain (0.04%). Anesthetic incidents (bradycardia and hypotension) occurred in 0.19% of cases.

Complications reported in the immediate postoperative period were mainly hemorrhagic (0.9% in total: subdural 0.3%, intraventricular 0.3%, intracerebral 0.2%, epidural hematomas 0.1%), infectious (1.8% in total, meningitis 1.7%, sepsis 0.1%), subdural collections, and CSF leak (others in total 2.3%).

The overall ETV-related mortality rate was 0.29% (8 patients). Six patients died postoperatively (2 due to sepsis, 3 because of hemorrhagic incidents, and 1 because of thalamic injury). There were two reports of delayed fatal acute deterioration (after 25 months and after 5 years), in two pediatric patients, resembling a so-called sudden death phenomenon. One of the patients had undergone a ventriculostomy at the age of 12 years, as a treatment of hydrocephalus caused by aqueductal stenosis. Twenty-five months later, he presented with rapid deterioration which led to his death. At autopsy, massive hydrocephalus due to stoma occlusion was found [11]. The second patient had been shunted as a neonate due to congenital hydrocephalus. At 4 years of age he underwent an ETV as treatment for shunt failure. Five years later, he presented an acute clinical deterioration and died. Massive hydrocephalus and stoma occlusion was the autopsy finding here also [20].

Morbidity rates were similar between short and long series (2.2% vs 2.1%). All deaths were reported in series with more than 100 patients operated. Technical and infectious complications were higher in series with fewer than 100 patients (1.41% vs. 1.03% and 1.9% vs. 1.8%, respectively), but these differences did not reach statistical significance. The comparison between adult and pediatric series yielded a slightly higher complication rate in all subcategories of the adult series.

Discussion

There is an important variation regarding the reported complication rate of ETV. In the included series this rate varies from 2.9% to 16.1%. The severity of the reported complications varies correspondingly. There is also confusion regarding the designation of intraoperative events (e.g., hemorrhage) as complications, and the correlation of certain complications with their clinical phenotype – namely, neurologic or hormonal morbidity. In this review, the overall complication rate was calculated at 8.8%. This rate corresponds to the rate of procedures that were complicated by any intraoperative, postoperative, or delayed adverse incident.

The permanent morbidity of the procedure is reported to be lower than 5% in a recent series. In our review this rate was 2.1% and was analyzed into two main categories: neurologic (1.2%) or hormonal (0.9%). This rate is comparable to the morbidity rates reported for shunt placement [5, 7], and thus it is justifiable to characterize ETV as a safe, low-morbidity procedure.

Regarding intraoperative incidents, there are three main categories reported: hemorrhagic, neurotraumatic, and anesthetic. Among all procedures, 3.9% were complicated by hemorrhagic incidents, 0.66% of them being severe. In four cases (0.14%) there was rupture of the basilar artery. Thus, the most feared of intraoperative complications of ETV is of very low incidence; nevertheless, it should always be kept in mind during the procedure.

Intraoperative neural trauma was reported in only 0.2% of the procedures, affecting periventricular structures. In all of the cases, injury was induced by the endoscope. The very low rate of reported trauma, compared with the rate of neurologic morbidity, implies that some cases of intraoperative injury were not appreciated.

Finally, anesthetic incidents, bradycardia and hypotension that necessitated the abandonment of the operation occurred in only 0.19% of cases.

In the immediate postoperative period, there were mainly hemorrhagic or infectious complications, reported in 0.9% and 1.8% of cases, respectively. The complication rate for subdural collections was reported to be 0.6%. This rate is probably an underestimation due to the fact that in only a few such cases was more drastic treatment needed. CSF leak was the most common isolated complication reported [21].

Eight patients were reported to have died as a result of a complication of the ETV itself (mortality 0.29%). None of them died during the operation. Six patients died in the immediate postoperative period due to sepsis (two), hemorrhagic incidents (three), and one after a thalamic infract.

The calculated rate of late sudden death, according to this review, was 0.07%. Until now, there are several case reports and short series reports of such incidents, without a valid estimation of the possibility of occurrence. Drake et al. have published two reports with 16 cases, in total, collected from various centers worldwide; according to them, a rapid and often lethal deterioration can occur from 5 weeks to 7.8 years after ETV, and the finding is almost always stoma occlusion [6, 14]. Given this possibly long delay until its occurrence, sudden death may have been underestimated in our study – its mean follow-up being 26 months. As a conclusion, this complication is very rare; however it should always be kept in mind, and patients and relatives should be informed about this possibility.

Simple statistics performed have shown that there is a slight difference regarding the complication and morbidity rates between shorter and longer series (cutoff: 100 patients), and between pediatric and adult series, with the rates of long and pediatric series being lower. These differences did not reach statistical significance, and conclusions relating center experience to complication rates (at least among centers which have achieved an experience level high enough to publish their results) cannot be drawn.

Conclusion

Overall, ETV can be regarded as a safe procedure with a low complication, permanent morbidity and mortality rate.

Conflicts of interest statement We declare that we have no conflict of interest.

References

1. Amini A, Schmidt R (2005) Endoscopic third ventriculostomy in adult patients. Neurosurg Focus 19(6):E9
2. Baldauf J, Oertel J, Gaab MR, Schroeder HWS (2006) Endoscopic third ventriculostomy for occlusive hydrocephalus caused by cerebellar infraction. Neurosurgery 59:539–544
3. Baykan N, Isbir O, Gercxek A, Dagcxınar A, Ozek MM (2005) Ten years of experience with pediatric neuroendoscopic third ventriculostomy: features and perioperative complications of 210 cases. J Neurosurg Anesthesiol 17:33–37
4. Brockmeyer D, Abtin K, Carey L, Walker ML (1998) Endoscopic third ventriculostomy: an outcome analysis. Pediatr Neurosurg 28(5):236–240
5. de Ribaupierre S, Rilliet B, Vernet O, Regli L, Villemure JG (2007) Third ventriculostomy vs ventriculoperitoneal shunt in pediatric obstructive hydrocephalus: results from a Swiss series and literature review. Childs Nerv Syst 23:527–533
6. Drake J, Chumas P, Kestle J, Pierre-Kahn A, Vinchon M, Brown J, Pollack IF, Arai H (2006) Late rapid deterioration after endoscopic third ventriculostomy: additional cases and review of the literature. J Neurosurg 105(2 Suppl):118–126
7. Drake JM, Kulkarni AV, Kestle J (2009) Endoscopic third ventriculostomy versus ventriculoperitoneal shunt in pediatric patients: a decision analysis. Childs Nerv Syst 25(4):467–472
8. Dusick JR, McArthur DL, Bergsneider M (2008) Success and complication rates of endoscopic third ventriculostomy for adult hydrocephalus: a series of 108 patients. Surg Neurol 69:5–15
9. Er ahin Y, Arslan D (2008) Complications of endoscopic third ventriculostomy. Childs Nerv Syst 24:943–948
10. Gangemi M, Maiuri F, Buonamassa S, Colella G, de Divitiis E (2004) Endoscopic third ventriculostomy in idiopathic normal pressure hydrocephalus. Neurosurgery 55:129–134
11. Garton HJL, Kestle JRW, Cochrane DD, Steinbok P (2002) A cost-effectiveness analysis of endoscopic third ventriculostomy. Neurosurgery 51:69–78
12. Gorayeb RP, Cavalheiro S, Zymberg ST (2004) Endoscopic third ventriculostomy in children younger than 1 year of age. J Neurosurg 100(5 Suppl Pediatrics):427–429
13. Grunert P, Charalampaki P, Hopf N, Filippi R (2003) The role of third ventriculostomy in the management of obstructive hydrocephalus. Minim Invasive Neurosurg 46(1):16–21
14. Hader WJ, Drake J, Cochrane D, Sparrow O, Johnson ES, Kestle J (2002) Death after late failure of third ventriculostomy in children. Report of three cases. J Neurosurg 97(1):211–215
15. Hader WJ, Walker RL, Myles ST, Hamilton M (2008) Complications of endoscopic third ventriculostomy in previously shunted patients. Neurosurgery 63(ONS Suppl 1):ONS170–ONS177
16. Hailong F, Guangfu H, Xiaoling L, Kai F, Haibin T, Hong P, Yong C, Weidong L, Dongdnog Z (2004) Endoscopic third ventriculostomy in the management of obstructive hydrocephalus: an outcome analysis. J Neurosurg 100:626–633
17. Hayhurst C, Javadpour M, O'Brien DF, Mallucci CL (2006) The role of endoscopic third ventriculostomy in the management of hydrocephalus associated with cerebellopontine angle tumours. Acta Neurochir (Wien) 148:1147–1150
18. Hopf NJ, Grunert P, Fries G, Resch K, Perneczky A (1999) Endoscopic third ventriculostomy: outcome analysis of 100 consecutive procedures. Neurosurgery 44(4):795–806
19. Jenkinson MD, Hayhurst C, Al-Jumaily M, Kandasamy J, Clark S, Mallucci CL (2009) The role of endoscopic third ventriculostomy in adult patients with hydrocephalus. J Neurosurg 110(5):861–866
20. Kadrian D, Gelder J, Florida D, Jones R, Vonau M, Teo C, Stening W, Kwok B (2005) Long-term reliability of endoscopic third ventriculostomy. Neurosurgery 56:1271–1278
21. Kurschel S, Ono S, Oi S (2007) Risk reduction of subdural collections following endoscopic third ventriculostomy. Childs Nerv Syst 23(5):521–526
22. Navarro R, Gil-Parra R, Reitman AJ, Olavarria G, Grant JA, Tomita T (2006) Endoscopic third ventriculostomy in children: early and late complications and their avoidance. Childs Nerv Syst 22:506–513
23. Ray P, Jallo GI, Kim RYH, Kim BS, Wilson S, Kothbauer K, Abbott R (2005) Endoscopic third ventriculostomy for tumor-related hydrocephalus in a pediatric population. Neurosurg Focus 19(6):E8
24. Ruggiero C, Cinalli G, Spennato P, Aliberti F, Cianciulli E, Trischitta V, Maggi G (2004) Endoscopic third ventriculostomy in the treatment of hydrocephalus in posterior fossa tumors in children. Childs Nerv Syst 20:828–833

25. Sacko O, Boetto S, Lauwers-Cances V, Dupuy M, Roux FE (2010) Endoscopic third ventriculostomy: outcome analysis in 368 procedures. J Neurosurg Pediatr 5(1):68–74
26. Santamarta D, Diaz Alvarez A, Goncalves JM, Hernandez J (2005) Outcome of endoscopic third ventriculostomy. Results from an unselected series with noncommunicating hydrocephalus. Acta Neurochir (Wien) 147:377–382
27. Schroeder HWS, Niedorf WR, Gaab MR (2002) Complications of endoscopic third ventriculostomy. J Neurosurg 96:1032–1040
28. van Beijnum J, Hanlo PW, Fischer K, Majidpour MM, Kortekaas MF, Verdaasdonk RM, Vandertop WP (2008) Laser-assisted endoscopic third ventriculostomy: long-term results in a series of 202 patients. Neurosurgery 62:437–444

Syndrome of Inappropriately Low-Pressure Acute Hydrocephalus (SILPAH)[1]

Mark G. Hamilton and Angel V. Price

Abstract *Introduction*: Most patients with acute hydrocephalus have ventriculomegaly and high intracranial pressure (ICP). However, there is a subset of patients who are symptomatic with acute ventriculomegaly and inappropriately low ICP.

Methods: Two patient groups were defined. Each patient presented with clinical deterioration that included a significant decrease in level of consciousness with new and significant ventriculomegaly. Patients in group 1 ($n=10$) were managed without endoscopic third ventriculostomy (ETV). Group 2 was a series of patients ($n=10$) managed with ETV.

Results: Treatment for both groups involved insertion of an external ventricular drain (EVD) with ICP <5 cmH$_2$O. Further treatment consisted of either neck wrapping with a tensor bandage and/or lowering the EVD to negative levels to facilitate drainage of cerebrospinal fluid (CSF), which resulted in clinical improvement and resolution of ventriculomegaly. All 20 patients had anatomical obstruction to CSF flow into the subarachnoid space (SAS) confirmed by magnetic resonance imaging (MRI) with cine MRI studies. Group 1 patients were treated until shunt revision/insertion was possible ($n=7$), ICP normalized, and the EVD could be removed ($n=2$), or death ($n=1$) occurred. Patients in group 2 all underwent ETV, and ICP patterns normalized in all. Group 2 patients were managed with an EVD until shunt revision/insertion was required ($n=2$), ICP normalized and the EVD could be removed ($n=7$), or death ($n=1$) occurred.

Discussion/Conclusions: The syndrome of inappropriately low-pressure acute hydrocephalus (SILPAH) is an important entity in both children and adults. A possible hypothesis invokes loss of an effective SAS. ETV reestablishes communication between the SAS and ventricles, producing a rapid return of normal ICP dynamics and a significant decrease in the number of shunt-dependant patients.

Keywords Hydrocephalus • Negative pressure • Inappropriate low-pressure hydrocephalus • SILPAH • Third ventriculostomy • ETV

Introduction

Acute hydrocephalus associated with ventriculomegaly on imaging studies usually presents with well-recognized symptomatology, initially including headaches, vomiting, abulia, cranial neuropathies, and increasing obtundation. If untreated, acute hydrocephalus may eventually culminate in coma or death. Ventriculostomy typically reveals that the intracranial pressure (ICP) in these patients is higher than normal. There is, however, a small subset of patients with progressive neurological deterioration, acute progressive ventriculomegaly, and ICP that is inappropriately low upon ventriculostomy. Pang and Altschuler have referred to this condition as the "low-pressure hydrocephalic state" [3]. We prefer to identify this disorder as the "syndrome of inappropriately low-pressure acute hydrocephalus (SILPAH)" to fully distinguish it from other low ICP states and normal pressure hydrocephalus (NPH). Patients with SILPAH behave very differently from patients with classic acute high-pressure hydrocephalus. They fail to respond with either clinical improvement or reduction in ventricular size, to standard external ventricular drainage protocols or to routine shunt revision.

In this paper we present our experience with SILPAH and propose a management algorithm for patients with SILPAH, an uncommon yet clinically important neurosurgical disorder.

---

[1]Previously known as negative-pressure hydrocephalus.

M.G. Hamilton (✉)
Division of Neurosurgery, Department of Clinical Neurosciences, University of Calgary, Calgary, Canada and
Foothills Hospital, Calgary, Canada
e-mail: mhamilto@ucalgary.ca

A.V. Price
Department of Pediatric Neurosurgery, Children's Medical Center Dallas, University of Texas Southwestern, Dallas, TX, USA

Materials and Methods

Patients from The Foothills Hospital and Alberta Children's Hospital in Calgary, Alberta, Canada, with SILPAH were identified between January 1997 and April 2010. This was a consecutive series of patients, not a clinical trial. A change in management was instituted after the first ten patients, and outcomes between the two groups were compared. Patients were included if they had (1) clinical neurological deterioration, (2) significant ventriculomegaly on either computed tomography (CT) or magnetic resonance imaging (MRI) head scan, and (3) insertion of an external ventricular drain (EVD) that demonstrated an intracranial pressure (ICP) of <5 cmH$_2$O, with unyielding ventriculomegaly and failure to respond clinically to normal EVD drainage protocols.

Results and Illustrative Cases

Two patient groups are presented. Each patient experienced clinical deterioration that included a significant decrease in level of consciousness with new and significant ventriculomegaly. Patients in group 1 ($n=10$; seven with shunts; three without shunts) were managed without endoscopic third ventriculostomy (ETV). Group 2 was a series of patients ($n=10$; seven with shunts; three without shunts) managed with ETV. There were two children and eight adults in each group (age range 2–65 years). Three case histories are presented to demonstrate pathophysiological and treatment issues, and outcomes are reviewed.

Illustrative Case 1

A 52-year-old man underwent a posterior fossa operation to remove a fourth ventricular tumor (ependymoma). An aberrant dural sinus present in the posterior fossa dura resulted in substantial blood loss. The patient remained hemodynamically stable throughout the operation, and a gross-total removal of tumor was accomplished. Postoperatively, the patient was kept intubated and ventilated in the intensive care unit. On the first postoperative day, his level of consciousness was significantly depressed (GCS=5) and a CT scan revealed significant ventriculomegaly and intraventricular blood. An EVD was placed and the ICP opening pressure was 5 cmH$_2$O and cerebrospinal fluid (CSF) would not flow without significant lowering of the EVD. The patient's neck was gently wrapped with a tensor bandage "tourniquet," CSF flowed readily and his level of consciousness rapidly improved. A head CT scan done within 4 h revealed resolution of the ventriculomegaly. The tensor bandage and the EVD were discontinued after 10 days, and a CT scan following this revealed normal size ventricles. A ventriculoperitoneal shunt was not required.

Commentary

This patient demonstrated striking inappropriately low ICP in the presence of significant ventriculomegaly and a very abnormal neurological exam (coma). His CT scan demonstrated intraventricular blood with obstruction of CSF outflow through the fourth ventricle. Note that while this patient (without a shunt) did not demonstrate negative opening pressures, the pressures were inappropriately low, and CSF would not flow through the drain using a normal drainage protocol. An additional important observation is that this patient did not require a ventriculoperitoneal shunt.

Illustrative Case 2

Patient 2 was a 48-year-old man who presented to hospital with altered level of consciousness (GCS=13) and a stiff neck. A CT scan was followed by a lumbar puncture (LP) to rule out meningitis. CSF analysis was consistent with meningitis and was suspicious for tuberculosis (TB). One day following the LP, the patient experienced a further significant deterioration in his level of consciousness (GCS=8), and a repeat CT scan demonstrated a significant increase in ventricular size. An external ventricular catheter was placed with an opening pressure of 4 cmH$_2$O. A gentle tensor bandage tourniquet was placed around the patient's neck with a subsequent clinical improvement, a decrease in ventricular size, and reexpansion of the cerebral mantle. Removal of the tensor bandage after 3 days of drainage resulted in a decreased level of consciousness and progressive ventriculomegaly. The EVD was lowered to a subzero level (i.e., −20 cmH$_2$O) to promote CSF drainage, and the patient improved clinically as well as demonstrating a decrease in ventricular size. A brain biopsy confirmed a diagnosis of TB meningoencephalitis. A ventriculoperitoneal shunt was inserted after 4 weeks when the patient's ICP dynamics normalized.

Commentary

This patient demonstrated striking inappropriately low ICP in the presence of significant ventriculomegaly and a very abnormal neurological exam. All of this developed after he had a LP. Note that while this patient (without a shunt) did not demonstrate negative opening pressures, the pressures

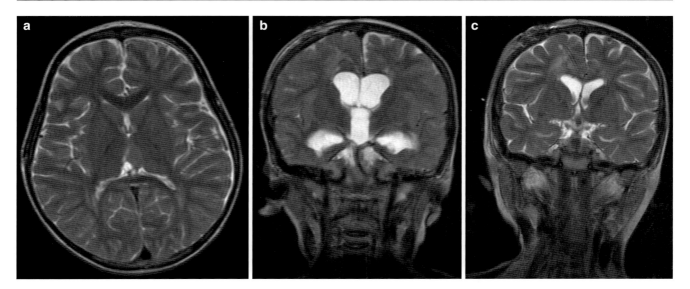

Fig. 1 (**a**) Axial T2 magnetic resonance imaging (MRI) scan showing slit ventricles. (**b**) Coronal T2 magnetic resonance imaging (MRI) scan showing large ventricles. (**c**) Coronal T2 magnetic resonance imaging (MRI) scan after endoscopic third ventriculostomy (ETV), showing reduction in ventricular size. Patient was clinically improved

were inappropriately low, and CSF would not flow through the drain with a normal drainage protocol. Both a neck wrap and lowering of the EVD to a subzero level were employed to normalize ventricle size and clinical function. This patient eventually required a ventriculoperitoneal shunt, although a prolonged period of time was required before ICP dynamics normalized enough to allow successful shunt function.

Illustrative Case 3

A 9-year-old girl had undergone treatment of a third ventricular ependymoma and insertion of a ventriculoperitoneal shunt 6 years earlier in another country. She presented with intractable headaches that were characterized as "low-pressure." There was no evidence of tumor recurrence, and she had slit-like ventricles on CT and MRI (Fig. 1a). Her mother provided a history that there were significant problems "making the shunt work" after it was first inserted. Her shunt system had no valve. She was admitted, and her shunt was externalized as an EVD. Early next morning she was unarousable with an ICP of only 1 cmH_2O. Her MRI demonstrated significant ventricular enlargement with obstruction of the aqueduct (Fig. 1b). Her EVD was lowered to a subzero level (-5 cmH_2O) to facilitate CSF drainage in a controlled fashion prior to undergoing an emergent ETV. After the ETV, she experienced an immediate normalization of her ICP dynamics, clinical improvement, and a reduction in the size of her ventricles (Fig. 1c). Her EVD was discontinued after 3 days, and she was discharged home.

Commentary

This patient number demonstrated striking inappropriately low ICP in the presence of significant ventriculomegaly and a very abnormal neurological exam (coma). Initial treatment involved lowering the EVD to a subatmospheric level (i.e. -5 cmH_2O) promoting CSF drainage in a controlled fashion to stabilize the patient and allow for the completion of an emergency ETV. The ICP findings associated with SILPAH immediately resolved after the ETV connected the ventricular system to the cortical subarachnoid space. The ETV thus quickly established effective CSF flow, and her hospital stay was significantly shorter in comparison with the previous patients.

Overall Treatment Results

Treatment for both groups involved insertion of an EVD with ICP <5 cmH_2O. Further treatment consisted of either neck wrapping with a tensor bandage and/or lowering the EVD to negative levels to facilitate drainage of CSF, which resulted in clinical improvement and resolution of ventriculomegaly. All 20 patients had suspected or confirmed obstruction of CSF flow into the subarachnoid space based on imaging studies (MRI and CT).

Group 1 patients were treated using an EVD until shunt revision/insertion was possible ($n=7$), ICP normalized, and the EVD could be removed ($n=2$), or death occurred ($n=1$). Patients in group 2 all underwent ETV, and ICP dynamics normalized in all. Group 2 patients were managed with an EVD until shunt revision/insertion was required ($n=2$), ICP normalized, and the EVD could be removed ($n=7$), or death occurred ($n=1$). Therefore, the requirement for use of a shunt decreased from 70% in the patient Group 1 to 20% in Group 2.

Discussion

Three patient cases have been presented that illustrate the issues associated with a small subset of patients with progressive neurological deterioration, *acute* progressive ventriculomegaly, and ICP that is inappropriately low when an EVD was inserted. The phrase *syndrome of inappropriately low-pressure acute hydrocephalus* (SILPAH) is used to label this group of patients. Previous authors have offered a variety of terms, including *negative-pressure hydrocephalus* [6, 7] and *low-pressure hydrocephalus* [2, 3] to describe these patients. Such terms are imprecise and fail to fully capture the true spectrum of ICP abnormalities in these patients. We suggest that the common finding identified in these patients is inappropriately low ICP, but not necessarily "negative" ICP. However, treatment with an EVD typically requires a "negative" (subzero) pressure gradient to create effective CSF drainage.

Two typical ICP scenarios were identified: (1) the shunted patient presenting with SILPAH typically has opening intracranial pressures (with an EVD or during shunt revision) that are <0 cmH$_2$O; while (2) the patient without a shunt presenting with SILPAH typically will have opening intracranial pressures (with an EVD) that are much lower than expected but rapidly become inappropriately low. In both scenarios, ICP is too low to allow drainage of CSF with normal EVD drainage protocols, and ventriculomegaly and clinical symptoms persist. Another important premise is that all patients have suspected or confirmed obstruction to CSF flow from the ventricles into the subarachnoid space.

The neurological symptoms experienced by patients with SILPAH can be attributed to two separate mechanisms: first through brain distortion, and second as a consequence of cortical ischemia occurring because of the severe ventricular distortion and elevated radial compressive stresses [1, 3]. Lesniak et al. suggested that stretched axonal fibers in the periventricular area result in slow progressive neurological dysfunction [1]. Vassilyadi et al. suggested that the signs and symptoms of SILPAH were secondary to the establishment of a craniovertebral pressure gradient that leads to altered brainstem function [7].

SILPAH is both uncommon, and we suspect, frequently not recognized by physicians. SILPAH is often unrecognized because of its enigmatic and counterintuitive nature.

Some investigators believe that "negative-pressure hydrocephalus" can only occur in patients with a ventriculoperitoneal shunt. Review of the relevant literature reveals a dearth of information on this topic, and the exact pathophysiology remains controversial. When SILPAH is unrecognized, treatment decisions are inappropriate. Patients may experience multiple shunt revisions, each with no obvious shunt obstruction identified; or patients may have acute non-shunt-related ventriculomegaly that does not respond to standard external ventricular drainage techniques or insertion of a ventriculoperitoneal shunt.

A clear understanding of the pathophysiology is important because it will determine effective treatment strategies. Some have attempted to define the pathophysiology of SILPAH with mathematical pressure volume models [1, 3–5]. The premise of these models is based on the mathematical derivation of the pressure-volume index of the brain. They suggest that these patients have experienced an alteration in the viscoelastic properties of the brain parenchyma, or brain turgor. Patients experiencing hydrocephalus with high ICP have ventriculomegaly secondary to increased CSF and the resulting pressure of this intraventricular fluid compressing the cerebral mantle. Patients experiencing ventriculomegaly with inappropriately low ICP have ventricular expansion secondary to decreased brain turgor. It was initially proposed that decreasing brain turgor resulted in a decrease in the size of the cerebral mantle, loss of an effective cortical subarachnoid space (CSAS) for CSF circulation and consequently ventricular expansion [3–5]. Our population of patients had a large age range (2–65 years), but only 20% were children. This conforms to a hypothesis that the mechanical conditions (i.e., that result in decreased brain turgor) that come into play to allow SILPAH are more likely acquired, not congenital. A decrease in brain turgor may occur secondary to potential insults such as infection, hemorrhage, tumors, cranial irradiation, and trauma.

All these previous models have failed to appreciate the importance of the relationship between the CSAS and the intraventricular obstructive hydrocephalus present in patients with SILPAH. Rekate et al. [6] recently presented a synthesis of these issues as the following hypothesis for the shunted patient: In the presence of a complete obstruction of CSF outflow from the ventricular system, the CSAS is subject to drainage due to a leak or through the dural venous system. Selective drainage of the CSAS, in the presence of low brain turgor results in a decrease in ICP, accumulation of CSF within, and resultant expansion of, the ventricles (the ICP is lower than the opening pressure of the shunt valve and therefore drainage does not occur). We suggest that the hypothesis of Rekate et al. is equally applicable to a patient with SILPAH who does not have a shunt. Patient 2 did not have a shunt, had isolation of his ventricular system from his CSAS, and experienced clinical deterioration (and the onset of SILPAH) after a LP.

An EVD is typically used as an initial therapy for all patients. Treatment of patients with SILPAH can then be directed at: (1) restoring brain turgor by increasing dural sinus pressure to inhibit drainage of CSF from the CSAS with either a gentle neck tourniquet or an abdominal binder; (2) "forced" drainage of the ventricular system by lowering an EVD to subzero pressures until normal ICP and cerebral mantle size is obtained; and (3) restoration of communication between the ventricular system and the CSAS by ETV.

The process to either reestablish a working shunt system or to wean the EVD can be protracted. In certain circumstances, a long ventricular drain (tunneled to the abdomen) can be used to allow a patient to mobilize until the ICP dynamics (SILPAH) is "correct." At that time, the EVD may potentially be weaned, or a ventriculoperitoneal or lumboperitoneal shunt inserted if indicated. Neck wrapping and abdominal binders likely increase both brain turgor and dural venous pressure, allowing distention of the CAS and reexpansion of the brain with flow of CSF out of the ventricle. A neck tourniquet or abdominal binder can also be used in the presence of a "working" shunt to facilitate drainage. Other methods to facilitate CSF drainage through a patent shunt system include: (1) shunt pumping; (2) raising the head of bed to 30-45°; (3) use of the lowest resistance shunt system possible or replacing the valve with a simple reservoir; and and (4) use of a ventriculopleural shunt (subzero intrathoracic pressures).

These strategies are however self-limited by their failure to correct the underlying pathophysiology. An appreciation of the observation that these patients typically have complete obstruction of CSF outflow from the ventricular system (as illustrated by Patient 3) was used to establish an alternative strategy for management of patients with SILPAH (i.e. reestablish communication between the CSAS and the ventricular system). This can be accomplished in many patients by performing an ETV. ICP dynamics are quickly reestablished, and in many patients the treatment is definitive and no shunt system is required. Furthermore, the treatment process is typically much faster, and hospital stay is reduced, in comparison with the non-ETV-treated patients with SILPAH. A limitation of this report is its lack of a randomized controlled clinical trial structure. However, the observation that the long-term requirement for a shunt was substantially lower in this ETV-treated population (20% vs. 70%) is clinically robust.

Conclusion

The syndrome of inappropriately low-pressure acute hydrocephalus (SILPAH) is a little recognized but clinically important clinical entity occurring in both adults and children. The pathophysiology likely involves isolation of the ventricular system from the CSAS, decreased brain turgor, and loss of an effective CSAS. Reestablishment of communication between the ventricular system and the CSAS has the potential to definitively correct ICP dynamics and reduce the probability that a shunt will be required.

Conflicts of interest statement We declare that we have no conflict of interest.

References

1. Lesniak MS, Clatterbuck RE, Rigamonti D, Williams MA (2002) Low pressure hydrocephalus and ventriculomegaly: hysteresis, non-linear dynamics, and the benefits of CSF diversion. Br J Neurosurg 16:555–561
2. Owler BK, Jacobson EE, Johnston IH (2001) Low pressure hydrocephalus: issues of diagnosis and treatment in five cases. Br J Neurosurg 15:353–359
3. Pang D, Altschuler E (1994) Low-pressure hydrocephalic state and viscoelastic alterations in the brain. Neurosurgery 35:643–655; discussion 655–646
4. Rekate HL (1992) Brain turgor (Kb): intrinsic property of the brain to resist distortion. Pediatr Neurosurg 18:257–262
5. Rekate HL (1994) The usefulness of mathematical modeling in hydrocephalus research. Childs Nerv Syst 10:13–18
6. Rekate HL, Nadkarni TD, Wallace D (2008) The importance of the cortical subarachnoid space in understanding hydrocephalus. J Neurosurg Pediatr 2:1–11
7. Vassilyadi M, Farmer JP, Montes JL (1995) Negative-pressure hydrocephalus. J Neurosurg 83:486–490

Lhermitte–Duclos Disease Presenting with Hydrocephalus

Mun Sul Yang, Choong Hyun Kim, Jin Hwan Cheong, and Jae Min Kim

Abstract Lhermitte–Duclos disease (LDD) is a rare cerebellar disorder characterized by diffuse or focal enlargement of cerebellar folia. Clinical manifestations are usually related to a mass effect and secondary obstructive hydrocephalus. Increased intracranial pressure symptoms and cerebellar symptoms are the most frequent patient complaints. We describe the case of a patient with LDD who developed secondary obstructive hydrocephalus. A 68-year-old woman was brought to the emergency room for sudden vertigo following several bouts of vomiting and headache. There were no external signs of trauma, serious illness or infection. On admission, the patient was alert and had no neurological deficits. Brain computed tomography (CT) and magnetic resonance imaging (MRI) showed hydrocephalus and a cerebellar mass in the right cerebellar hemisphere compressing the fourth ventricle. Suboccipital craniotomy and subtotal removal of the mass was performed. Pathological study of the surgical specimen showed abnormal ganglionic neurons and an enlarged molecular layer compatible with dysplastic gangliocytoma. Cytoreduction can achieve improvement in symptoms caused by mass effect, but postoperative swelling may aggravate obstructive hydrocephalus. Therefore, if symptoms still remain after removal of the mass, an additional shunting procedure may be needed as a further management option.

Keywords Gangliocytoma • Lhermitte–Duclos disease • Hydrocephalus • Cerebellar signs • Shunt

M.S. Yang, C.H. Kim (✉), J.H. Cheong, and J.M. Kim
Department of Neurosurgery, Hanyang University Guri Hospital,
Guri, South Korea
e-mail: kch5142@hanyang.ac.kr

Introduction

Since Lhermitte and Duclos reported the first case of Lhermitte–Duclos disease (LDD) in 1920, various synonymous descriptions, such as diffuse gangliocytoma of the cerebellar cortex, benign hypertrophy of the cerebellum, Purkinjeoma and hamartoma of the cerebellum have been used to describe this lesion [10, 12, 16]. LDD has benign pathological findings, but its pathophysiology has not been established definitively. LDD has been considered to be a congenital and genetic malformation or hypertrophy of the cerebellar cortex, but recurrent cases have prompted questions regarding a neoplastic etiology [5, 8, 10]. Clinical symptoms are mainly the results of two pathogenetic mechanisms. One is the gradual increase of intracranial pressure due to mass effect and secondary obstructive hydrocephalus, and the other is cerebellar dysfunction. Most patients complain of long-standing or slowly aggravating symptoms such as occipital headache, vertigo, cranial nerve palsies, and cerebellar ataxia.

LDD was difficult to diagnose before the development of neuro-imaging modalities, and patients with LDD had very poor prognoses. About one-third of patients in the approximately 90 reported cases died due to mass effect [10, 17]. Utilization of magnetic resonance (MR) imaging facilitated the correct preoperative diagnosis and enabled more accurate procedures in surgical treatment. Although LDD is benign in nature, many concomitant diseases have been described in LDD patients, such as cutaneous lesions, dysmorphic features, and tumors of other organs. Furthermore, association with genetic syndromes such as Cowden syndrome, Proteus syndrome, and Bannayan–Riley–Ruvalcaba syndrome – all PTEN hamartoma tumor syndromes – have not been clarified [7, 10, 17, 19]. Among the several PTEN mutation syndromes, Cowden syndrome is the most commonly cited disease that is speculated to be related to LDD. Simultaneous occurrence and similar clinical manifestations are described in many case reports. Moreover, Williams et al. suggested that LDD could be a component of Cowden syndrome [15, 18].

In our report, we describe a rare case of an elderly patient with a dysplastic gangliocytoma in the right cerebellar hemisphere combined with obstructive hydrocephalus. Diagnostic and therapeutic modalities as well as pathological findings are discussed through our experience and literature review.

Case Report

A 68-year-old woman visited the emergency room presenting with sudden paroxysmal vertigo, nausea, vomiting, and loss of consciousness. The patient had never suffered from these symptoms before the attack. She recovered, and left-beating nystagmus was the only residual abnormal finding detected by cranial nerve examination on admission. Cerebellar function tests showed a positive Romberg sign and cerebellar dysfunction. Computed tomography (CT) scans showed a large mass in the right cerebellar hemisphere combined with amorphous calcifications. The mass compressed the fourth ventricle, and secondary obstructive hydrocephalus was noted. MR images showed cortical thickening with subcortical high signal intensity on T2-weighted images. Change in the cerebellar cortex similar to the so-called tiger-striped appearance pattern was observed, and gadolinium-enhanced images showed subtle enhancement of the lesion (Fig. 1). The tumor was immediately removed via a right suboccipital osteoplastic craniotomy. Because the margins of the mass were not clearly demarcated in the surgical field, as much of the mass as possible was removed, avoiding damage to the vermis or cerebellar peduncle. Histological examination showed areas of increased dysplastic ganglion-like cells of the cortex. An enlarged molecular layer with dysplastic ganglion-like cells and a hypertrophied granular layer were observed with hematoxylin and eosin staining, but no mitotic, atypical, or pleomorphic features or other invasive behaviors were noticed microscopically. The dysplastic ganglion cells were diffusely positive for synaptophysin and neurofilament on immunohistochemical analysis (Fig. 2). The patient's slight drowsiness and confused mental state continued for a week after surgery. Postoperative CT scanning was performed, and slightly aggravated hydrocephalus due to cerebellar swelling was noticed despite medication for increased intracranial pressure. An additional shunt operation was considered, but the patient's cerebellar swelling was becoming slowly controlled, and her symptoms were getting better after a week following surgery. Her obstructive hydrocephalus spontaneously improved on serial radiological examination, and regrowth of the tumor or development of hydrocephalus did not recur.

Discussion

LDD exhibits different radiological and pathological features from other neoplastic lesions of the brain. MRI findings in this rare cerebellar disorder include a striated and laminar pattern of the cerebellar cortex, especially well manifested on T2-weighted imaging. Gadolinium-enhanced T1-weighted images usually show scanty enhancement of the lesion and, to our knowledge, peritumoral invasion or necrotic changes have not been observed in reported cases [1, 2, 9]. Histopathological examination of LDD shows thickening of cerebellar folia due to a hypertrophied molecular layer composed of hypertrophic myelinated and non-myelinated axons originating from underlying abnormal ganglionic cells. In contrast, the Purkinje cell layer and granular layer are replaced and expanded by large neurons with vesicular nuclei and prominent nucleoli [10, 11, 14]. These dysplastic cells seem to be derived from granular cells for the most part, but several Purkinje-cell-specific antibodies are labeled by immunohistochemical staining. Our results from microscopic examination and immunohistochemical staining were not different from those in previous case reports. In spite of some reported late recurrences, histological and immunohistochemical studies of recurrent cases did not reveal proliferative activity [4, 5, 8]. As evidence supporting a congenital etiology for LDD, association of LDD with chromosomal mutation also suggests genetic control of the dysplasia [14, 19, 20]. PTEN gene mutations are representatively related to this genetic disorder. Mutations in this region can promote proliferation and invasion as well as inhibit apoptosis, and the mutated allele has been shown to be expressed in 83% of pathological specimens [14, 21]. Mutation in the PTEN gene has a tendency to produce dysplastic-hyperplastic lesions and neoplasms in the skin, gonads, thyroid, and colon. These kinds of mutation are also observed in Cowden disease. Padberg et al. postulated that Cowden disease and LDD could be related to each other, and that LDD could be one of the central nervous system manifestations associated with Cowden disease, among others such as megalencephaly, mental impairment, and seizure [13]. After the description by Padberg et al., many coincident cases have been reported of these two rare diseases [3, 13, 14, 17]. Case reports of isolated LDD patients, in contrast, have also been described. Our patient had no clinical or radiological evidence satisfying the criteria for Cowden disease (except LDD) and also had no familial history. According to some case reports, however, LDD patients frequently develop other central nervous system manifestations as well as skin and soft-tissue lesions such as trichilemmomas, angiomas, lipomas, and café au lait spots, in addition to dysmorphic anomalies such as large hands or feet and polydactyly. Neoplastic lesions of the thyroid, breast, and gastrointestinal tract have also been reported in patients with LDD. Approximately 50% of case reports describe these concomitant abnormalities [3, 6, 10, 11, 14, 17]. Physicians should always consider a diagnosis of Cowden disease or other concomitant diseases in patients with LDD, considering the reported cases.

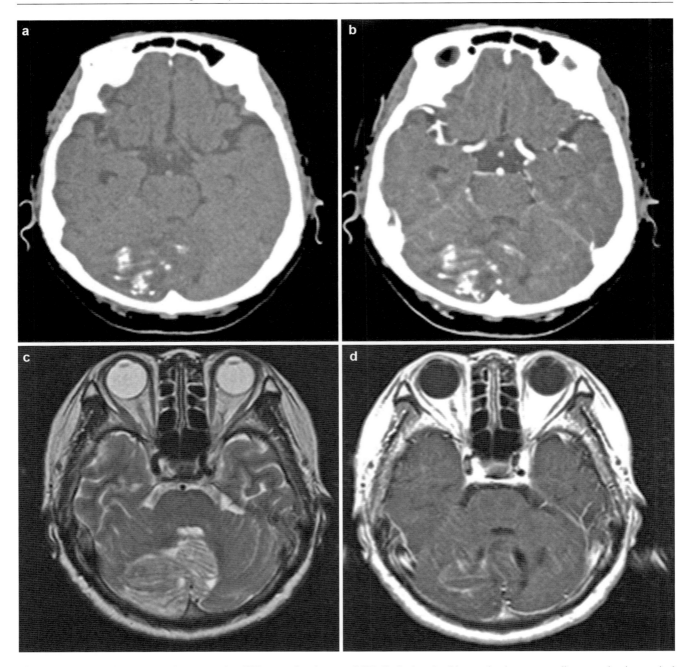

Fig. 1 (**a**) Preoperative computed tomography (CT) scan showing a large mass (3.7×5.7×3.5 cm) in the right cerebellar hemisphere with amorphous calcifications. (**b**) Postcontrast CT scan demonstrating the subtle enhancement of the tumor. (**c**) Preoperative T2-weighted axial MRI displaying the "tiger-striped appearance" pattern that is a typical finding in Lhermitte–Duclos disease. (**d**) Preoperative T2-weighted axial magnetic resonance imaging (MRI) demonstrating secondary hydrocephalus

Our patient was not a typical case considering her old age, paroxysmal symptoms, and absence of other clinical symptoms and signs occasionally related to LDD, but the diagnosis of this rare cerebellar disorder was not difficult, due to pathognomonic MRI findings. In actuality, the development of imaging modalities such as CT and MRI has simplified both the diagnosis and the decision process regarding a therapeutic plan. Focal or diffuse thickening of the cerebellar cortex without enhancement is a characteristic MRI finding in patients with LDD and is common to most reported cases [1, 9, 10, 14].

Complete excision of the hypertrophied lesion is the treatment of choice, but total excision destroying important adjacent structures is unnecessary, because of the benign nature of LDD, especially in elderly patients. Compression of the fourth ventricle is a cause of obstructive hydrocephalus and syringomyelia in LDD patients. Excision of the cerebellar mass mostly resolves the compression and can

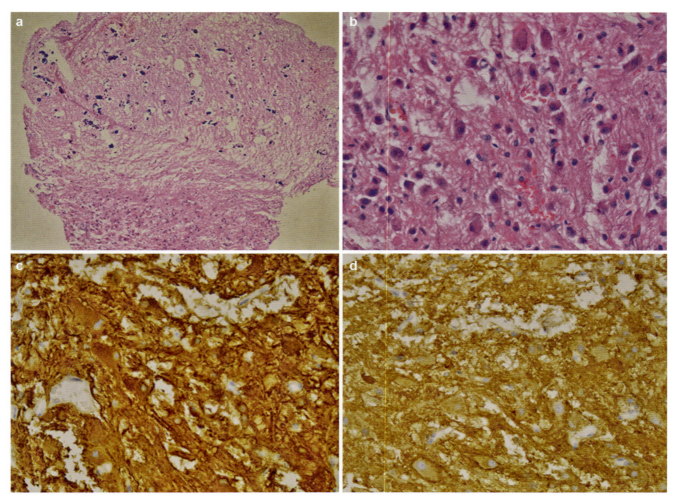

Fig. 2 Microscopic examination of the tumor specimen. (**a**) Photomicrograph showing an enlarged molecular layer with dysplastic ganglion-like cells (hematoxylin and eosin stain [H & E], magnification × 100). (**b**) Abnormal ganglion-like neurons showing eosinophilic cytoplasm and large nuclei; no findings suggestive of neoplasia were noticed (H & E, × 400). Immunohistochemical study of the speciemen: Dysplastic ganglion cells were diffusely stained by neurofilament (**c**) and synaptophysin (**d**)

slowly reduce intracranial pressure and ventricle size. Longstanding hydrocephalus or syringomyelia, however, may not be affected by decompression. Postoperative swelling may aggravate the symptoms, so if severe swelling and aggravated symptoms are observed after surgery, an additional shunting procedure or temporary drainage of cerebrospinal fluid should be considered.

Conclusion

LDD has a benign pathological finding. However, in symptomatic case, cytoreduction can improve symptoms caused by mass effect. If symptoms still remain after removal of the mass, an additional shunting procedure should be required.

Acknowledgements This study was supported by the research fund of Hanyang University (HY-2006-C).

Conflict of interest statement We declare that we have no conflict of interest.

References

1. Ashley D, Zee C, Chandrasoma P, Segall H (1990) Lhermitte-Duclos disease: CT and MR findings. J Comput Assist Tomogr 14:984
2. Carter J, Merren M, Swann K (1989) Preoperative diagnosis of Lhermitte-Duclos disease by magnetic resonance imaging. J Neurosurg 70:135–137
3. Derrey S, Proust F, Debono B, Langlois O, Layet A, Layet V, Longy M, Freger P, Laquerriere A (2004) Association between Cowden syndrome and Lhermitte-Duclos disease: report of two cases and review of the literature. Surg Neurol 61:447–454

4. Hair L, Symmans F, Powers J, Carmel P (1992) Immunohistochemistry and proliferative activity in Lhermitte-Duclos disease. Acta Neuropathol 84:570–573
5. Hashimoto H, Iida J, Masui K, Nishi N, Sakaki T (1997) Recurrent Lhermitte-Duclos disease–case report. Neurol Med Chir (Tokyo) 37:692–696
6. Hobert JA, Eng C (2009) PTEN hamartoma tumor syndrome: an overview. Genet Med 11:687–694
7. Lynch NE, Lynch SA, McMenamin J, Webb D (2009) Bannayan-Riley-Ruvalcaba syndrome: a cause of extreme macrocephaly and neurodevelopmental delay. Arch Dis Child 94:553–554
8. Marano SR, Johnson PC, Spetzler RF (1988) Recurrent Lhermitte-Duclos disease in a child. Case report. J Neurosurg 69:599–603
9. Meltzer C, Smirniotopoulos J, Jones R (1995) The striated cerebellum: an MR imaging sign in Lhermitte-Duclos disease (dysplastic gangliocytoma). Radiology 194:699
10. Nowak DA, Trost HA (2002) Lhermitte-Duclos disease (dysplastic cerebellar gangliocytoma): a malformation, hamartoma or neoplasm? Acta Neurol Scand 105:137–145
11. Nowak D, Trost H, Porr A, Stolzle A, Lumenta C (2001) Lhermitte-Duclos disease (Dysplastic gangliocytoma of the cerebellum). Clin Neurol Neurosurg 103:105–110
12. Oppenheimer DR (1955) A benign tumour of the cerebellum; report on two cases of diffuse hypertrophy of the cerebellar cortex with a review of nine previously reported cases. J Neurol Neurosurg Psychiatry 18:199–213
13. Padberg G, Schot J, Vielvoye G, Bots G, De Beer F (2004) Lhermitte-Duclos disease and Cowden disease: a single phakomatosis. Ann Neurol 29:517–523
14. Prez-Nez A, Lagares A, Bentez J, Urioste M, Lobato RD, Ricoy JR, Ramos A, Gonzlez P (2004) Lhermitte-Duclos disease and Cowden disease: clinical and genetic study in five patients with Lhermitte-Duclos disease and literature review. Acta Neurochir (Wien) 146:679–690
15. Rainov N, Holzhausen H, Burkert W (1995) Dysplastic gangliocytoma of the cerebellum (Lhermitte-Duclos disease). Clin Neurol Neurosurg 97:175–180
16. Roski RA, Roessmann U, Spetzler RF, Kaufman B, Nulsen FE (1981) Clinical and pathological study of dysplastic gangliocytoma. Case report. J Neurosurg 55:318–321
17. Vinchon M, Blond S, Lejeune J, Krivosik I, Fossati P, Assaker R, Christiaens J (1994) Association of Lhermitte-Duclos and Cowden disease: report of a new case and review of the literature. Br Med J 57:699
18. Williams DW, Elster AD, Ginsberg LE, Stanton C (1992) Recurrent Lhermitte-Duclos disease: report of two cases and association with Cowden's disease. AJNR Am J Neuroradiol 13:287–290
19. Yachnis A, Rorke L, Trojanowski J (1994) Cerebellar dysplasias in humans: development and possible relationship to glial and primitive neuroectodermal tumors of the cerebellar vermis. J Neuropathol Exp Neurol 53:61
20. Yachnis A, Trojanowski J, Memmo M, Schlaepfer W (1988) Expression of neurofilament proteins in the hypertrophic granule cells of Lhermitte-Duclos disease: an explanation for the mass effect and the myelination of parallel fibers in the disease state. J Neuropathol Exp Neurol 47:206
21. Zhou X, Marsh D, Morrison C, Chaudhury A, Maxwell M, Reifenberger G, Eng C (2003) Germline inactivation of PTEN and dysregulation of the phosphoinositol-3-kinase/Akt pathway cause human Lhermitte-Duclos disease in adults. Am J Hum Genet 73:1191–1198

Atypical Meningioma in the Posterior Fossa Associated with Colpocephaly and Agenesis of the Corpus Callosum

Jin Hwan Cheong, Choong Hyun Kim, Mun Sul Yang, and Jae Min Kim

Abstract Colpocephaly is an abnormal enlargement of the occipital horns, i.e., the posterior or rear portions of the lateral ventricles of the brain, and is associated with several other brain abnormalities. Colpocephaly is occasionally misdiagnosed as hydrocephalus, and various etiologies have been postulated, including genetic disorders and errors of morphogenesis. Meanwhile, chromosomal losses including 22q and rarely 21q are observed in malignant and atypical meningiomas. We report an uncommon case of a 67-year-old woman with colpocephaly and an atypical meningioma in the posterior fossa. There were no neurological deficits or family history of hereditary neuropsychiatric disorders. Brain magnetic resonance (MR) images showed bilateral enlarged occipital horns, agenesis of corpus callosum, and a cerebellar mass in the right cerebellar hemisphere. Right suboccipital craniotomy was performed, and the tumor was resected totally. Pathological study of the surgical specimen showed findings of atypical meningioma, and the postoperative course was uneventful until hydrocephalus developed. At 36th day after tumor removal, the patient undertook an external ventricular drainage followed by replacement of the ventriculoperitoneal shunt. We discuss the importance of colpocephaly in terms of the differential diagnosis for hydrocephalus and review the pertinent literature.

Keywords Atypical meningioma • Colpocephaly • Hydrocephalus • Corpus callosum

J.H. Cheong, C.H. Kim (✉), M.S. Yang, and J.M. Kim
Department of Neurosurgery, Hanyang University Guri Hospital, Guri, South Korea
e-mail: kch5142@hanyang.ac.kr

Introduction

Colpocephaly is a congenital enlargement of the occipital horns of the lateral ventricles [1] and is associated with a number of other central nervous system malformations, including agenesis of the corpus callosum, neuronal migration disorders, schizencephaly, microcephaly, meningomyelocele, and hydrocephalus [4, 11, 14]. There are a variety of possible etiologies for colpocephaly including intrauterine infection, intrauterine growth retardation, maternal drug ingestion (corticosteroids, salbutamol, and theophylline), perinatal anoxic-ischemic encephalopathy, and chromosomal abnormalities such as deletion of chromosome 21 [8, 9]. On the other hand, meningiomas comprise up to 30% of intracranial neoplasms. Approximately 10–40% of meningiomas correspond to atypical (World Health Organization grade II) and anaplastic (grade III) subtypes [3, 6, 15]. Meanwhile, frequent chromosomal losses including 22q and 1p have been detected in malignant and atypical meningiomas [5]. We report an unusual case of colpocephaly with an atypical meningioma, and also emphasize the importance of colpocephaly in terms of the differential diagnosis for hydrocephalus and review the pertinent literature.

Case Report

A 67-year-old woman presented with a 4-month history of headache and dizziness. There was no family history of hereditary neuropsychiatric disorders. On neurological examination, no significant abnormalities were found, and cerebellar dysfunction was not disclosed. Brain magnetic resonance imaging (MRI) showed a well-enhanced mass in the posterior fossa that was approximately 3.7×3.5×3.3 cm in size, bilateral enlarged occipital horns, and agenesis of corpus callosum (Fig. 1). We performed a total surgical resection of the tumor via suboccipital craniotomy. The mass adjacent to the cortex was fragile, and its margin was poorly

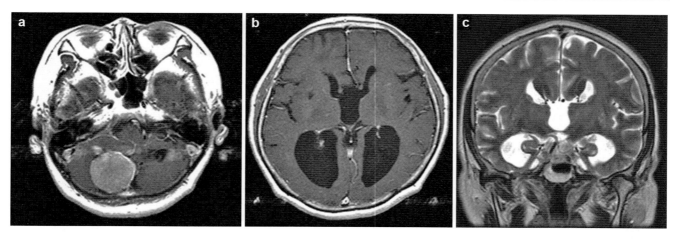

Fig. 1 Preoperative brain magnetic resonance (MR) images. (**a**) Gadolinium (Gd)-enhanced axial MRI showing a large, homogeneous hyperintense mass (3.7×3.5×3.3 cm in size) in right cerebellar hemisphere and vermis. (**b**) Gd-enhanced axial MRI revealing enlargement of both occipital horns and normal size of bilateral frontal horns. (**c**) Coronal MRI scan demonstrating abnormal enlargement of temporal horns and agenesis of the corpus callosum

defined, while the deep portion of the mass was of firm consistency. Histopathological examination of the tumor revealed the whorl patterns of spindle-shaped cells which showed hyperchromatism, hypercellularity, and four mitoses in ten high-power fields (HPFs). Immunohistochemical study showed 9% in Ki-67 labeling index. These findings were compatible with atypical meningioma (Fig. 2).

On the 36th day after the operation, the patient complained of headache and poor oral intake, and ultimately deteriorated into a stuporous state despite conservative management. Follow-up brain computed tomography (CT) scans were performed and revealed a marked enlargement of the ventricles and swelling of the entire brain parenchyma. An external ventricular drainage was performed immediately, and 7 days later the ventriculoperitoneal shunt with a programmable valve was replaced. After this procedure, the postoperative course was uneventful, and a follow-up CT examination 1 month later revealed a markedly decreased size of bilateral ventricles and resolving cerebral gyral effacement (Fig. 3). The patient recovered, and the headache gradually improved after the second operation. She was discharged home without neurological deficits.

Discussion

Colpocephaly is an abnormal enlargement of the occipital horn of the lateral ventricles, and is also described as persistence of the fetal configuration of the lateral ventricles. Colpocephaly is a disorder of multiple and diverse etiologies, including (1) chromosomal anomalies such as trisomy 8 mosaicism and trisomy 9 mosaicism, (2) intrauterine infection such as toxoplasmosis, (3) perinatal anoxic-ischemic encephalopathy, and (4) maternal drug ingestion during early pregnancy, such as corticosteroids, salbutamol, and theophylline [8, 9]. Familial occurrence of colpocephaly has been noted in many reports. Early reports suggested that the ventricular enlargement in colpocephaly is caused by white matter development arrest occurring between the middle of the second month to the fifth month of fetal life [2, 9]. More recent publications have favored the idea that colpocephaly may result from an anatomic malformation of genetic origin with an autosomal or X-linked recessive inheritance [2, 7]. Some authors have suggested that brain abnormalities with overlapping deletions of chromosome 21 include cortical dysplasia consisting of pachygyria, polymicrogyria, and colpocephaly; hypoplasia of the corpus callosum; cerebellar hypoplasia; and enlargement of the ventricular system [7].

Agenesis of the corpus callosum is the most frequently associated malformation. Unfortunately, the congenital dilatation of the occipital horns of the lateral ventricles, a striking feature in this case, is often misdiagnosed as hydrocephalus. Colpocephaly is accurately diagnosed when signs of mental retardation, microcephaly, and seizures are present [13]. While there is no definite treatment, anticonvulsant medication and the prevention of contractures (shortening of muscles) are essential for the care of patients with colpocephaly.

Meningiomas are common brain tumors and approximately 10–40% of meningiomas have atypical or anaplastic characteristics. Atypical and anaplastic meningiomas are associated with less favorable clinical outcomes [10, 12, 15]. Meningiomas are among the most studied human solid tumors by karyotype analysis, and among the characteristic genetic alterations, the loss of chromosome 22 is

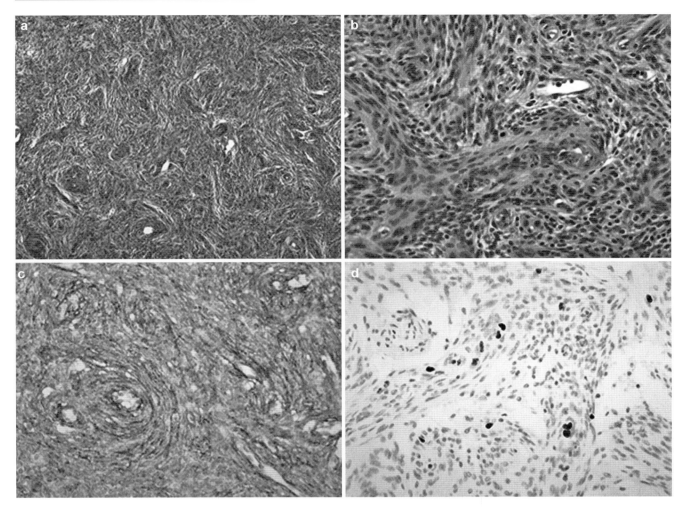

Fig. 2 Microscopic examination of tumor specimens. (**a**) Photomicrograph showing whorls and sheet-like growth pattern of spindle shaped cells (hematoxylin and eosin stain [H & E], magnification × 200). (**b**) Picture displaying the prominent and hyperchromatic nuclei and hypercellularity with a few mitoses (3–4 cells/10 high-power fields) (H & E, × 400). Tumor specimen shows a diffuse immunoreactive to epithelial membrane antigen (EMA) (**c**) and Ki-67 (**d**) (magnification × 400)

commonly reported [16]. Meanwhile, high proportions (85%) of atypical meningiomas exhibit the loss of 22q. The second most frequent regions of loss are confined to the short arm of chromosome 1, particularly subbands 1p33-p36.2 (70%) and 1p13.2 (64%) [3]. However, chromosome 21 abnormality has been observed very rarely [5]. Because there is a paucity of data evaluating the clinical correlation and significance of genetic abnormalities in atypical meningiomas and colpocephaly with agenesis of the corpus callosum, this report provides clues to the possible relationships among the colpocephaly, callosal agenesis, and atypical meningioma, even though this case with atypical meningioma and colpocephaly may be a coincidental association.

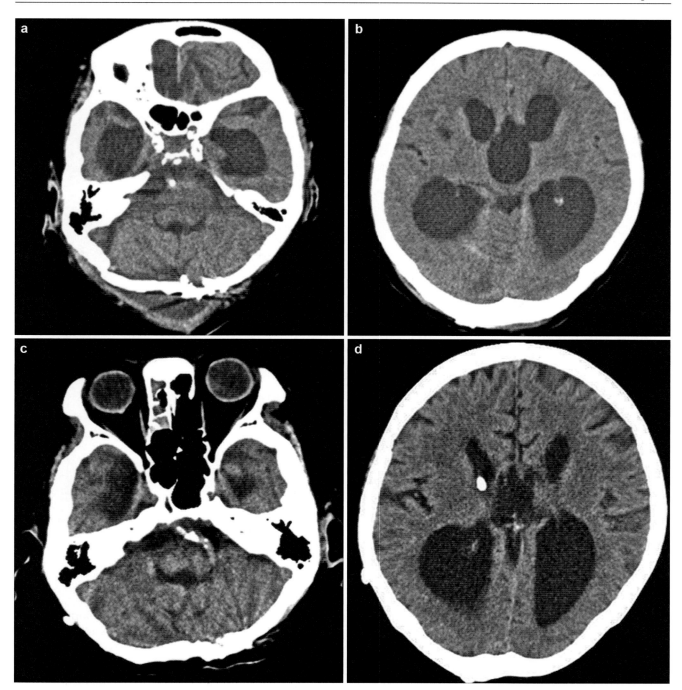

Fig. 3 Postoperative brain computed tomography (CT) scans. (**a**) Brain CT scan taken at 36th day after tumor resection showing total removal of tumor in the right cerebellar region, prominent temporal horns, and pseudomeningocele. (**b**) Brain CT scan demonstrating markedly enlarged ventricles and effacement of the gyral markings. (**c**) Brain CT scan obtained after shunt procedure revealing disappearance of pseudomeningocele and reduced size of temporal horns. (**d**) Brain CT scan taken after shunt procedure displaying the decreased size of ventricles and prominent sulcal marking

Conclusion

Colpocephaly is often misdiagnosed as hydrocephalus, and when ventriculomegaly is present, it is important to differentiate whether it is due to obstructive hydrocephalus or colpocephaly. A correlation between colpocephaly with callosal agenesis and atypical meningioma is poorly established at present, and we suggest that further study is necessary to determine whether atypical meningioma is a coincidental finding or whether it represents de novo cancerogenesis.

Conflicts of interest statement   We declare that we have no conflict of interest.

References

1. Bodensteiner J, Gay CT (1990) Colpocephaly: pitfalls in the diagnosis of a pathologic entity utilizing neuroimaging techniques. J Child Neurol 5:166–168
2. Cerullo A, Marini C, Cevoli S, Carelli V, Ontagna P, Tinuper P (2000) Colpocephaly in two siblings: further evidence of a genetic transmission. Dev Med Child Neurol 42:280–282
3. Dziuk TW, Woo S, Butler EB, Thornby J, Grossman R, Dennis WS, Lu H, Carpenter LS, Chiu JK (1998) Malignant meningioma: an indication for initial aggressive surgery and adjuvant radiotherapy. J Neurooncol 37:177–188
4. Ferrie CD, Jackson GD, Giannakodimos S, Panayiotopoulos CP (1995) Posterior agyria-pachygyria with polymicrogyria: evidence for an inherited neuronal migration disorder. Neurology 45:150–153
5. Gabeau-Lacet D, Engler D, Gupta S, Scangas GA, Betensky RA, Barker FG 2nd, Loeffler JS, Louis DN, Mohapatra G (2009) Genomic profiling of atypical meningiomas associates gain of 1q with poor clinical outcome. J Neuropathol Exp Neurol 68:1155–1165
6. Goyal LK, Suh JH, Mohan DS, Prayson RA, Lee J, Barnett GH (2000) Local control and overall survival in atypical meningioma: a retrospective study. Int J Radiat Oncol Biol Phys 46:57–61
7. Guimei Y, Xiao-Ning C, Laura FS, Gillian MB, Giandomenico P, John BM, Barbara M, Richard PM, Julie RK (2006) Deletion of chromosome 21 disturbs human brain morphogenesis. Genet Med 8:1–7
8. Herskowitz J, Rosman NP, Wheeler CB (1985) Colpocephaly: clinical, radiologic, and pathogenetic aspects. Neurology 35:1594–1598
9. Landman J, Weitz R, Dulitzki F, Shuper A, Sirota L, Aloni D, Bar-Ziv J, Gadoth N (1989) Radiological colpocephaly: a congenital malformation or the result of intrauterine and perinatal brain damage. Brain Dev 11:313–316
10. Milker-Zabel S, Zabel A, Schulz-Ertner D, Schlegel W, Wannenmacher M, Debus J (2005) Fractionated stereotactic radiotherapy in patients with benign or atypical intracranial meningioma: long-term experience and prognostic factors. Int J Radiat Oncol Biol Phys 61:809–816
11. Noorani PA, Bodensteiner JB, Barnes PD (1988) Colpocephaly: frequency and associated findings. J Child Neurol 3:100–104
12. Palma L, Celli P, Franco C, Cervoni L, Cantore G (1997) Long-term prognosis for atypical and malignant meningiomas: a study of 71 surgical cases. J Neurosurg 86:793–800
13. Puvabanditsin S, Garrow E, Ostrerov Y, Trucanu D, Ilic M, Cholenkeril JV (2006) Colpocephaly: a case report. Am J Perinatol 23:295–297
14. Utsunomiya H, Ogasawara T, Hayashi T, Hashimoto T, Okazaki M (1997) Dysgenesis of the corpus callosum and associated telencephalic anomalies: MRI. Neuroradiology 39:302–310
15. Willis J, Smith C, Ironside JW, Erridge S, Whittle IR, Everington D (2000) The accuracy of meningioma grading: a 10-year retrospective audit. Neuropathol Appl Neurobiol 31:141–149
16. Zang KD (2001) Meningioma: a cytogenetic model of a complex benign human tumor, including data on 394 karyotyped cases. Cytogenet Cell Genet 93:207–220

Management of Intraventricular Hemorrhage in Preterm Infants with Low Birth Weight

Takayuki Inagaki, Takuya Kawaguchi, Takahiro Yamahara, Naoyuki Kitamura, Takashi Ryu, Yo Kinoshita, Yasuo Yamanouchi, Kazunari Kaneko, and Keiji Kawamoto

Abstract The management of posthemorrhagic hydrocephalus is difficult and not well standardized. We evaluated our management protocol for infants with intraventricular and/or periventricular hemorrhage (IVH and PVH, respectively). There were four deaths and two significant treatment-related complications in our series. We also observed two cases of isolated ventricle in patients treated with reservoir placement. After evaluating our series, we modified our protocol from reservoir placement to either cerebrospinal fluid (CSF) drainage or ventriculosubgaleal shunt directly. We will reevaluate this new protocol in the near future.

Keywords Preterm infant • Low birth weight • Intra- and periventricular hemorrhage • Hydrocephalus • Isolated ventricle

Introduction

Intraventricular hemorrhage (IVH) and periventricular hemorrhage (PVH) and resultant hydrocephalus are common causes of neonatal morbidity and mortality among preterm and low-birth-weight infants. The management of posthemorrhagic hydrocephalus is difficult and not well standardized. In this study, we aimed to determine the incidence of hydrocephalus after IVH and the associated risk factors for surgical intervention in those patients treated in our institute.

Materials and Methods

Between January 1998 and September 2005, 18 premature babies were reported as suffering from IVH. The number of the patients admitted to our neonatal intensive care unit in the same period was 1,346. The diagnosis of IVH and/or PVH was made with echogram via anterior fontanel, and the grading system for IVH was adapted from that described by Papile et al. [6] Our treatment strategy during that period was (1) close observation of the patient's condition, (2) cerebrospinal fluid (CSF) withdrawn via lumbar tap, (3) reservoir placement, and (4) ventriculoperitoneal (V-P) shunt placement (Fig. 1). Criteria for surgical intervention were continuously enlarging ventricle, tense anterior fontanel, and/or enlarging head size more than 2 mm/day. V-P shunt was placed after the body weight reached approximately 2,000 g. We retrospectively analyzed birth weight, gestational age, and patient's condition both before and after discharge.

Results

The mean birth weight was 969.1 g varying from 466 to 2,190 g. Mean gestation age was 27.7 weeks (range 23.4–36.5 weeks). The Apgar score of these patients varied from 0 to 10 for 1 min and 1 to 10 for 5 min. The IVH and/or PVH

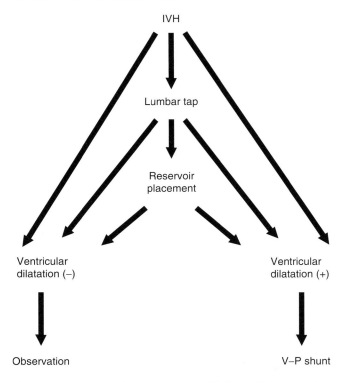

Fig. 1 Previous protocol for management of infants with intraventricular hemorrhage (IVH)

were noticed between days 1 and 25. More than 82% of cases were detected within 72 h after birth. Seven patients were classified as grade II, five patients were grade III, and two patients were grade IV, while the remaining four patients were grade I. Three out of 18 patients required a lumbar tap. Four patients required reservoir placement. Two patients required V-P shunt placement eventually. Four patients died, but the cause of death was not related to the IVH. The body weights of those who died were 666, 636, 609 and 892 g, and their grades were IV, III, II, and III, respectively.

When the management for each grade was analyzed, the treatment seemed to be diverse. One out of two patients with grade IV IVH required reservoir placement; however, the second patient with grade IV died before treatment. Two out of five patients with grade III IVH required reservoir placement, and the other two patients with grade III required a lumbar tap. The remaining patient with grade III eventually needed shunt placement. Only one out of seven patients with grade II IVH required shunt placement.

The complications varied from severe to mild, while two patients developed severe and one patient developed mild morbidity. Additionally, two patients who required reservoir placement developed a so-called isolated ventricular system. The isolated ventricular system was observed in these cases due to inadequate CSF removal. The condition of one of them had deteriorated severely, and the family of the patient refused further treatment. The other patient required neuroendoscopic surgery. The remaining patients developed normally according to their correct age.

Discussion

From around 1970 to the early 1980s, the incidence of the IVH was more than 30%. At the end of the 1990s, the incidence declined to approximately 10%. The reason for this decline was thought to be the advent of new instruments and improvement of total neonatal care by attending physicians [1, 3]. The incident of IVH in this study was around 1.3%. No grade I patient needed surgical intervention. In those with grade II, one out of seven patients required V-P shunt placement. In those with grade III, two patients needed CSF withdrawal via lumbar tap, two patients required reservoir placement, and one patient required V-P shunt placement. In those with grade IV, one patient required reservoir placement. Because of the continuous ventricular enlargement in this last patient, we thought shunt placement was suitable. But the parents of this patient did not want further surgical intervention. So 2 patients out of 13 survivors required shunt placement eventually. This rate is relatively low compared with that in previous reports. There was a correlation between severity of hemorrhage and treatment outcome. The higher the volume of IVH, the more severe the developmental delay became. The mortality rate in our series was approximately 22.2%. Even though there was no direct connection between the cause of death and IVH in this series, the rate was considered high [7]. One reason for this was that the average weight of these patients was fairly low (mean 700 g).

Until now, there is still no established treatment protocol for these patients. The indication for the necessity of a surgical intervention in our institute was a combination of the following: (1) tense fontanel, (2) enlarging head circumference, by approximately 1.5 cm/week, (3) increasing ventricular size at the level of the third ventricle and foramen of Monro (larger than 1.5 cm) [2, 4]. We prefer to place a V-P shunt when the patient is heavier than 2,000 g.

Although there are no data indicating whether repeated lumbar taps prevent V-P shunt placement or not [5, 8], we performed lumbar taps for a few days during which a plentiful amount of CSF was withdrawn. When it was difficult to withdraw CSF via lumbar tap, we placed a reservoir for further CSF removal. We performed CSF removal once or twice a day based upon the ventricular size and/or head circumference. Only in a few cases, were multiple CSF removals per day required because of suspected high intracranial pressure. The CSF production and absorption in the infants at this period varied, based not only on the patients' weight and age, but also on their condition. Therefore, it was difficult to estimate how many milliliters of CSF should be removed each time.

We found that an isolated ventricular system was observed in two cases, because an inadequate amount of CSF was withdrawn in these patients. Two cases also developed severe morbidity. Due to multiple operations and possible developmental delay in one patient, the parents did not want further treatment, as described earlier. The other patient developed severe mental delay. She only spoke a few words at the age

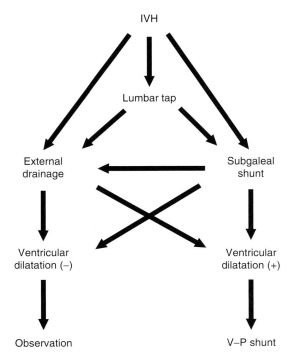

Fig. 2 New protocol for management of infants with intraventricular hemorrhage (IVH)

of 4 years. Her whole body was also insensitive to any kind of pain. One patient who had an isolated fourth ventricle treated with both V-P shunt and neuroendoscopic aqueductal plasty had mild spasticity in his lower extremities. The morbidity in this series was not very high compared with the previous reported series.

After evaluating these patients, we have changed our protocol from reservoir placement to CSF drainage or ventriculosubgaleal shunt insertion (Fig. 2). We will reevaluate this to see if there is a statistical difference in our new protocol regarding the patients requiring surgical intervention and their corresponding outcomes.

Conclusion

The management of posthemorrhagic hydrocephalus is difficult and not well standardized. From our own experience, we described our current treatment strategies for those patients.

Conflicts of interest statement We declare that we have no conflict of interest.

References

1. Ahman PA, Lazzara A, Kykes FD, Brann AW Jr, Schwartz JF (1980) Intraventricular hemorrhage in the high-risk preterm infant: incidence and outcome. Ann Neurol 7:118–124
2. Allan C, Philip JH, Sawyer LR, Tito AM, Meade SK (1982) Ventricular dilation after neonatal ventricular-intraventricular haemorrhage. Am J Dis Child 136:589–593
3. Ment LR, Ehrenkranz RA, Duncan CC, Scott DT, Taylor KJW, Katz KH, Schneider KC, Makuch RW, Oh W, Vohr B, Philip AG, Allan W (1994) Low-dose indomethacin and prevention of intraventricular hemorrhage: a multicenter randomized trial. Pediatrics 93:543–550
4. Müller WD, Urlesberger B (1992) Correlation of ventricular size and head circumference after severe intra-periventricular haemorrhage in preterm infants. Childs Nerv Syst 8:33–35
5. Müller WD, Urlesberger B, Maurer U, Kuttnig-Haim M, Reiterer F, Moradi G, Pichler G (1998) Serial lumbar taping to prevent post-haemorrhagic hydrocephalus after intracranial haemorrhage in preterm infants. Wien Kin Wochenschr 110:631–634
6. Papile LA, Burstein J, Burstein R, Koffler H (1978) Relationship of intravenous sodium bicarbonate infusions and cerebral intraventricular hemorrhage. J Pediatr 92:529–534
7. Ventriculomegaly Trial Group (1990) Randomised trial of early tapping in neonatal posthaemorrhagic ventricular dilatation. Arch Dis Child 65:3–10
8. Whitelaw A (2001) Repeated lumbar or ventricular punctures in newborns with intraventricular hemorrhage (Review). Cochrane Database Syst Rev. 1–14

Pathophysiology of Brainstem Lesions Due to Overdrainage

Sebastian Antes, Regina Eymann, Melanie Schmitt, and Michael Kiefer

Abstract Overdrainage in hydrocephalus therapy is a common shunt complication responsible for many different side effects. Especially an association with an impairment of upper brainstem structures causing symptoms of a dorsal midbrain syndrome (DMS) has already been described. Yet apart from these known mesencephalic lesions, we found several more brainstem signs and symptoms resulting from overdrainage. Parinaud's syndrome was diagnosed in all six patients examined; moreover, parkinsonism, memory disturbances, fluctuations in the level of consciousness, and hypothalamic dysfunctions could be detected in five of six patients. In addition hypersalivation combined with peripheral facial nerve palsy and blepharospasm occurred in two patients each, respectively. We postulate an upward herniation of the midbrain into the tentorial notch causing a secondary aqueductal stenosis as causal. An obstructed Sylvian aqueduct and the occurrence of shunt failure can lead to a bulging or enlargement of the third ventricle resulting in diencephalic lesions. If combined with fourth ventricle outlet occlusion, secondary aqueductal stenosis aggravates the situation with a fourth ventricle entrapment. Symptomatology and proposed pathophysiology are presented.

Keywords Hydrocephalus • Overdrainage • Brain stem lesions • Upward herniation • Dorsal midbrain syndrome • Fourth ventricle entrapment • Parinaud's syndrome • Hypersalivation • Blepharospasm • Facial nerve palsy

S. Antes (✉), R. Eymann, M. Schmitt, and M. Kiefer
Department of Neurosurgery, Medical School,
Saarland University, Homburg-Saar, Germany
e-mail: sebastian.antes@uks.eu

Introduction

Dorsal midbrain syndrome (DMS), also known as Parinaud's syndrome, Pretectal syndrome, Sylvian aqueduct syndrome, or Koerber–Salus–Elschnig syndrome [9], is a common clinical entity associated with hydrocephalus and shunt malfunction: Overdrainage as well as underdrainage can both be responsible for typical eye movement abnormalities and pupil dysfunctions [1, 2, 9, 15]. In constract, DMS combined with more complex clinical signs such as parkinsonism, mental disturbances, and fluctuations in the level of consciousness – a constellation called global rostral midbrain dysfunction [1, 2, 16] – has not yet been described as a consequence of overdraining shunts. Hypothalamic disorders and deeper brainstem lesions such as cranial nerve failures [6] have not so far been mentioned in the literature either.

The initial pathophysiological event is a brainstem upward herniation due to overdrainage resulting in direct lateral midbrain compression in the tentorial notch [4, 5]. The direct impact leads to mesencephalic lesions, and further augmented reduction of cerebrospinal fluid (CSF) can cause a secondary aqueductal stenosis [7]. Such preconditions combined with shunt failure – e.g., ventricular catheter obstruction resulting from overdrainage [1, 2, 8, 12, 15] – may result in a third ventricle enlargement. If an obstruction of fourth ventricle outlets (foramina of Luschka and Magendie) also emerges (e.g., congenitally or functionally) [3], its entrapment [3, 6, 10, 11, 13] could be the logical consequence resulting in direct compression on nearby brainstem structures.

Materials and Methods

During the past 10 years we have observed six shunt-treated adults with typical signs of DMS. For clinical work-up, high-resolution magnetic resonance imaging (MRI) with CSF flow-sensitive sequences, bicompartimental intracranial pressure (ICP) monitoring, and the DaTSCAN™ technique were performed. Depending on the findings, different therapeutic strategies were indicated: To overcome the underlying

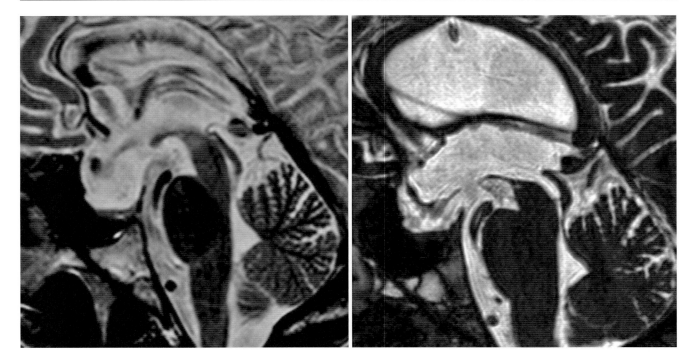

Fig. 1 *Left* Sagittal T2-weighted magnetic resonance (MR) image showing an upward herniation of the brainstem into the tentorial notch with secondary aqueductal stenosis and mesencephalic edema before treatment. *Right* After endoscopic third ventriculostomy (ETV), proximal aqueductal stenosis and dislocation of the brainstem could be reversed

pathophysiological phenomenon of overdrainage, the implantation of gravitational shunts had been the first measure. If clinical symptoms did not improve thereafter, and mesencephalic fixation in the tentorial notch had to be assumed, endoscopic third ventriculostomy (ETV) was necessary to eliminate an inverse supratentorial/infratentorial pressure gradient. In cases of a fourth ventricle entrapment, decompression of the posterior fossa to reestablish the communication of all CSF compartments was performed. Furthermore, symptomatic and supportive treatment (e.g., dopamine agonists, hydrocortisone, amitriptyline, botulinum toxin, and hormone substitution) was provided. Patients were followed up annually.

Results

All six patients showed symptoms of a DMS with typical eye movement abnormalities (e.g., upward gaze palsy) and pupil dysfunctions (Argyll Robertson pupils). Beyond typical DMS signs, parkinsonism, short-term memory deficits, and fluctuations in the level of consciousness could be observed in five of six patients. These persons presented with brainstem upward herniation into the tentorial notch leading to a compression of the proximal Sylvian aqueduct as could be seen on MRI (Fig. 1): Hyperintensity on T2-weighted imaging in the upper brainstem region points to direct mesencephalic damage. Interestingly, an inverse supratentorial/infratentorial pressure gradient typically did not exceed figures of 7–12 mmHg (after correction for hydrostatic pressure differences). In patients suffering from parkinsonism, the DaTSCAN™ technique revealed lower radionuclide (^{123}I-ioflupane) uptake in the caudate nucleus (about 50–60% compared with normal values), while enhancement in putamen amounted to normal values. Consequently the C/P quotient was about 0.5 (in healthy persons 1.0) indicating disturbed dopamine metabolism. Endocrine dysfunctions were diagnosed in five patients resulting from shunt failure. The MRI (Fig. 1) showed a clear deformation and downward bulging of the third ventricle, implying hypothalamic structures and mamillary bodies; in some cases, a kinking of the pituitary stalk could be observed too. Two of the six patients developed further symptoms of brainstem lesions: One presented a peripheral facial nerve palsy combined with hypersalivation, another suffered from severe blepharospasm. Imaging revealed a significant fourth ventricle enlargement in both.

Treatment of all patients consisted of multimodal, individualized therapeutic approaches combining causal and symptomatic strategies. Retrospectively, duration of treatment including surgical and drug therapy to achieve convalescence amounted to 1–3 years. All symptoms except for blepharospasm, which required further treatment, could be totally cured.

Discussion

Lesions of the dorsal midbrain resulting from shunt malfunction in hydrocephalus therapy have already been described in the literature [2, 8, 9, 15, 17]. And those combined with overdrainage have been mentioned as well [9]. Many authors refer to an inverse pressure gradient as the cause for midbrain dysfunctions [2, 9, 16]. Contrary to the earlier interpretations of the underlying pathomechanisms, we postulate that the pathophysiology of all sequels emerges from the discrepancy between the maximal flow rate of overdraining shunts and that of the small Sylvian aqueduct. This difference must result in underdrainage of the fourth ventricle (during each episode of shunt overdrainage in supratentorial compartments). A consequence of relative fourth ventricle underdrainage can be the mass displacement of hindbrain structures [13] effectuating midbrain upward herniation into the tentorial notch: On the one hand, sharp tentorial edges cause direct damage to lateral mesencephalic structures, while on the other hand, compression affects the more medially located structures – e.g., by cerebral blood flow reduction [12, 17]. Resulting compressive forces [13] on the brain stem, the occurrence of periaqueductal edema [14] or a collapse of the aqueduct due to a reduction of intracranial CSF [7] may be the reason for secondary aqueductal stenosis. Whether a measured inverse pressure gradient (7–12 mmHg) is sufficient to cause shear and distortion leading to such serious mesencephalic damage remains questionable.

Many different theories about the pathophysiology of parkinsonian symptoms due to shunt malfunction have been described in the literature [2, 12, 16, 17]. Lateral midbrain damage may affect the substantia nigra. Our theory is supported by the anatomical relation between the location of the substantia nigra and the more medial red nucleus. While signs of red nucleus damage were not seen, parkinsonism occurred in all patients with brainstem upward herniation. Therefore we hypothesize that direct lateral mesencephalic lesions caused by sharp tentorial edges play a significant causative role in the pathophysiology of parkinsonism in an overdrainage situation. In contrast, compressive effects on central midbrain structures – e.g., the nuclei of Darkschewitsch and Cajal, posterior commissure, nuclei of the posterior commissure, and the interstitial nucleus of the medial longitudinal fasciculus [2] – may result in Parinaud's syndrome (e.g., due to regional blood flow reduction) and aqueductal stenosis as mentioned above.

In cases of shunt malfunction due to an obstruction of the ventricular catheter, memory disturbances and fluctuations in the level of consciousness have been described in the literature [1, 2, 15, 16]. The underlying pathophysiology for these symptoms is still under discussion: A huge enlargement of the third ventricle may cause a malfunction of the mamillary bodies and a stretching of the columns of the fornix leading

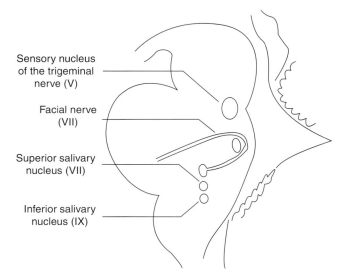

Fig. 2 The anatomical relationship between the bottom of the fourth ventricle and superficially located neuronal structures which may be responsible for blepharospasm, peripheral facial nerve palsy, and hypersalivation in cases of an entrapped ventricle

to the observed memory deficits. Direct compressive stress on the upper midbrain may be responsible for fluctuations in the level of consciousness. The same pathological mechanisms may have resulted in endocrine disorders in our patients: Enlargement and compression can affect the bottom of the third ventricle leading to an impairment of hypothalamic structures or the pituitary stalk (e.g., by kinking).

Two patients of our group who presented an entrapment of the fourth ventricle suffered from blepharospasm or peripheral facial nerve palsy combined with hypersalivation. An association between fourth ventricle entrapment and overdrainage have been previously described in the literature [10, 11, 13]. Such an enlargement causes compressive stress on neuronal structures which are in close contact with the bottom of the fourth ventricle (Fig. 2). Sialorrhea and tetraventricular hydrocephalus emerging from direct involvement of the superior and inferior salivary nuclei have been described [6]. Extrapyramidal pharyngeal dysfunction in patients suffering from parkinsonism may aggravate this symptomatology. The discussed direct compressive stress on the rhomboid fossa can also be responsible for other clinical signs: Impairment of the inner genu of the seventh cranial nerve may effectuate peripheral facial nerve palsy and probably blepharospasm too. Yet the latter could also be a result of an affection of the sensory nucleus of the trigeminal nerve. In our cases, it remains unclear whether the obstruction of the fourth ventricle outlets has simply been the underlying reason for hydrocephalus – e.g., congenital or inflammatory [3] – or brainstem shifting has caused a functional occlusion. Yet congenital or early acquired outlet blockage may remain asymptomatic as long as no secondary aqueductal stenosis due to overdrainage occurs.

Conclusion

Several brainstem signs and symptoms in shunt-treated hydrocephalus patients may arise from CSF overdrainage. We postulate a midbrain upward herniation into the tentorial notch to be the preliminary pathophysiological event initiating a complex impairment of adjacent neuronal structures

Conflicts of interest statement R.E. and M.K. have received some financial support during the past for other research, from Raumedic AG, Helmbrecht, Germany. M.S. and S.A. have received financial support for purposes of education from Codman (Johnson & Johnson), Raynham, MA, USA, and Aesculap AG (Miethke), Tuttlingen, Germany.

References

1. Barrer SJ, Schut L, Bruce DA (1980) Global rostral midbrain dysfunction secondary to shunt malfunction in hydrocephalus. Neurosurgery 7:322–325
2. Cinalli G, Sainte-Rose C, Simon I, Lot G, Sgouros S (1999) Sylvian aqueduct syndrome and global rostral midbrain dysfunction associated with shunt malfunction. J Neurosurg 90:227–236
3. Dandy WE (1921) The diagnosis and treatment of hydrocephalus due to occlusions of the foramina of Magendie and Luschka. Surg Gynecol Obstet 32:112–124
4. Emery JL (1965) Intracranial effects of long-standing decompression of the brain in children with hydrocephalus and meningomyelocele. Dev Med Child Neurol 7:302–309
5. Faulhauer K, Schmitz P (1978) Overdrainage phenomena in shunt treated hydrocephalus. Acta Neurochir (Wien) 45:89–101
6. Filippi S, Monaco P, Godano U, Calbucci F (1994) Sialorrhea from fourth ventricle hydrocephalus. J Neurosurg 81:297–298
7. Foltz EL, Shurtleff DB (1966) Conversion of communicating hydrocephalus to stenosis or occlusion of the aqueduct during ventricular shunt. J Neurosurg 24:520–529
8. Gruber R (1987) Das Schlitz-Ventrikel-Syndrom, 1st edn. Hippokrates Verlag GmbH, Stuttgart, pp 44–50
9. Maroulis H, Halmagyi GM, Heard R, Cook RJ (2008) Sylvian aqueduct syndrome with slit ventricles in shunted hydrocephalus due to adult aqueduct stenosis. J Neurosurg 5:939–943
10. Oi S, Matsumoto S (1985) Slit ventricles as a cause of isolated ventricles after shunting. Childs Nerv Syst 1:189–193
11. Oi S, Matsumoto S (1986) Pathophysiology of aqueductal obstruction in isolated IV ventricle after shunting. Childs Nerv Syst 2:282–286
12. Racette BA, Esper GJ, Antenor J, Black KJ, Burkey A, Moerlein SM, Videen TO, Kotagal V, Ojemann JG, Perlmutter JS (2004) Pathophysiology of parkinsonism due to hydrocephalus. J Neurol Neurosurg Psychiatry 75:1617–1619
13. Raimondi AJ, Samuelson G, Yarzagaray L, Norton T (1969) Atresia of the foramina of Luschka and Magendie: the Dandy-Walker cyst. J Neurosurg 31:202–216
14. Raimondi AJ, Clark SJ, McLone DG (1976) Pathogenesis of aqueductal occlusion in congenital murine hydrocephalus. J Neurosurg 45:66–77
15. Shallat RF, Pawl RP, Jerva MJ (1973) Significance of upward gaze palsy (Parinaud's syndrome) in hydrocephalus due to shunt malfunction. J Neurosurg 38:717–721
16. Yomo S, Hongo K, Kuroyanagi T, Kobayashi S (2006) Parkinsonism and midbrain dysfunction after shunt placement for obstructive hydrocephalus. J Clin Neurosci 13:373–378
17. Zeidler M, Dorman PJ, Ferguson IT, Bateman DE (1998) Parkinsonism associated with obstructive hydrocephalus due to idiopathic aqueductal stenosis. J Neurol Neurosurg Psychiatry 64:657–658

Dynamics of Cerebrospinal Fluid Flow in Slit Ventricle Syndrome

Regina Eymann, Melanie Schmitt, Sebastian Antes, Mohammed Ghiat Shamdeen, and Michael Kiefer

Abstract *Introduction*: Although slit ventricle syndrome (SVS) is identified as a serious complication in shunt-treated hydrocephalus, cerebral spinal fluid (CSF) flow via external ventricular drainage (EVD) or shunts in SVS have not been studied up to now.

Material and methods: A new apparatus (LiquoGuard®; Möller-Medical, Fulda, Germany) was used for EVD in a child with SVS. The LiquoGuard actively controls CSF drainage, based on intracranial pressure (ICP).

Results: To achieve well-tolerated clinical conditions, an ICP level of 4 mmHg was necessary; realizable by drainage rates between 0 and 35 mL/h. Drainage rate variations typically occurred with repetitive time intervals of 2 h causing a "saw tooth" shaped CSF flow pattern throughout 24 h.

Discussion: SVS seems to be characterized largely by quickly varying CSF drainage demands. Whether this is a general phenomenon or just true for this case has still to be studied and needs further clarification.

Keywords Slit ventricle syndrome • Hydrocephalus • Intracranial pressure • Cerebrospinal fluid • CSF • Complication • ICP measurement • CSF flow rates

R. Eymann (✉), M. Schmitt, S. Antes, and M. Kiefer
Department of Neurosurgery, Medical School, Saarland University,
Homburg-Saar, Germany
e-mail: regina.eymann@uks.eu, reginaeymann@web.de

M.G. Shamdeen
Department of General Pediatrics and Neonatology, Medical School,
Saarland University, Homburg-Saar, Germany

Introduction

Slit ventricle syndrome (SVS) is a serious, potentially suddenly life-threatening complication of long-term (many years) overdrainage in shunted children [2, 17]. Especially when shunting occurs before fontanelle and suture closure, the risk can amount to 20% according to some reports in the literature [17]. Hence true SVS prevalence is still under debate as a consequence of diverging definitions: Some sources do not differentiate between pure imaging morphology of slit ventricles with and without accompanying clinical symptoms.

Given low intracranial pressure (ICP) due to chronic overdrainage, the driving force for head growth deficiency, resulting in microcephalus, premature suture ossification and fontanelle closure, causing typical scaphocephalic head deformity [4]. The craniospinal compliance becomes in this way osseously fixed and reduced that some milliliters of CSF more or less can decide a patient's clinical state.

Reduced compliance and cerebrospinal fluid (CSF) overdrainage go along with venous overdrainage due to a lack of the Starling effect on the bridging veins, resulting in crushing of the superficial and the inner cerebral veins which normally forms one of the major intracranial buffering capacities. As a consequence, the shearing and compressing stress on the brain parenchyma increases during the systolic capillary loading. Periventricular gliosis, as seen in animal models [5, 13, 15], might be related to chronic tissue damage [9]. The periventricular accentuation of such effects can easily be understood as being the result of the differently shaped inner and outer CSF–brain interface. The application of such simple (oversimplifying) physical laws as Pascal's and Laplace's predicts a much higher impact on the inner compared with the outer brain surface [1, 9]. Whether the periventricular gliosis and/or purely the consequences of physics cause what has been termed "stiff ventricles" remains a matter of debate. This being the situation, *noncompliant ventricle syndrome* might be a much more accurate term for what is typically termed SVS [14].

Accordingly, slit ventricles require enormous intraventricular pressure (IVP) before enlarging [9] as a simple physical principle, and given that they lack ventricular enlargement during shunt failure [1], the enlargement must be not just because of microcephalus.

Another pathophysiological concept of SVS is that shunt-related idiopathic intracranial hypertension (IIH) due to increased sagittal sinus venous pressure [17] appears as an excellent completion of the aforementioned: The osseous skull base deformation in scaphocephalous due to SVS also reduces the jugular veins' outlets on the skull base increasing the pressure in the intracranial venous sinus and amplifies the missing Starling effect on the bridging veins while increasing the inner veins' diameter. The latter mimics conditions similar to those in benign intracranial hypertensions (BIH) (yet restricted to the inner brain tissue) and in parallel, due to increased venous pressure, reduces CSF absorption capacity.

Based on ICP and clinical symptoms (headache) Rekate (1993) [16] established a new SVS classification to facilitate individual treatment, separating:

- Intermittent extremely low pressure headaches
- Intermittent proximal obstruction of ventricle catheter
- Shunt failure with small ventricles (normal volume hydrocephalus [NVH])
- Intracranial hypertension with working shunts (hydrocephalic BIH)
- Headaches unrelated to shunt function.

Even when combining all these pathophysiological concepts, the CSF hydrodynamics of SVS has not been fully understood. To provide some further insight into that complexity, we studied the circadian CSF flow dynamics in SVS during external CSF drainage.

Materials and Methods

A 12-year-old girl (body mass index 23 kg/m^2, height 159 cm, distance from foramen of Monro to diaphragm 39 cm) suffered amnesia for about 5 h in an upright position, as a result of suffering from orthostatic headache for several years. At the age of 2 weeks, an adjustable shunt had been inserted with an initially setting of 8 cm H$_2$O to treat her diagnosed hydrocephalus. As she had not been treated in our department before, the initial setting had not changed during follow-up to compensate for the increasing hydrostatic pressure due to her growing.

She was actually operated on for appendicitis causing peritonitis in another hospital 4 h before her first admission to our department. During the appendectomy, the peritoneal catheter was externalized by the general surgeon.

On admission she complained of severe headache while cranial computed tomography (CCT) revealed very small ventricles (frontal occipital horn ratio: 0.33). To treat the initially suspected retrograde shunt infection with meningitis, the remaining parts of the shunt were explanted immediately. The explanted catheter and CSF samples were examined for bacteria and other signs of intracranial infection. According to Rekate's recommendations [16] an external drainage with features to measure ICP was implanted. Assuming dramatically reduced craniospinal compliance in this child, an extremely precise CSF drainage, avoiding both overdrainage and underdrainage seemed mandatory. The new Möller-Medical LiquoGuard® (Möller-Medical, Fulda, Germany) device appeared most suitable for that purpose, allowing an ICP-controlled automated external CSF drainage. Built-in algorithms avoid unintended overdrainage during coughing and other Valsalva maneuvers that might provoke overdrainage in a conventional external ventricular drainage (EVD) that uses drip chambers for controlling the targeted IVP. The drainage speed can be controlled by preselecting drainage rates between 0 and 50 mL/h, while the drainage volume is ICP-controlled. The device allows predefining an ICP level between 2 and 30 cm H$_2$O, which is maintained by automatically varying drainage at the preset drainage speed. When ICP is lower than the preset maximally tolerated ICP, no drainage occurs. If ICP exceeds the critical limit, then CSF is drained until the preset level is regained. In this way, the ICP level can be controlled perfectly constantly over time. All data (time stamps, ICP, drainage rate, drainage speed, drainage volume, and presettings) are electronically stored at a sampling rate of 1 Hz. Data can be transferred to Microsoft Excel® (as we did) or other software for further analysis.

External CSF drainage was performed for 7 days before a new shunt was inserted.

Results

No bacteria were detected from the culture of CSF samples collected daily or from the entire hardware of the removed shunt, nor were there any further signs of general infection. In parallel, clinical signs of meningitis did not occur.

The headache on admission was due to underdrainage and consequent increased ICP as could be seen by the fact that it vanished immediately after CSF drainage. The initial conventional EVD proved unsuitable, as the girl suffered some hours later from severe position-dependent headache. As clinical signs of meningitis were absent, the drained CSF volume was comparatively greater, so that the underlying reason for headache seemed to be overdrainage. This could be well understood, because, as a consequence of some pain and vomiting due to the preceding abdominal operation and peritonitis, short episodes of Valsalva maneuvers occurred causing overshooting of CSF drainage with conventional EVD. Therefore precise, ICP-controlled EVD using the LiquoGuard device seemed reasonable, as it avoids unnecessary CSF

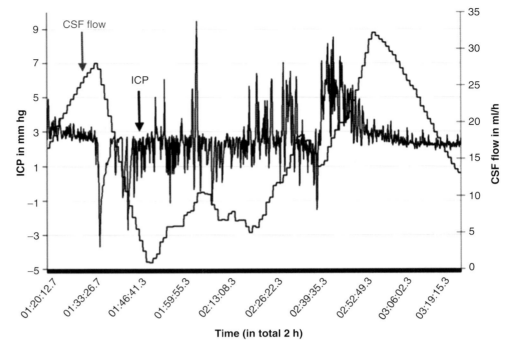

Fig. 1 Two-hour chart of intracranial pressure (ICP) (*black*) and cerebrospinal fluid (CSF) drainage (*gray line*) demonstrating clearly the variability of the drainage rates with 45-min cycles

drainage during Valsalva maneuvers. It took some effort to establish the most suitable presetting. The optimum value for the ICP was found to be 4 mmHg as with this setting the girl remained free of headache. However, identification of the proper drainage speed was still challenging: If set too low, underdrainage and headache might occur again, if set too high, ventricular collapse and overdrainage-related headache might result (Fig. 1). Using, as is normal when applying the LiquoGuard, a constant preset CSF drainage speed proved to be insufficient (Fig. 2). The drainage had to be precisely controlled according to circadian variations, ranging between 25 and 35 mL/h, so that the drainage speed maintained a constant ICP level of 4 mmHg. An appropriate pattern of CSF drainage rates was found (Fig. 2) for a time period of 120–180 min. During these time slices, the CSF drainage requirement normally increased steadily from nearly 0 ml/h up to 35 mL/h within 60–90 min. Thereafter, the drainage requirement again decreased to the starting level within the same duration, thus forming a sine-shaped cyclic CSF drainage requirement over time. The CSF volume drained per time unit at a given preset drainage speed to maintain the desired ICP level was automatically adapted by the LiquoGuard. When maximal CSF delivery was necessary, the device drained permanently. Eventually, as the drainage requirement was reduced, the periods of drainage became shorter. In this way constant ICP at the desired level could be maintained. Only one or two times a day, the drainage speed had to be adjusted. By day, a drainage speed of 25 mL/h was normally the best, while a setting of 35 mL/h was necessary at night.

As no episodes of damped ICP pulse amplitude occurred it can be assumed that the measured ICP was reliable and ventricular collapse could be forestalled.

Discussion

As conventional EVD, using hydrostatic pressure defined by the height of a dripping chamber over the foramen of Monro, has many drawbacks, more sophisticated concepts for ICP-controlled EVD have been explored recently [19]. The LiquoGuard® is the first commercially available device providing ICP-controlled, artifact-adjusted, "intelligent" EVD. Physicians predefine the desired ICP setting, and the drainage speed and the CSF volume drained per time period is automatically controlled by a closed-loop ICP-regulated control cycle. Any accidentally or naturally occurring disturbances (e.g., coughing or other Valsalva maneuvers), which typically result in hydraulic mismanagement in conventional EVD therapy, can be eliminated. In this way, a reliable and precise ICP-controlled EVD can be maintained. The importance of such perfectly controlled EVD becomes obvious with the clinical preconditions discussed.

In this child, an inadequate craniospinal compliance as a consequence of chronic overdrainage, must be assumed, because minimally higher or lower drainage rates promptly resulted in underdrainage and overdrainage symptoms, respectively.

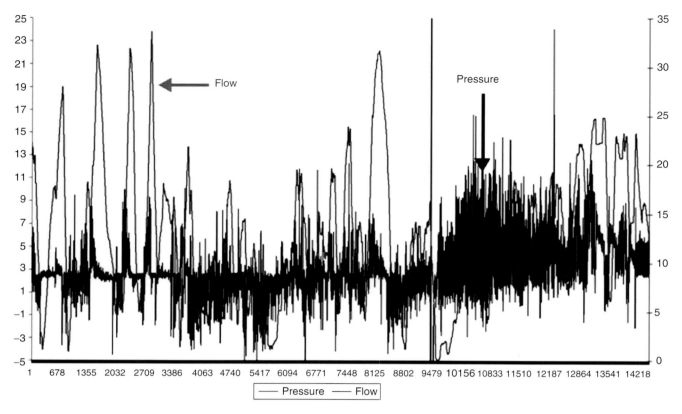

Fig. 2 Twenty-four-hour overview of drainage rate (*gray line*) and intracranial pressure (ICP), demonstrating that ICP remained within the physiological range, while drainage rates clearly varied, which excludes ICP as a major influencing factor in CSF production rate

Textbooks still claim that CSF production rates are constant at about 20 mL/h. For the last two decades, however, there has been some evidence of circadian rhythms controlled mainly by the autonomic nervous system [3, 6, 7, 10–12], which cause lower CSF production rates during the day (range 7–30 mL/h) and higher production rates at night (30–70 mL/h) as we (unpublished data) and others have found [6]. Extremes can typically be found at midnight to 2 a.m. and at 4–6 p.m. Hence, CSF production rate variations at short intervals have been observed only once before with quite similar time periods as those we have observed [12], though never before in SVS. The exceptional nature of our observations lead us to suppose that inadequate craniospinal compliance as measured by the CSF drainage rates can be assumed to reflect the rhythmicity of CSF production too. The variation range (0–35 mL/h) within 2–3 h, by far exceeds the variations attributable to the state of the autonomous nervous system, as the rhythmicity and range of variation remain nearly the same by day and night and have also been proven to be independent of alertness. Recently there is some evidence that further influencing factors such as age and ICP level might affect CSF production rates [18]. In the case presented here, we assume that ICP may be one of the most influential variables regulating CSF production. In such cases of SVS with extremely reduced craniospinal compliance, minimal variations of CSF production must significantly change ICP. The constant phase shift between ICP and CSF drainage rates (Figs. 1 and 3) supports these conclusions.

However, a precondition for claiming that the CSF drainage rates reflect its production rate is that the resistance to CSF outflow (Rout) remains constant during 24 h and unaffected by the ICP level. Figure 2 might suggest that there is no circadian rhythm to CSF absorption. The influence of ICP on Rout is vigorously being debated [12]. Since Rout might change rapidly as the response to ICP increases or decreases, this might introduce some bias when concluding that the observed drainage rates reflect CSF production rates. While ICP-induced Rout variations are mild to moderate at ICP levels <20 mmHg (depending on the hydrodynamic model), significant Rout increase is predicted by all models if ICP exceeds 30 mmHg. As ICP never reached such a level during the observation period, bias due to ICP-induced Rout variations can be assumed to be mild in the given case. Therefore our assumption of the ICP role in CSF production rates appears reasonable for the observed rhythmicity. And yet, even now, unknown factors affecting CSF production rate cannot be ruled out.

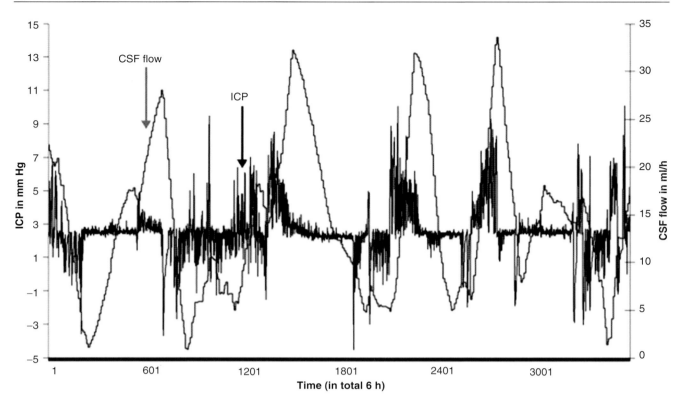

Fig. 3 Three-hour chart of intracranial pressure (ICP) (*black*) and cerebrospinal fluid (CSF) drainage rate (*gray line*) probably suggesting with some phase shift a correlation between ICP and drainage rate

Conclusion

The case presented here, moreover, demonstrates how quickly and precisely shunts have to control CSF drainage in SVS, as maintenance of a preset ICP level with minimal hysteresis is of utmost importance. Accordingly, any influence of hydrostatic pressure alterations must be excluded too, to achieve reasonable quality of life. In the presented case, an adjustable gravitational shunt seemingly provided such preconditions, as the girl remained free of any symptoms after the implant of an adjustable shunt design, in significant contrast to her complaints with the formerly implanted simple differential pressure valve.

Conflicts of interest statement This scientific work has been sponsored in part by a grant from the German Federal Ministry of Education and Research (BMBF). R.E. and M.K. have received some financial support in the past for other research work, from Raumedic AG (Helmbrechts, Germany). Further they have received honoraria and financial support for attending scientific congresses, from Codman & Shurtleff Inc. (Raynham, MA, USA), a division of Ethicon (Somerville, NJ, USA) and Johnson & Johnson (New Brunswick, NJ, USA) and Aesculap AG (Tuttlingen, Germany), a division of B. Braun Melsungen AG (Melsungen, Germany). M.S. and S.A. have received financial support for educational purposes from Codman & Shurtleff Inc. (Raynham, MA, USA), a division of Ethicon (Somerville, NJ, USA) and Johnson & Johnson (New Brunswick, NJ, USA) and Aesculap AG (Tuttlingen, Germany), a division of B. Braun Melsungen AG (Melsungen, Germany).

References

1. Albright AL, Tyler-Kabara E (2001) Slit-ventricle syndrome secondary to shunt-induced suture ossification. Neurosurgery 48:764–770
2. Da Silva PS, Suriano IC, Neto HM (2009) Slitlike ventricle syndrome: a life threatening presentation. Pediatr Emerg Care 25:674–676
3. Davson H, Hollingsworth JG, Carey MB, Fenstermacher JD (1982) Ventriculo-cisternal perfusion of twelve amino acids in the rabbit. J Neurobiol 13:293–318
4. Faulhauer K, Schmitz P (1978) Overdrainage phenomena in shunt treated hydrocephalus. Acta Neurochir (Wien) 45:89–101
5. Goldstein I, La Marca V, Abbott R, Jallo GI (2001) Slit ventricle syndrome: overview of pathophysiology and treatment. Internet J Neurosurg 1; article 2
6. Hara M, Kadowaki C, Konishi Y, Ogashiwa M, Numoto M, Takeuchi K (1983) A new method for measuring cerebrospinal fluid flow in shunts. J Neurosurg 58:557–561
7. Haywood JR, Vogh BP (1979) Some measurements of autonomic nervous system influence on production of cerebrospinal fluid in the cat. J Pharmacol Exp Ther 208:341–346
8. Kiefer M (2006) Chronic hydrocephalus in adults: computerized assessment of CSF hydrodynamics and treatment using gravitational valves. Post-Doctoral thesis, Saarland University, Medical School, pp 1–12
9. Lindvall M, Owman C (1984) Sympathetic nervous control of cerebrospinal fluid production in experimental obstructive hydrocephalus. Exp Neurol 84:606–615
10. McComb JG, Davson H, Hyman S, Weiss MH (1982) Cerebrospinal fluid drainage as influenced by ventricular pressure in the rabbit. J Neurosurg 56:790–797

11. Minns RA, Brown JK, Engleman HM (1987) CSF production rate: "real time" estimation. Z Kinderchir 42(Suppl 1):36–40
12. Oi S, Matsumoto S (1987) Infantile hydrocephalus and the slit ventricle syndrome in early infancy. Childs Nerv Syst 3:145–150
13. Olson S (2004) The problematic slit ventricle syndrome. A review of the literature and proposed algorithm for treatment. Pediatr Neurosurg 40:264–269
14. Pudenz RH, Folta EL (1991) Hydrocephalus: overdrainage by ventricular shunts: a review and recommendations. Surg Neurol 35:200–212
15. Rekate HL (1993) Classification of slit-ventricle syndromes using intracranial pressure monitoring. Pediatr Neurosurg 19:15–20
16. Rekate HL (2004) The slit ventricle syndrome: advances based on technology and understanding. Pediatr Neurosurg 40:259–263
17. Sood S, Kumar CR, Jamous M, Schuhmann MU, Ham SD, Canady A (2004) Pathophysiological changes in cerebrovascular distensibility in patients undergoing chronic shunt therapy. J Neurosurg 100(5 Suppl Pediatrics):447–453
18. Walter M, Kiefer M, Leonhardt S, Steudel WI, Isermann R (2002) Online analysis of intracranial pressure waves. Acta Neurochir Suppl 81:161–162

Quality and Safety of Home ICP Monitoring Compared with In-Hospital Monitoring

Morten Andresen, Marianne Juhler, and Tina Nørgaard Munch

Abstract *Introduction*: Intracranial pressure (ICP) monitoring is usually conducted in-hospital using stationary devices. Modern mobile ICP monitoring systems present new monitoring possibilities more closely following the patients' daily life. We reviewed patient safety, quality of technical data, and adequacy for clinical evaluation in ICP monitoring in the home setting versus in-hospital monitoring.

Methods: Patients were divided into two subgroups (home or hospital monitoring). We noted technical curve quality and clinically useful parameters for both subgroups.

Results: Forty-four patients (aged 1–55 years) were included in this survey, with 50 sessions (home/in-hospital monitoring: 21/29). No difference was found in technical curve quality by comparing number of interruptions ($p=0.22$), percentage of measurement duration with valid curve ($p=0.57$), or the ability to perform adequate clinical evaluation of the data ($p=0.52$). No clinically detectable complications were encountered in either group.

Conclusion: We propose home ICP monitoring as a feasible and safe alternative to in-hospital monitoring in select cases where the patient's caregiver – with prior meticulous instructions – can adequately observe the patient during the monitoring session.

Keywords Hydrocephalus • Intracranial pressure • Intraparenchymal • Patient monitoring

Introduction

Intracranial pressure (ICP) monitoring is a useful diagnostic tool in complex cases of shunt dysfunction with questionable clinical and/or radiological findings. There is no particular requirement for the length of time the device has to remain in place. The added value of overnight monitoring sessions, as opposed to daytime measurements, has become apparent [6], as some patients display a normal diurnal ICP curve, but an abnormal nocturnal curve. Curve analysis comprises an estimation of average baseline pressure and analysis of the curve waveform. The normal supine baseline is assumed to be between 10 and 15 mmHg, and a baseline in the upright position between 0 and 10 mmHg [5]. Analysis of the curve usually includes description of the waveform, amplitude, and occurrence of abnormal pressure waves, known as A and B waves. A waves are always pathological and require intervention or further investigation. However, the clinical and physiological significance of B waves is much less clear. They may be normal and show a possible correlation with REM sleep [10], or they could reflect abnormal compliance or defective autoregulation [4]. Thus, analysis of the curve is often a valuable adjunct to the clinical symptoms of abnormal intracranial pressure.

ICP monitoring sessions are usually conducted in-hospital using a stationary device, which places restrictions on the mobility of the patient for the duration of the test. It is our experience that patients would be more likely to remain in bed when using the stationary ICP monitoring system. This behavior reduces the chances of observing abnormal ICP curves during activity, and presents concerns that the monitoring session may fail to accurately mirror the patients' special daily and nightly routines. Modern mobile ICP monitoring systems present new possibilities for monitoring, including during the patient's routine and daily life – thus allowing us access to an ICP curve that is potentially more true to life. The aim of this study was to evaluate if the quality of technical and clinical data obtained by home ICP

M. Andresen (✉), M. Juhler, and T.N. Munch
Clinic of Neurosurgery, Copenhagen University Hospital,
Copenhagen, Denmark
e-mail: andresen@gmail.com

monitoring sessions equaled those obtained in-hospital, and consequently if the advantages of a mobile ICP monitoring system could be exploited outside the confines of the hospital with proper respect for patient safety.

Materials and Methods

Patient Selection and Subgroups

Our survey included all patients – pediatric as well as adult – requiring nonemergency ICP monitoring in our department from June 2007 until November 2009. All sessions were reviewed along with clinical data based on a review of the patients' charts. Clinical information included demographic data, the indication for ICP registration, the treatment consequences of ICP monitoring, and complications.

Patients were divided into two groups according to the location of the monitoring session: hospital or at home/outside the hospital. The decision was made by the attending physician based on the patient's neurological status, and an assessment of the family's skills in safely observing the patient outside the hospital for the duration of the session. Individual instructions were given to make sure the patient was safely cared for during the monitoring period.

Postoperative Observation

Following insertion of the ICP measurement probe, patients were observed postoperatively for at least 6 h before going home on leave or being transferred to a non-intensive-care ward, as surgical hematomas are most likely to occur within this timeframe [9]. As many of the patients have undergone numerous radiological examinations over the years, with potentially harmful radiation exposure, we do not routinely perform postoperative computed tomography (CT) to exclude a surgical hematoma. None of the patients in this study exhibited clinical signs of complications after insertion of the probe.

ICP Measurement Probe

The Raumedic NEUROVENT-P intraparenchymal ICP monitoring system (Raumedic AG®, Münchberg, Germany) was used. This system allows the patient to move about freely with the measurement probe attached to a mobile datalogging system in a shoulder bag or strap, with minimal discomfort [2, 3, 7]. After completing the ICP measurement, the data is extracted to a Windows PC for postprocessing and archiving in the data analysis software.

Curve Evaluation

All monitoring sessions were reviewed for their technical quality and clinically useful parameters. To assess technical quality, we noted the number of interruptions in the curve-registration and the percentage of the monitoring session containing a valid curve. Multiple short sessions lasting between a few seconds and a few minutes, because of repeated resetting of the device, were classified as a single longer lasting interruption. To assess clinically useful parameters, all ICP curves were reviewed for variations of mean ICP between daytime and nighttime, percentage of the curve containing B waves, number of episodes with raised ICP, and duration of the longest lasting episode with raised ICP.

For each of these parameters, it was noted whether a satisfactory assessment could be made. For monitoring sessions lasting more than 24 h, we reviewed the second day and night of the session for the above clinical parameters.

Statistics

Statistical analysis was carried out using PASW Statistics package v18.0 (SPSS Inc., Chicago, IL, USA). The Mann–Whitney U test was used to compare ICP measurement time and number of interruptions between home and in-hospital monitoring groups. Values of $p<0.05$ were considered statistically significant.

Results

Forty-four patients were included, presenting 50 monitoring sessions. Six patients were monitored more than once. A single patient was excluded from the study: Upon waking from surgery, this severely autistic patient removed the ICP measurement probe, and no new measurement attempts were made. Twenty-one patients were outside the neurosurgical department during the ICP monitoring session (and thus placed in the Home group). Twenty-nine patients were admitted for the duration of the monitoring session (In-hospital group).

When looking at indications for ICP measurement, diagnostic procedures to uncover idiopathic intracranial hypertension (IIH), shunt dysfunction, or hydrocephalus were the most common indications (Fig. 1). No significant age difference was noted between the two subgroups (Table 1; $p=0.86$).

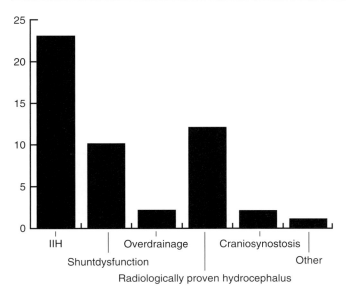

Fig. 1 Indications for intracranial pressure (ICP) measurement. The frequency of clinical indications listed for ICP measurement. The "Other" category consists of a single patient with atypical facial pains following shunt removal

Table 1 Age of participating patients

	Mean (years)	Range (years)	SD (years)	Median (years)	p value
Home group	15.14	1–43	11.47	12	0.86
In-hospital group	17.07	1–55	15.27	12	

Mean patient age was slightly lower for the patient group monitored in the home setting, but the groups showed identical medians

Technical Curve Evaluation

Curve evaluations are summarized in Table 2, and show that the Home group participated in longer monitoring sessions than the In-hospital group ($p=0.01$). No differences were found when comparing the percentage of curve containing valid data ($p=0.57$), the number of technical interruptions in the curve data ($p=0.22$), or the sessions that were interrupted ($p=0.35$).

Clinical Curve Evaluation and Results of Monitoring

When comparing clinical parameters for the two subgroups, no difference was noted in the ability to verify required clinical parameters (Table 3; $p=0.52$). Setting the equipment in long play mode provides only information on mean ICP without wave details. This was the case in almost all cases where curve details were unavailable.

When looking at the clinical consequences of ICP monitoring, further clinical action was taken in 20 cases, and there was no significant difference between the two subgroups (Table 4; $p=0.73$).

Discussion

Our results show home ICP monitoring to be a safe and reliable addition to the existing toolkit used in diagnosing

Table 2 Length and technical quality of ICP monitoring sessions

	Mean	Range	SD	Median	p value
[a] Length of ICP measurement					
• All patients	38.4 h	3–98 h	23.5 h	29 h	0.01
• Home group	47.9 h	5–95 h	25.3 h	44 h	
• In-hospital group	31.5 h	3–98 h	19.8 h	24 h	
[b] Length of ICP measurement with valid curve					
• All patients	37.2 h	3–97 h	23.6 h	26.5 h	–
• Home group	46.7 h	5–94 h	26.0 h	44 h	
• In-hospital group	30.4 h	3–97 h	19.5 h	24 h	
[c] Part of curve with valid measurement					
• All patients	96.80%	57–100%	9.2%	100%	0.57
• Home group	96.10%	63–100%	10.2%	100%	
• In-hospital group	97.20%	57–100%	8.7%	100%	
[d] Number of interruptions					
• All patients	1.2	0–6	1.8	0	0.22
• Home group	1.5	0–6	1.9	1	
• In-hospital group	1.0	0–6	1.8	0	

Row 'a' shows home sessions to be significantly longer than in-hospital sessions. This is not surprising as the group consisted of more difficult cases requiring longer monitoring. Rows 'b' and 'c' show the sessions to be of a consistent quality, regardless where the session took place. Row 'd' shows a slightly higher – but not significant – frequency of interruptions in the home group
ICP intracranial pressure

Table 3 Clinical curve evaluation

	Mean ICP		Percentage of curve with B waves		No. episodes with raised ICP		Duration of longest episode with raised ICP	
	Day	Night	Day	Night	Day	Night	Day	Night
Parameter measurable								
• All patients	48/50	46/50	42/50	43/50	39/50	43/50	41/50	43/50
• Home group	20/21	20/21	15/21	17/21	16/21	18/21	17/21	18/21
• In-hospital group	28/29	26/29	27/29	26/29	23/29	25/29	24/29	25/29
Parameter not measurable								
• All patients	2/50	4/50	8/50	7/50	11/50	7/50	9/50	7/50
• Home group	1/21	1/21	6/21	4/21	5/21	3/21	4/21	3/21
• In-hospital group	1/29	3/29	2/29	3/29	6/29	4/29	5/29	4/29

For each monitoring session we noted whether the selected clinical parameters were measurable and thus of sufficient quality to be used for clinical decisions. If the answer was no to just one of the clinical parameters, we flagged the session as being of inadequate quality

ICP intracranial pressure

Table 4 Clinical result of ICP measurement

	No action	Shunt insertion	Shunt revision	Medical treatment	Decompressive surgery	Shunt removal	Other	Total
Home group	12	2	6	0	0	1	0	21
In-hospital group	18	5	1	1	2	1	1	29
Total	30	7	7	1	2	2	1	50

Decompressive surgery' concerns two cases with craniosynostosis, requiring frontal advancement of the cranium. The 'Other' group contains a single patient who underwent third ventriculostomy with good clinical effect

ICP intracranial pressure

conditions related to abnormal ICP. In this study, placement in either the home or the in-hospital subgroup was based solely on the clinical assessment of the attending physician. To standardize future use of home ICP monitoring, we recommend establishing working criteria for the routine use of monitoring in the home setting. Based on our experiences with home ICP monitoring, a large group of patients can safely be discharged from the hospital to a monitoring session in the home setting. The limitations of this method are primarily competing medical disorders, surgical risks, and problems with inadequate observation by the patient's caregiver at home.

Safety

Other studies have shown varying complication rates. By performing routine postimplantation imaging, the occurrence of radiologically detected surgical hematomas may be as high as 10% without clinical implications or symptoms resulting from this [1, 8]. Most studies have been carried out in patient populations with head injuries, different from the patients of this study.

Following 6-h postoperative observation, there were no clinical symptoms compatible with complications in either group. We consider the procedure safe only if postoperative observation has been completely uneventful, and the patient's caregiver is capable of observation at home. The mean age of patients in the home group was slightly lower than in the in-hospital group, which we attribute to easier access to a competent adult caregiver for the duration of the monitoring session in the pediatric patient subgroup.

Data Quality

For this study we kept a narrow focus on whether the gathered data was of sufficient quality for clinical decisions. Typical ICP wave oscillations were present throughout the duration of all measurement periods (Table 2; part of curve with valid measurement). Our findings are consistent with frequently observed ICP ranges in the daily clinical setting. We did not ask patients to register postural changes during the day, but consistent with previous results [10] diurnal ICP values were lower than nocturnal values, and values in shunted patients were 10–20 mmHg lower than in nonshunted patients depending on the type of shunt.

We found no differences in the number of interruptions of the curve, the percentage of the curve with valid data, or possibility to sufficiently assess selected clinical curve parameters. Therefore there should be no reservations regarding the quality of the home ICP monitoring sessions compared with in-hospital sessions.

Several patients presented with a normal diurnal curve, but showed abnormal nocturnal activity, highlighting the need for overnight ICP monitoring sessions. Furthermore, in most patients we observed clustering of the ICP elevations during phases of REM sleep, consistent with other reports [10].

The treatment decision following in-hospital monitoring was mostly primary shunt insertion, whereas shunt revision usually occurred after home monitoring (Table 4). We feel this highlights the potential of home ICP monitoring in clinically difficult cases, where several diagnostic as well as treatment procedures had previously failed.

Conclusion

Based on our results, we propose home-ICP monitoring as a feasible and safe alternative to in-hospital monitoring in select cases where the patient's caregiver – with prior meticulous instructions – can adequately observe the patient during the monitoring session.

Acknowledgments The authors received research grants from The Aase og Ejnar Danielsen Fund, The Augustinus Fund, and The Beckett Fund. We are grateful for their help and their support of this study.

Conflicts of interest statement We declare that we have no conflict of interest.

References

1. Blaha M, Lazar D, Winn RH, Ghatan S (2003) Hemorrhagic complications of intracranial pressure monitors in children. Pediatr Neurosurg 39(1):27–31
2. Citerio G, Piper I, Chambers IR, Galli D, Enblad P, Kiening K et al (2008) Multicenter clinical assessment of the Raumedic Neurovent-P intracranial pressure sensor: a report by the BrainIT group. Neurosurgery 63(6):1152–1158; discussion 1158
3. Citerio G, Piper I, Cormio M, Galli D, Cazzaniga S, Enblad P et al (2004) Bench test assessment of the new Raumedic Neurovent-P ICP sensor: a technical report by the BrainIT group. Acta Neurochir 146(11):1221–1226
4. Czosnyka M, Brady K, Reinhard M, Smielewski P, Steiner LA (2009) Monitoring of cerebrovascular autoregulation: facts, myths, and missing links. Neurocrit Care 10(3):373–386
5. Czosnyka M, Czosnyka Z, Momjian S, Pickard JD (2004) Cerebrospinal fluid dynamics. Physiol Meas 25(5):R51–R76
6. Schuhmann MU, Sood S, McAllister JP, Jaeger M, Ham SD, Czosnyka Z et al (2008) Value of overnight monitoring of intracranial pressure in hydrocephalic children. Pediatr Neurosurg 44(4):269–279
7. Stendel R, Heidenreich J, Schilling A, Akhavan-Sigari R, Kurth R, Picht T et al (2003) Clinical evaluation of a new intracranial pressure monitoring device. Acta Neurochir 145(3):185–193; discussion 193
8. Tamburrini G, Di Rocco C, Velardi F, Santini P (2004) Prolonged intracranial pressure (ICP) monitoring in non-traumatic pediatric neurosurgical diseases. Med Sci Monit 10(4):53–63
9. Taylor WA, Thomas NW, Wellings JA, Bell BA (1995) Timing of postoperative intracranial hematoma development and implications for the best use of neurosurgical intensive care. J Neurosurg 82(1):48–50
10. Yokota A, Matsuoka S, Ishikawa T, Kohshi K, Kajiwara H (1989) Overnight recordings of intracranial pressure and electroencephalography in neurosurgical patients. Part II: changes in intracranial pressure during sleep. J UOEH 11(4):383–391

Author Index

A
Agarwal-Harding, K.J., 9
Ameli, P.A., 59
Ampertos, N., 119, 141
Andresen, M., 187
Antes, S., 87, 109, 177, 181
Arai, H., 91, 97, 103
Aygok, G.A., 1

B
Balédent, O., 43, 65
Bohle, R.M., 87
Borgarello, S., 123
Bouramas, D., 135
Bouras, T., 149
Bouzerar, R., 65
Brotis, A.G., 25

C
Chan, Sic L., 59
Charalambides, C., 83
Cheong, J.H., 161, 167
Chigurupati, S., 59
Chrissicopoulos, C., 119, 141
Czosnyka, M., 9, 43, 65, 71
Czosnyka, Z., 9, 65, 71

D
Demura, K., 29
Deramond, H., 43

E
Ebner, F.H., 143
Elixmann, I.M., 77
Eymann, R., 87, 109, 177, 181

F
Fayeye, O., 33
Fezoulidis, I., 39
Fichten, A., 43
Filippidis, A.S., 51, 55
Flint, G., 33
Fountas, K.N., 25, 39, 129

G
Gan, Y.C., 33
Gatos, H., 25
Gekas, N., 135
Gondry-Jouet, C., 43

H
Hadjigeorgiou, G.M., 129
Hagiwara, Y., 97
Hamilton, M.G., 155
Hara, M., 29
Hattori, M., 29

I
Inagaki, T., 173

J
Juhler, M., 187

K
Kalamatianos, T., 115
Kalani, M.Y.S., 51, 55
Kaneko, K., 173
Kapsalaki, E., 39
Kapsalaki, E.Z., 129
Kasai, H., 29
Kawaguchi, T., 173
Kawamoto, K., 173
Kiefer, M., 77, 87, 109, 177, 181
Kim, C.H., 161, 167
Kim, J.M., 161, 167
Kim, Y.-J., 87
Kinoshita, Y., 173
Kirgiannis, K., 119, 141
Kitamura, N., 173
Kitchen, N.D., 21
Klinge, P.M., 1
Kobayashi, K., 97
Kombogiorgas, D., 33
Koutsarnakis, C., 115
Kouzelis, K., 1
Kouzounias, K., 135
Kunichika, M., 91

L
Lee, G.P., 129
Legars, D., 43
Leonhardt, S., 77
Loufardaki, M., 115

M
Madan, M., 59
Mase, M., 29
Menger, M.D., 87
Miyajima, M., 91, 97, 103

Miyati, T., 29
Mourgela, S., 119, 141
Mpakopoulou, M., 25
Munch, T.N., 187
Murphy, H., 33

N
Naddeo, M., 123
Nagel, C., 143
Nakajima, M., 91, 97, 103
Nakamura, S., 91

O
Ogino, I., 91, 97, 103
Osawa, T., 29

P
Paidakakos, N., 123, 135
Papadopoulos, M.C., 21
Paterakis, K., 25
Paterakis, K.N., 129
Pattisapu, J.V., 59
Petritsis, K., 119, 141
Pickard, J.D., 9, 71
Pollay, M., 1, 47
Price, A.V., 155

R
Rekate, H.L., 1, 51, 55
Ryu, T., 173

S
Sakas, D.E., 115
Sakellaropoulos, A., 119, 141
Schmitt, M., 87, 109, 177, 181

Schuhmann, M.U., 143
Segawa, T., 97
Sgouros, S., 83, 149
Shamdeen, M.G., 181
Shibamoto, Y., 29
Shimoji, K., 103
Sklavounou, M., 135
Sotiriou, F., 135
Spanos, A., 119, 141
Stapleton, S., 21
Stavrinou, L., 115
Stoquart-El Sankari S., 43
Stranjalis, G., 115
Svolos, P., 39

T
Tamangani, J., 33
Tarnaris, A., 33
Tatagiba, M., 143
Theodorou, K., 39
Toma, A.K., 21
Tsougos, I., 39

W
Walter, M., 77
Watanabe, M., 91, 97, 103
Watkins, L.D., 21
Williams, M.A., 15

Y
Yamada, K., 29
Yamahara, T., 173
Yamanouchi, Y., 173
Yang, M.S., 161, 167
Yu, A., 59

Subject Index

A

Acetazolamide (AZA)
    adenylyl cyclase, soluble, 62
    AQP1 protein expression, 60–61
    CP tissue culture, 60
    CSF production, 62
    effect, AQP–1, 4
    fluid assay, 60, 62
    fluid transport, 60–61
    immunoblot, 60
    immunocytochemistry, 60
    mRNA expression, 60–61
    reverse transcriptase polymerase chain reaction, 60
Acute hydrocephalus, 155
Alzheimer's disease (AD)
    idiopathic normal pressure hydrocephalus, 46
    treatment, 3
Apparent diffusion coefficient (ADC), 29–32
Aquaporin (AQP)
    fluid management, 4
    types, 59
Aquaporin–1 (AQP1)
    choroid plexus tumor, 52
    CSF production, 53
    feedback mechanisms, 53
    hydrocephalic rats, 52
    mice
        CSF production, 51–52
        lower central venous pressure, 52
Aquaporin–4 (AQP4)
    aqueductal stenosis development, 56
    brain water content, 56
    CSF production and absorption, 57
    overexpression, 56
    up-regulation, 57
Aqueductal stenosis (AS)
    anatomical distortion, 142
    clinical history, 141
    primary and secondary, 141–142
    shunt placement, 142
Arachnoid villi (AV), 47–48
Arterial vasogenic component, 13
Artificial cerebrospinal fluid
    astrocytes, morphological characterization, 104
    DNA array gene expression analysis, 105
    history, 103
    materials and methods, 104
    saline solution, 106
    volcano plot analysis, 105, 106
AS. *See* Aqueductal stenosis
AZA. *See* Acetazolamide

B

Benign cerebral aqueductal stenosis, 141–142
Biocompatibility, of implants, 87
Brain fluid dynamics model. *See* Electromechanical shunt, simulation model
Brainstem lesions pathophysiology, 177–180

C

Carbonic anhydrase (CA) inhibitor, 59
Cerebral aqueductal stenosis, benign, 141–142
Cerebrospinal fluid (CSF)
    dual outflow system
        absorption site, 48
        cranial villi, 48
        drainage dynamics, 49
        history, 47
        lymphatic system, 48
        morphologic changes, 48–49
        spinal arachnoid villi, 47–48
    dynamics modeling, mathematical model
        bolus injection, 11–12
        clinical applications, 9, 13
        constant rate infusion test, 12
        CSF production, 10
        electrical circuit, 9, 10
        identification methods, 11
        slit ventricle syndrome, 181–185
        storage, CSF, 10
    flow quantification
        cerebral aqueduct values, 41
        cerebral blood flow, 39
        PC-cine MRI, 41
        region-of-interest, 40
        stroke volume and peak velocities value, 41
        T1 FLAIR imaging, 40
    shunt valve deposits examination, 83–85
    tap test
        vs. CSF aqueductal stroke volume, 43–46
        idiopathic normal pressure hydrocephalus, 29–30
Choroid plexus tumor, 4, 52

Colpocephaly
    chromosome abnormality, 169
    computed tomography, 168
    diagnosis, 167–168
    etiology, 167
    magnetic resonance imaging, 168
    microscopic examination, 169
    postoperative brain computed tomography, 170
    symptoms, 167
Corpus callosum, agenesis, 167–171
Cortical subarachnoid space (CSAS), 158
Cranial villi, 48
Craniospinal hydrodynamics
    cerebral volume and intracranial pressure, 65
    CSF and blood flow measurement, 66, 68
    intracranial pressure, 67
    phase-contrast MRI, 65
    physical phantom, 66
    pressure measurements, 68
    signals measurement, 67
CSF. See Cerebrospinal fluid

D
Dorsal midbrain syndrome (DMS)
    diagnosis, 177
    endocrine dysfunctions, 178
    fourth ventricle, 179
    magnetic resonance imaging, 178
    mesencephalic lesions, 177
    midbrain damage, 179
    shunt malfunction, 179
    symptoms, 178
    treatment, 178
    ventricle enlargement, 177

E
Electromechanical shunt, simulation model
    advantages, 78
    A and B wave simulation, 79–80
    craniospinal volume, 77
    evaluation, 80
    ICP oscillation, 77
    intracranial pressure dynamics, 78
    monoexponential pressure-volume, 77
    P-V flow characteristics, 78
    tube squeezer, 79
Endoscopic third ventriculostomy (ETV)
    complications
        clinical factors assessment, 149, 150
        intraoperative issues, 151
        morbidity and mortality, 150, 151
        pathology, 150–151
        postoperative issues, 151
        sporadic incidents, 149–150
        sudden death, 152
    normal pressure hydrocephalus, 4–5, 123–127, 129–132
    obstructive hydrocephalus, 135–138
    treatment efficacy, 2–3
Ethical considerations
    adults
        cognitive impairment, 18
        consent and assent, 17
    children, 17
    clinical care vs. research, 16
    innovation, 16–17
    stem cells implantation, 15–16

ETV. See Endoscopic third ventriculostomy
EVD. See External ventricular drain
External lumbar drainage (ELD), 124
External ventricular drain (EVD)
    ICP measurement, 109
    slit ventricle syndrome, 182–183
    syndrome of inappropriately low-pressure acute
        hydrocephalus, 157–159

F
FA. See Fractional anisotropy
Fixed-pressure and programmable valve treatment
    cerebrospinal fluid, 25
    complications, 26, 27
    lumboperitoneal shunt, 26
    neurological examination, 26
    patient history, 25–26
    pressure adjustment, 26
    shunt implantation, 25, 27
    surgical revision, 26, 27
Fractional anisotropy (FA), 3, 29–32

G
Gangliocytoma, 162

H
High mobility group box–1 protein (HMGB–1)
    cerebellum, 92
    functions, 91
    hippocampus, 92
    hydrocephalic H-Tx rats, 91
    immunostaining, 92–95
    mRNA expression, 92
    neuronal cell damage, 96
    neuron development, 91
    reverse transcriptase polymerase chain
        reaction, 91–92
    secretory mechanisms, 92–93
    Western blot, 92
Hydrocephalic edema, 56, 57

I
ICP. See Intracranial pressure
Idiopathic normal pressure hydrocephalus (INPH)
    conservative vs. surgical management
        assessment, 22
        clinical evidence, 22
        clinical history, 21
        diagnosis, 22
        gait and mental function improvement, 22
        shunt insertion, 22
        shunt valve system, 23
        valve opening pressure, 23
    demographic characteristics, 117
    diagnosis, 29, 115
    fractional anisotropy and apparent diffusion coefficient
        clinical trial, 30
        CR location, 30
        FA values, 30, 32
        regions of interest, 30, 31
        tap test, 29–30
        water diffusion, 31–32
    patient identification, 115, 116
    postoperative shunt-related complications, 116
    shunt type, 116
    surgical management, 117

Subject Index

tap test *vs.* CSF aqueductal stroke volume
    Alzheimer's disease, 46
    clinical evaluation, 44
    negative tap test, 45
    patients, 44
    phase-contrast MRI, 44, 45
    positive tap test, 45
    risk factors, 46
    statistical analysis, 44
Virchow-Robin spaces
    anatomical region, 35
    classification, 35
    dementia patients, 34
    epidemiological characteristics, 35
    imaging techniques, 34
    incidence of, 35–36
    interstitial fluid, 36
    MR imaging, 33–34
    syndrome development, 33
Infancy, treatment complication, 5
INPH. *See* Idiopathic normal pressure hydrocephalus
International Society for Hydrocephalus and Cerebrospinal Fluid Disorders (ISHCSF), 6
Intracranial pressure (ICP)
  CSF dynamics modeling, 11, 12
  electromechanical shunt, simulation model, 77–80
  measurement, telemetric device
    bony layer, macroscopic finding, 112
    computed tomography, 109, 111
    conventional method, 109
    histopathological examinations, 110
    materials and methods, 110
    Rautel, 109
  monitoring
    advantages, 187
    clinical data evaluation, 189, 190
    curve evaluation, 188
    data quality, 190–191
    indications, 189
    measurement probe, 188
    patient selection and subgroups, 188
    postoperative observation, 188
    safety, 190
    stationary device, 187
    statistical analysis, 188
    technical quality evaluation, 189
  pressure volume index, 2
Intraventricular hemorrhage (IVH) management
  Apgar score, 173–174
  complications, 174
  diagnosis, 173
  mortality rate, 174
  neonatal care, 174
  protocol, 175
  treatment strategy, 173
  ventricular system, 174–175
IVH. *See* Intraventricular hemorrhage (IVH) management

K
Kaolin injection, 56
Koerber-Salus-Elschnig syndrome. *See* Dorsal midbrain syndrome (DMS)

L
Lactated Ringer's solution, 104
L-α-lysophosphatidylcholine (LPC) stearoyl injection, 56

Laser-assisted techniques. *See* 2-Micron continuous wave laser, neuroendoscopic procedures
LDD. *See* Lhermitte-Duclos disease
Leucine-rich alpha–2-glycoprotein (LRG)
  antibody staining, 98
  anti-myelin basic protein, 99
  autopsied brain specimens, 97–98
  cerebral cortex, expression in, 98
  expression changes, with age, 100
  Olig2, and GLUT5 immunostaining, brain, 99
  reverse transcriptase polymerase chain reaction, 98, 100
Lhermitte–Duclos disease (LDD)
  clinical findings, 161
  computed tomography, preoperative, 163
  diagnosis, 161
  gangliocytoma, 162
  histological examination, 162
  imaging, 162
  microscopic examination, tumor, 164
  obstructive hydrocephalus, 162
  PTEN gene, 162
  symptoms, 163
Low-pressure hydrocephalus, 158
LRG. *See* Leucine-rich alpha–2-glycoprotein
Lumboperitoneal (LP) shunt, 26, 117

M
Magnetic resonance imaging (MRI)
  colpocephaly, 168
  dorsal midbrain syndrome (DMS), 178
  idiopathic normal pressure hydrocephalus, 33–34
  research tool, 3–4
Mathematical modeling, CSF, 10–13
2-Micron continuous wave laser, neuroendoscopic procedures
  application, 146
  characteristics, 146
  clinical study, 143
  endoscopic procedure, 145
  flexible laser fiber, 144
  postoperative CT scan, 145
  surgical technique, 144
  technical description, 144
Mini-Mental State Examination score, 17

N
Negative-pressure hydrocephalus, 158
Neuroendoscopic surgery
  artificial cerebrospinal fluid role, 103–106
  2-micron continuous wave laser, 143–146
Normal pressure hydrocephalus (NPH)
  clinical findings, 119
  computed tomography, 119
  CSF flow parameters, 121
  diagnosis and management, 2
  endoscopic third ventriculostomy
    Black's scale, 125
    clinical evaluation, 130, 131
    cognitive impairment assessment, 124
    CSF outflow resistance, 126
    efficacy of, 132
    external lumbar drainage, 124, 126
    gait disturbance, 125
    imaging techniques, 124
    infusion tests, 125
    lumbar Rout values, 124–125
    patient identification, 123–124

Normal pressure hydrocephalus (NPH) (cont.)
  patient population, 130–131
  postoperative evaluation, 131
  preoperative evaluation, 130–131
  Rout calculation, 124
  surgical technique, 124, 131
  symptomatology, 130
  symptoms duration, 132
 pathological characterization, 120–121
 radionuclide cisternography, 120
 subdural hematoma, computed tomography, 120
 ventricular system, 120
NPH. See Normal pressure hydrocephalus

O

Obstructive hydrocephalus
 endoscopic third ventriculostomy
  complications, 138
  etiology, 135–136
  imaging, 136
  postoperative evaluation, 137, 138
  safe and effective, 137
  stoma occlusion, 136
  surgical technique, 136
  venous bleeding, 137
 Lhermitte–Duclos disease, 162

P

Parinaud's syndrome. See Dorsal midbrain syndrome (DMS)
Parkinsonism, 178
Phase-contrast MRI
 craniospinal hydrodynamics, 65
 CSF flow quantification, 41
 idiopathic normal pressure hydrocephalus, 44, 45
Posterior fossa, meningioma, 167–171
Pressure volume index (PVI), 2
Pretectal syndrome. See Dorsal midbrain syndrome (DMS)
ProGAV shunt valve, 22, 23, 74
Programmable shunt assistant (ProSA) test
 CSF drainage, 71
 disadvantage, 71
 experimental setup, 72
 functions, 72, 73
 parameters, normal conditions, 73
 physical methods, 72
 programmable valve, 72
 programming, 74, 75
 properties, 74
 statistical methods, 73
 valve functions, 73–74
 valve's stability, 71
PTEN gene, 162

R

Randomized controlled trial (RCT), 2–3, 17
Research ethics. See Ethical considerations
Reverse transcriptase polymerase chain reaction (RT-PCR)
 acetazolamide effect, 60
 high mobility group box–1 protein expression analysis, 91–92
 leucine-rich alpha–2-glycoprotein localization, 98, 100

S

Scanning electron microscopy, shunt valve deposits examination
 abnormal deposits, 84
 energy-dispersive X-ray microanalysis, 84
 experimental setup, 83–84
 inorganic crystals, 85
 Medos programmable valves, 83
 protein accumulation, 85
 shunt malfunction, 85
 synthetic ruby ball, 84
 ventricular catheter occlusion, 83
Silicone catheters
 animal model, 88
 biocompatibility, of implants, 87
 collagen fiber-rich capsule, 89
 histopathological findings, 88–89
 intraperitoneal occlusions, 89
 light-optical microscope imaging, 89
 shunted patients, 87–88
 validity and reliability, 88
SILPAH. See Syndrome of inappropriately low-pressure acute hydrocephalus
Slit ventricle syndrome (SVS)
 benign intracranial hypertensions, 182
 diagnosis, 182
 drainage rate, 183–185
 external ventricular drainage, 183
 idiopathic intracranial hypertension, 182
 intracranial pressure, 181, 183, 184
 intraventricular pressure, 181–182
 periventricular gliosi, 181
 symptoms, 182
Spinal arachnoid villi, 47–48
Subdural/intraparenchymal placement, 109–112
SVS. See Slit ventricle syndrome
Sylvian aqueduct syndrome. See Dorsal midbrain syndrome (DMS)
Syndrome of inappropriately low-pressure acute hydrocephalus (SILPAH)
 clinical deterioration, 156
 cortical subarachnoid space, 158
 EVD, 159
 initial treatment, 157
 low ICP, 157, 158
 neurological exam, 156–157
 pathophysiology, 158
 patients, 156
 shunt system, 159
 symptoms, 155
 treatment, 157–158
 ventricular catheter, 156
 ventriculomegaly, 156
 ventriculostomy, 155

V

Ventriculomegaly, 91, 120, 156, 158
Ventriculoperitoneal (VP) shunt, 116
Ventriculostomy, 138, 155. See also Endoscopic third ventriculostomy (ETV)
Virchow-Robin spaces, 33–36

Printing: Ten Brink, Meppel, The Netherlands
Binding: Stürtz, Würzburg, Germany